Frontiers of Radiation Therapy and Oncology

Vol. 23

Series Editors
Jerome M. Vaeth, San Francisco, Calif.
John L. Meyer, San Francisco, Calif.

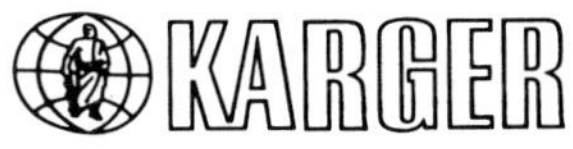

Basel · München · Paris · London · New York · New Delhi · Bangkok · Singapore · Tokyo · Sydney

Radiation Tolerance of Normal Tissues

23rd Annual San Francisco Cancer Symposium, San Francisco, Calif., March 4–5, 1988

Radiation Tolerance of Normal Tissues

Volume Editors
Jerome M. Vaeth, San Francisco, Calif.
John L. Meyer, San Francisco, Calif.

83 figures and 96 tables, 1989

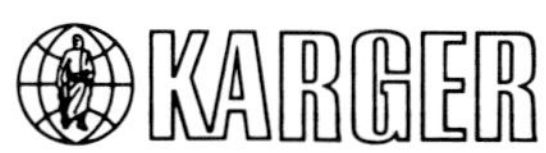

Basel · München · Paris · London · New York · New Delhi · Bangkok · Singapore · Tokyo · Sydney

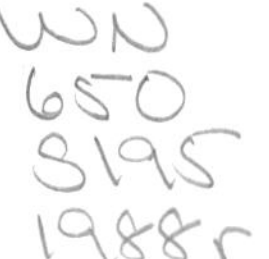

Frontiers of Radiation Therapy and Oncology

Library of Congress Cataloging-in-Publication Data
San Francisco Cancer Symposium (23rd: 1988)
Radiation tolerance of normal tissues / 23rd Annual San Francisco Cancer Symposium, San Francisco, Calif., March 4 and 5, 1988 ;
volume editors, Jerome M. Vaeth, John L. Meyer.
p. cm. – (Frontiers of radiation therapy and oncology ; vol. 23)
Includes bibliographical references.
1. Cancer – Radiotherapy – Complications and sequelae – Congresses.
2. Radiation tolerance – Congresses. 3. Cells – Effects of radiation on – Congresses.
I. Vaeth, Jerome M., 1925– . II. Meyer, John, 1949– . III. Title. IV. Series.
[DNLM: 1. Radiation Effects – congresses. 2. Radiation Tolerance – congresses.]
ISBN 3–8055–4837–0

Bibliographic Indices
This publication is listed in bibliographic services, including Current Contents® and Index Medicus.

Drug Dosage

The authors and the publisher have exerted every effort to ensure that drug selection and dosage set forth in this text are in accord with current recommendations and practice at the time of publication. However, in view of ongoing research, changes in government regulations, and the constant flow of information relating to drug therapy and drug reactions, the reader is urged to check the package insert for each drug for any change in indications and dosage and for added warnings and precautions. This is particularly important when the recommended agent is a new and/or infrequently employed drug.

Printed in Switzerland by Thür AG Offsetdruck, Pratteln
ISBN 3–8055–4837–0

Contents

To my daughter, Cullyn, and wife, Aurore, whose dedication and efforts contributed so much to this successful twenty-third symposium.

Foreword

In 1970, our 6th San Francisco Cancer Symposium and the subsequent volume 6 of *Frontiers of Radiation Therapy and Oncology* addressed the subject of the effects of ionizing radiations on normal tissues. The volume was enthusiastically received and quickly became the reference text for radiation tolerance. Much in addition to time has elapsed in that 18 years. Prior to 1970, most of the concepts of irradiated normal-tissue tolerance were based on 'so-called' conventional treatment schemes – 6,000 rad in 6 weeks, delivered daily five times weekly. In today's treatment programs, 'six in six' is almost the exception. Even established concepts of tolerance must now be reexamined in the light of new knowledge of the immune system, sensitizers, modifiers, chemotherapy, and altered fractionation schemes. We have yet to develop a vocabulary for defining and comparing the quality and quantity of normal-tissue tolerance. There is now an accumulation of both basic and clinical data enabling us to reexamine the older concepts and formulate the new. On March 4 and 5, 1988, a distinguished faculty, many of whom addressed the 6th San Francisco Symposium, joined us in San Francisco and addressed this challenge. The presentations assembled in this 23rd volume of this series are vital to the safe utilization of radiations in the treatment of cancers.

The symposium was produced under the auspices of the St. Mary's Foundation, in association with St. Mary's Hospital and Medical Center, San Francisco, Calif., USA.

Jerome M. Vaeth

Acknowledgements

The production of this year's symposium, leading to the 23rd volume of this series, was assisted by the generosity of donations made by Alpha Omega Services, Inc., Biotherapeutics, CIS-US, CliniTherm, Computerized Medical Systems, Dianon Systems, Inc., Gammex, Inc., Haynes Radiation, Northern California Radiation Therapists and Oncologists, Inc., Radiation Measurements, Inc., Reactor Experiments, Inc., Mary Roy, Siemens Corp., Therogenics Corp., Varian, Victoreen, and Wyeth Laboratories.

Vaeth JM, Meyer JL (eds): Radiation Tolerance of Normal Tissues.
Front Radiat Ther Oncol. Basel, Karger, 1989, vol 23, pp 1–6

Historical Perspective of Normal Tissue Tolerance or Stumbling Along the Pathway of Dose Response to Necrosis and Back

William Moss

Department of Radiation Therapy, Oregon Health Sciences University, Portland, Oreg., USA

From the historical perspective, there has been concern for normal tissue tolerance from the time radium was discovered and the X-ray tube was invented. Drury [8] described radiation necrosis of the skin produced by X-rays in 1896. Becquerel and Curie [2] produced a radionecrosis of their own skins in 1901 using radium. The first record I could find of a malpractice suit for therapeutic overdosage of the skin was filed when a physician was sued for irradiating a patient for cancer of the tongue, but seriously damaged the overlying skin [14] in 1903. Our problems are not new! The first human reported killed by total-body radiations was a radiologist who practiced 14 years with no protection. He died of severe anemia in 1916 [5].

Patients irradiated from the turn of the century until about 1920 were treated with a very poor quality of X-rays produced at 100–120 KV. The low output of the machines required that the patient be treated close to the X-ray tube and with little or no filtration. A Dr. Reavan stated that his X-ray beam had an 'effectual ray for 1 cm depth' [1]. After having vigorously treated the most superficial 1 cm, of a breast or skin cancer, he would wait until that 1 cm sloughed and then vigorously irradiate the next cm and so on until the cancer was removed, a sort of fractionation in space or the radiation oncologist's Moh's technique.

Attempts to treat any tissue other than skin with X-rays were virtually certain to lead to overdose of the skin. It was obvious, even at this point, that skin tolerances had to be defined as a prerequisite to a successful practice of X-ray therapy. This limitation of external irradiation sparked continued efforts to develop brachytherapy techniques. The long, almost uninterrupted search for tolerance data has continued to the present, and the need to preserve superficial tissues triggered research for better equipment and alternate techniques. Many different fractionation schemes were already in use. However, standardization of treatment factors was impractical. Techniques varied widely. The unit of dose at that time was not sharply defined, nor was the dose readily measurable. For this reason, the tolerance doses which were available were inconsistent and often unreliable. In the literature there are several definitions for normal-tissue tolerance dose, and this also led to confusion. For example, some have defined normal-tissue tolerance as the maximum dose one can deliver to a normal tissue and yet have that tissue remain virtually structurally sound or perform its essential function in a satisfactory manner. Perhaps a more contemporary definition might state that the tolerance dose of a given tissue is the maximum dose which can be given to a tissue without producing an unacceptable proportion of serious defects. In this definition the term 'dose' is used in a broad sense to include fraction size, number of fractions, overall time, volume, etc. This definition recognizes that there will be variation in response of patients. It allows the production of an agreed upon proportion of serious high-dose effects. The seriousness and number of defects which are acceptable or unacceptable will vary with anatomic site and with the alternatives promised by delivering the higher or lower dose. The determination of 'acceptability of sequelae' is a consensus reached over time by patients, not by radiation oncologists. In this sense, the normal tissue tolerance dose does not correspond to the optimum dose, except that the cancer in question may require a dose in the range of the normal tissue tolerance. For the most part, tissue tolerances were established empirically and without an understanding of the basic mechanisms involved. Lacking a knowledge of these basic mechanisms, early radiation oncologists were lucky if they had one reliable point on a single isoeffect curve. Thus, early radiation oncologists, i.e., up until about 1930, stumbled blindly along this dose-response path, overirradiating and underirradiating until enough clinical disasters were produced to define the upper limits of dose in a few clinical situations. During this period, the French, with the knowledge that cell killing could be selective [3] and with the fractionation patterns of Coutard [7], led the way in defining skin, mucosa, bone, cartilage, and vasculoconnective tissue tolerance using orthovoltage beams for cancers of the head and neck. The Scandinavians contributed heavily to our knowledge of tolerance of bowel and bladder. The concept of isoeffect curves, of the importance of volume, and a separation of acute and late effects were yet to come.

This was essentially the status of affairs until 1944 when Strandquist [16] crystallized the understanding at that time in the form of isoeffect curves, showing the relationship of total skin dose to duration of treatment. I cannot tell you what a tremendous impact his paper had on radiation oncologists of the late 1940s and early 1950s. Like magic, it brought some order to the fraction dose-total dose relationship. These curves were reproduced and glued or pasted in radiation therapy departments in the United States and in Europe in order that they might serve as dosage guides. They were misused as guides for tolerance of *all* normal tissues and for total doses for curative irradiation, even though they were never intended for such use. Four years later Paterson [12] published isoeffect curves for skin tolerance which incorporated field size and number of fractions as he had experienced them in clinical orthovoltage therapy. Refinements were added by von Essen in 1963 [18]. It was about this same time that Ellis [9], after studying the slope of a variety of these types of curves, developed his NSD concept and formula for normal tissue tolerance. Virtually everyone but Ellis knew something was wrong with the NSD concept, but most of us did not know why he was wrong. The curve just did not fit when we needed it most. However, we had nothing better. Remember the NSD slide rule which every resident used? Despite its faults, the NSD concept proved useful. It provoked vigorous renewed interest in the elements of fractionation, especially as related to normal tissue tolerance. Our contemporary concepts were born in the discussions and studies which followed.

The definition of tolerance of normal tissues, other than skin, did not await the development of megavoltage or cobalt beams. Before 1920 there were many small series of patients reported with late rectal radiation injuries from intravaginal and intrauterine brachytherapy. Shortly thereafter, tolerances of the normal rectum for both the Paris and Stockholm techniques were expressed in terms of milligram hours or millicuries destroyed. In 1938 Tod and Meredith [17] established the classical reference point 'A' in the paracervical triangle. Rectal tolerance was established as related to the dose at point 'A'. With all of its shortcomings, point 'A' retains much of its popularity and continues to be one of the most commonly used indicators of central dose. It is only recently, using computer-aided techniques as described by the International Commission on Radiation Units and Measurements (ICRU) [11], that the calculation of the rectal dose has been more or less standardized (Pourquier).

In the 1940s, Boden [4] in Manchester, UK, used a three-field technique with orthovoltage (a parallel opposed pair of lateral beams and a direct posterior beam) to irradiate cancers of the head and neck. The spinal cord was cross-fired by these three beams. In retrospect, it appears an ideal cord-damaging technique. Boden [4] described changes produced and the dose delivered in 8 patients who developed spinal cord damage. Unfortunately, this remarkable paper was not widely read. Cord damage continued to appear. This was aided by the appearance of megavoltage beams. With their increased depth dose and skin sparing, even a nonradiologist could deliver an excess dose. In addition, wide-field irradiation for Hodgkin's disease was popularized and led to an increased number of carelessly overlapped beams. We are still haunted by the possibility of these types of accidents.

Earlier, I cited the malpractice suit against a physician in 1903. Though I have been unable to track the course of malpractice suits during these early days, there is no question but that they plagued these early workers and played a substantial role in the establishment of tolerance doses of normal tissues. This has been particularly true for critical tissues such as the spinal cord, the brain, optic nerve, optic chiasm, and the kidneys etc. For these tissues virtually any high-dose effects have been difficult to justify. For these critical tissues the fear of litigation prompted both early and recent radiation oncologists to set 'tolerance doses' sufficiently low to assure near-zero complications. The impact of potential litigation in the establishment of tolerance doses of other normal tissues has varied with the alternative forms of treatment and the seriousness of the associated radiation-induced disabilities.

The critical tissue response with which we are concerned is, of course, dose related and, more often than not, is on the steep part of the dose-response curve. Small changes in dose generally result in substantial changes in high-dose effects. Let us look briefly at some illustrations of this.

Tolerance doses were initially established using orthovoltage beams. The dose was recorded in roentgens along the central axis in the tissue in question. In the late 50s cobalt beams became available. It was felt by radiobiologists that with the decrease in the relative biological effectiveness of ^{60}Co beams, the tolerance doses and tumor doses could be increased by 15% as compared to the conventional tumor doses given with orthovoltage beams. This was a vague recommendation from the radiation biologist and was not uniformly put into clinical practice. It resulted in much uncertainty as to tolerances. In any case, the skin sparing of ^{60}Co beams encouraged administration of increased tissue doses which overshadowed any differences in the relative biological effectiveness. The tolerances of subcutaneous and deep tissues had to be reestablished with ^{60}Co beams. About this same time we were asked to switch from the roentgen to the rad. In doing so, the *numerical value* of the tolerance dose had to be reduced by 5–10%. This reduction in the *numerical value* of dose was not uniformly carried out. Initially, at least, the same numerical value was often used. Only the label was changed. Thus, 5–10% higher doses were commonly given. Stockbine et al. [15] from the M. D. Anderson Hospital published that they observed an increased incidence of complications as a result of this apparent innocuous change of labels. The rest of us did not dare publish our mistakes.

About 1970, in our efforts to assure adequate irradiation of the cancer, many of us changed to recording the minimum dose in the target volume, but carried the 90% or even the 85% isodose curve to a dose which previously had been given only to the central axis. In effect, this resulted in a 10–15% increase in dose over that which had been previously been given. Here again there was an increase in high-dose effects. The ICRU [10], in 1978, recommended a format for reporting dose to minimize the risk of misunderstanding. There are, no doubt, other less widespread technical changes which also have continuously confirmed the criticality of the tolerance dose. Computer-aided dosimetry, which became available in the early to the mid-1970s, added precision to our dosage calculations and precision to our determination of tolerance doses. To summarize, I like the four periods of understanding described by Buschke [6] in 1971.

(1) During the early years, radiations were used as a caustic agent. The selectivity of cell killing was not fully appreciated and was not exploited. For therapy, very high fractions were the rule.

(2) In the 1920s, the selective killing effects of radiations were beautifully illustrated by the experiment of Regaud and Blanc [13] with the ram's testicles. Also, during this period, the critical role of the vasculoconnective tissue was revealed. Efforts to exploit the selective destructive effects of radiations flourished, especially by Coutard [7].

(3) During the early 1940s, 50s, and 60s, accurate treatment planning was developed, especially by the British. Special techniques were devised for accurate beam alignment and careful tumor localization to minimize the dose to normal structures.

(4) From the early 1960s to the present, the clinical and basic scientists have given our specialty a firm scientific basis, refined the concepts of acute and late reactions, and triggered trials using different fractionation schedules.

The history of defining normal tissue tolerance is a large part of the history of radiation oncology. It has been a slow and painful empirical process of recognizing our mistakes and adjusting our techniques to avoid them in the future. While families of curves of tolerances for all of the different technical factors and clinical situations would be optimum, at present we must settle for a few well-recognized points on these curves to serve as our guidepost. The variation in tolerances from patient to patient demands that we share our valued judgments with each patient. Normal tissue tolerance doses have acquired medical, ethical, and medicolegal implications which make it essential that these doses be established by consensus. The establishment of such dose levels is critical for optimization of treatment.

References

1 Allen, C. W.: Radiotherapy, phototherapy, radium and high frequency currents, p. 175 (Lea Brothers, New York 1904).
2 Becquerel, H.; Curie, P.: Action physiologique des rayons du radium. C.r. Acad. Sci., Paris *132:* 1289 (1901).
3 Bergonie, J.; Tribondeau, L.: Action des rayons X sur le testicule du rat blanc. C.r. Seánc. Soc. Biol., Paris *57:* 522 (1904); *58:* 156 (1905).
4 Boden, G.: Radiation myelitis of the cervical spinal cord. Br. J. Radiol. *21:* 464–469 (1948).
5 Bruwer, A. J.: Classic descriptions in diagnostic roentgenology, vol 1 (Thomas, Springfield, 1964).
6 Buschke, F.: Radiation therapy – historical perspective. Radiol. clin. biol. *40:* 217–220 (1971).
7 Coutard, H.: Roentgen therapy of epitheliomas of the tonsillar region, hypopharynx and larynx from 1920 to 1926, Am. J. Roentg. *28:* 313–331 (1932).
8 Drury, H.: Dermatitis caused by roentgen X-rays. Br. med. J. *ii:* 1377 (1896).
9 Ellis, F.: Dose-time and fractionation. A clinical hypothesis. Clin. Radiol. *20:* 1–7 (1969).
10 International Commission on Radiation Units and Measurements: Dose specification for reporting external beam therapy with photons and electron. ICRU Rep. No. 29 (National Institutes of Health, Bethesda 1978).
11 International Commission on Radiation Units and Measurements: Dose and volume specification for reporting intracavitary therapy in gynecology. ICRU Rep. No. 38 (National Institutes of Health, Bethesda 1985).
12 Paterson, R.: The treatment of malignant disease by radium and X-rays, p. 39 (Arnold, London, 1948).
13 Regaud, C.; Blanc, J.: Action des rayons X sur les diverses générations de la lignée spermatique. Extrême sensibilité des spermatogonies à ces rayons. C.r. Seánc. Soc. Biol., Paris *41:* 163 (1906).
14 Shelby vs. Dr. G. W. Spohn: Review of reviews, April 25, (1903).
15 Stockbine, M. F.; Hancock, J. E.; Fletcher, G. H.: Complications in 831 patients with squamous cell carcinoma of the intact cervix treated with 3,000 rad or more whole pelvis irradiation. Am. J. Roentg. *108:* 293–304 (1970).
16 Strandquist, M.: Time-dose relationships. Acta radiol., suppl. 55, p. 1 (1944).
17 Tod, M. C.; Meredith, W. J.: A dosage system for use in the treatment of cancer of the uterine cervix. Br. J. Radiol. *40:* 132 (1938).
18 Essen, C. F. van: A spatial model of time-dose-volume relationships in radiation therapy. Radiology *81:* 881–883 (1963).

William Moss, MD, Department of Radiation Therapy,
Oregon Health Sciences University, Portland, OR 97201 (USA)

Vaeth JM, Meyer JL (eds): Radiation Tolerance of Normal Tissues.
Front Radiat Ther Oncol. Basel, Karger, 1989, vol 23, pp 7–40

Law and Order of Radiation Sensitivity

Absolute versus Relative[1]

Philip Rubin

Department of Radiation Oncology, University of Rochester Cancer Center, Rochester, N. Y., USA

Introduction

There is an order of radiation sensitivity of normal tissues, and this order, in a general sense, applies to tumors derived from these tissues. The concept that tissue/organs have different tolerances to irradiation was the basis of my presentation more than a decade ago [13]. At the time, the sensitivity of each tissue/organ was ordered in terms of the dose required to induce organ failure and categorized each according to the potential for such failure to lead to life-threatening circumstances. The tolerance doses for 5 versus 50% complication rates within 5 years ($TD_{5/5}$ and $TD_{50/5}$; fig. 1) described the dose-response curves for severe radiation-induced lesions and, in fact, determined the ordering (fig. 2). The origin of the order of tissue/organ radiation sensitivity was rooted in radiation physiopathology. Based on the classic morphologic analysis of irradiated tissues by Casareet [2], we [14] provided a definition of normal-tissue radiosensitivity based on observed cellular depletion 2 months after exposure. Again, different normal tissues and organs in the body have different tolerance doses, with the most resistant tolerating doses 20-fold greater than the most sensitive.

It appeared to follow that tumors arising from radiosensitive tissues were radiosensitive and those arising from radioresistant tissues radioresistant (table I). For example, the tests and ovaries are extremely sensi-

[1] This work was supported in part by the Clinical-Experimental Radiation Research Interface Study (CERRIS) Grant No. CA11051-18 (National Cancer Institute).

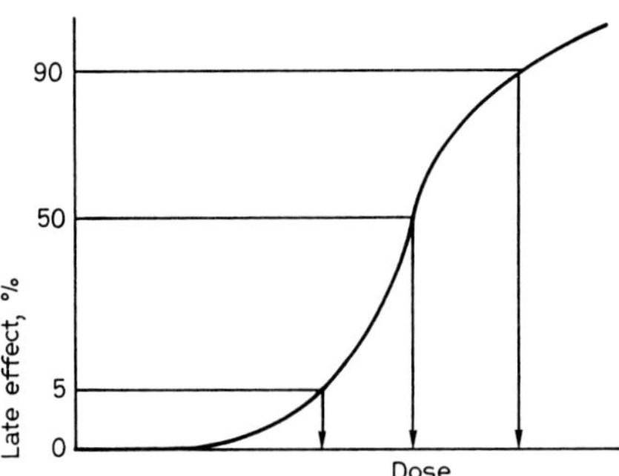

Fig. 1. Tolerance dose definitions. $TD_{5/5}$ is the tolerance dose representing the 5% complication rate 5 years after irradiation. The $TD_{50/5}$ represents the 50% complication level, and the $TD_{90/5}$ is the 90% complication rate accumulated within/5 years of radiation treatment. Taken together, these clinical data, when available, constitute the basis for forming dose-response curves.

Table I. Various tumors and tissues in decreasing order of radiosensitivity [modified from ref. 14, with permission]

Tumors	Relative radiosensitivity	Tissues of origin
Lymphoma, leukemia, seminoma, dysgerminoma	high	lymphoid, hematopoietic (marrow) spermatogenic epithelium, and ovarian follicular epithelium
Squamous cell cancer of the oropharynx, glottis, bladder skin, and cervical epithelia; adenocarcinomas of the alimentary tract	fairly high	oropharyngeal stratified epithelium, sebaceous gland epithelium, urinary bladder epithelium, optic lens epithelium, gastric gland epithelium, colon epithelium, and breast epithelium
Vascular and connective tissue elements of all tumors; secondary neurovascularization and astrocytomas	medium	ordinary interstitial tissue, neuroglial tissue (connective tissue of the nervous system), fine vasculature, and growing cartilage or bone tissue
Salivary gland tumors, hepatomas, renal cancer, pancreatic cancer, chondrosarcoma, and osteogenic sarcoma	fairly low	mature cartilage or bone tissue, salivary gland epithelium, hepatic epithelium, chondrocytes, and osteocytes
Rhabdomyosarcoma, leiomyosarcoma, and ganglioneurofibrosarcoma	low	muscle tissue and neuronal tissue

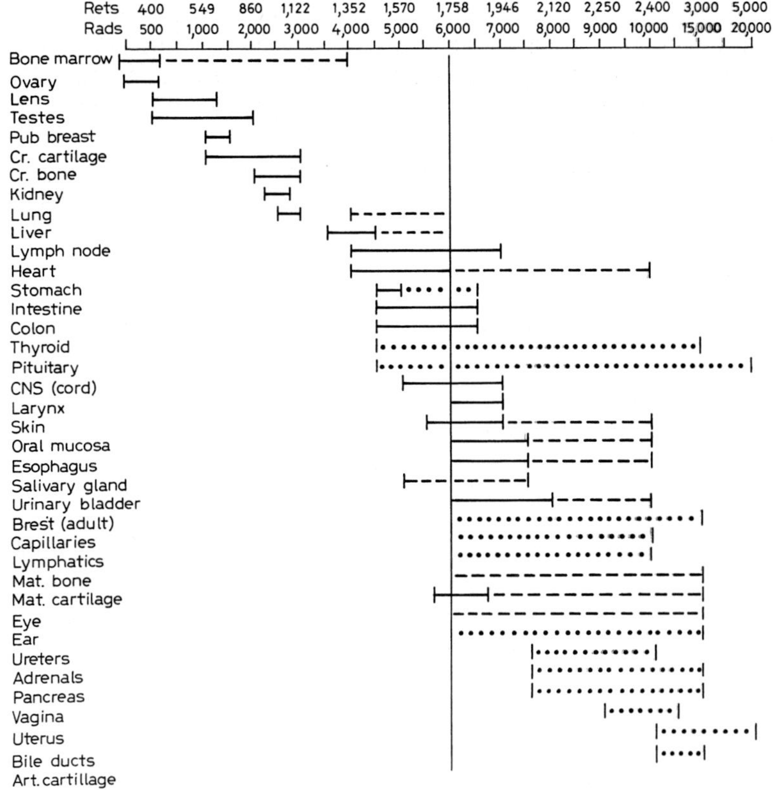

Fig. 2. Tolerance dose plot. The dose-response curves for every major organ is plotted as a linear fashion. The shorter the line, the steeper the dose-response curve. Modification of values according to volume was made. For many organ systems, particularly more radioresistant organs, the data are sparse and are estimated. Note key. [From ref. 73, with permission.]

tive as are the lymphoid and bone marrow systems, translating into a similar sensitivity for the derivative tumors, such as the seminoma, dysgerminomas, lymphomas, and leukemias. Nervous tissue, bone and cartilage, endocrine organs, and kidney are radioresistant tissues and so are their derivative tumors: glioblastoma multiforme, osteogenic sarcoma, adrenal carcinomas, and renal cancers. Between these extremes are the epithelial and glandular tissues which line the aerodigestive passages, the urinary tract, and the skin with the accompanying wide variety of squamous cell cancer and adenocarcinomas. The vascular connective tissue stroma is central in its radiation response and radiation sensitivity [14].

In the 60s, the world of radiation oncology was as orderly as the world of Newtonian physics and Darwinian biology. The order of tissue/organ/tumor radiation sensitivity was inherently logical and reasonable if not axiomatic and a law of radiation oncology. These concepts of radiation sensitivity were the foundation of our practice patterns [15]. We ablated radiosensitive tissues and their derivative tumors, such as seminomas of the testes, with doses as low as 2,000–3,000 cGy and similarly lymphocytes, lymphoid tissues, bone marrow, and their derivative neoplasmas – lymphomas and Hodgkin's Disease – with moderate doses of 3,000–4,500 cGy. Ablation of glioblastoma multiforme was difficult, since it came from the radioresistant nervous tissue which could withstand larger doses of 6,000–8,000 cGy. The occasional contradictory observations regarding the sensitivity of a tissue and its tumor could be explained by whether cells were proliferating or mature. The law of Bergonie and Tribondeau [1] defined radiosensitivity in terms of a tissue's proliferative capacity and its mitotic potential; i.e., adult nerve, bone and cartilage, muscle, and endocrine organs were resistant, but in the infant or child, where these tissues are rapidly proliferating, the neural tissues for growing bone, cartilage, muscle, and the thyroid are all vulnerable [16].

Today, the radiation oncologist is even more uncertain as to whether the dose prescribed is within tolerance. The concept of treating to the limits of tissue/organ tolerance is modified by the shifting of organ tolerance, resulting from the impact of numerous new variables [17]. Currently, the order of radiosensitivity of tissues/organs is clearly not absolute or fixed, but relative and changing, much as the world based upon Einstein's theory of relativity and Watson and Crick's model of DNA and molecular biology. In fact, in our current multimodal era, there are no safe or tolerance doses as I previously described in the 60s and 70s. The list of $TD_{5/5}$ and $TD_{50/5}$ must be modified. The cellular heterogeneity of tumors which confounds delivering a fixed curative dose in all circumstances applies to normal tissues and organs. As many as 20–50 different cell types compose different organ systems, although the clonogenic stem cell populations are more limited. The ability of irradiation to defunctionalize or devitalize an organ depends upon the vulnerability of a critical stem cell subpopulation and the cell cycle time for renewal before the injury expresses itself.

One of the limitations of mathematical modeling for predicting severe early and late effects is that it must encompass a variety of cell subpopulations in an organ: epithelial, parenchyma, connective tissue stroma, endothelial. The concept for a derived tolerance dose based on isoeffect lines melding fractionation and time-dose factors into a formula is confounded by the cellular heterogeneity of normal tissues in addition to variations in repair and repopulation mechanisms. With a known range of doses, intrapolation is possible, but exterpolation and predictions are unreliable. Depending on the intensity of the dose, the size of the fraction, and the time of delivery, each cell subpopulation in an organ responds differently and each have different regeneration capacities. Thus, establishing a model for an entire organ such as spinal cord, brain, lung, heart, and kidney is fraught with limitations. The end point of organ failure can be arrived at by different pathophysiologic mechanisms, since different critical cells or mircostructures are effected by irradiation. Thus, nominal single dose, time-dose fractionatioin, cumulaltive radiation effect, and new computer-based formulations are of value, but are not without boundaries [5, 10, 11]. The α/β ratio and linear quadratic equation are applicable to cellular subpopulations [28], but do not provide guidelines to safe doses for *in vivo* organ tolerances. An organ can decompensate as a result of different cellular mechanisms, and, more importantly, the interaction of multiple cellular events is the basis of the complex series of pathophysiologic alterations producing late effects.

Changing Order of Radiosensitivity

In this multimodality era, there are many factors effecting our concepts of radiosensitivity resulting from the rapid advances of radiation oncology and its science of radiation biology and radiation physics and from new modalities that are being introduced as well as the more standard treatments of chemotherapy and surgery. As concise review of the more common factors related to therapy in contrast to the host is briefly enumerated. Although the radiation tolerance doses (TD_5 and TD_{50}) are valuable guides, their applicability has changed as a result of the large armamentarium of new agents, drugs, modalities, and their concurrent and subsequent employment to irradiation; thus, these doses should not be naively viewed as 'safe' doses. Sufficient experience has been gained with seemingly 'safe' doses for each of the two modes of treatment, i.e., radiation versus drugs, that, when combined, lead to severe late effects with regard to different vital organs [10].

Therapy Factors

Dose. There is no absolute or fixed dose that ablates a normal tissue, because $TD_{5/5}$ and $TD_{50/5}$ are dependent on dose/time factors.

Fractionation. The fraction size of radiation and time interval are major determinates of both early and late effects. With alternate fractionation regimens under investigation, the $TD_{5/5}$ and $TD_{50/5}$ will shift for different organs in the ordering sequence. Hyperfractionation and hypofractionation will have different effects on tolerence doses.

Volume. A major factor in tolerance dose is whether the whole organ or a partial organ volume is exposed to irradiation. With the more widespread use of TBI and IORT techniques, the order of organ radiation sensitivity changes as a function of whole-organ or partial-organ irradiation and single versus fractionated exposures.

Time. The time to expression of the effect is related to the cell kinetics of different subpopulations within a tissue/organ. Whether there are differences between early or late effects depends on many factors: total dose/total time for irradiation delivery and the addition of other modalities, such as chemotherapy.

Chemotherapy. Of the various modalities, the addition of chemotherapy initially planned in a simultaneous or sequential fashion has a major impact on organ sensitivity. The use of an agent may dramatically effect either the same cell or a different cell subpopulation which leads to lower threshold doses for organ injury. The most common factor altering the tolerance dose concepts of normal tissues is the widespread use of drugs.

Innovations. The new modalities, hyperthermia, radiozensitizers and radioprotectors, and immunological and biologic response modifiers, may all or each alter late effects.

Patient Factors

Age. Proliferation and rapid renewal of all cells in an organ system lead to its vulnerability to irradiation, particularly during the fetal and the immediate postnatal years and again at puberty. The order of organ radiosensitivity in a child is different from adults.

Host. There are different altered physiopathologic states that can alter the radiation response, such as anemia, infection, diabetes, and arteriosclerosis. The baseline or reserve of cell repopulation varies with different diseases.

Trauma. Any kind of trauma inflicted upon an irradiated organ will lead to tissue breakdown, particularly surgical interventions. Pre- or post-operative irradiation and wound healing need to be considered.

Tumor Factors

These are: (1) *direct tissue effects:* extent of invasion into normal tissue and vessels; (2) *systemic effects:* systemic effects of organ dysfunction or chemical secretion, and (3) *indirect mechanical effects:* indirect mechanical effects, such as hydronephrosis from an obstructed ureter.

Changing Order of Radiosensitivity as a Function of Dose

The concept of an optimal dose that will provide maximal cures and minimal complications is and has been the basis of varying fractionation schedules [4, 13, 14, 17] (table II). The Strandqvist lines or isoeffect plots, based upon varying dose-time regimens, suggested that an optimal zone

Table II. Tolerance doses ($TD_{5/5}$–$TD_{50/5}$)

	Single dose Gy		Fractionated dose Gy
Lymphoid	2–5	Testes	1–2
Bone marrow	2–10	Ovary	6–10
Ovary	2–6	Eye (lens)	6–12
Testes	2–10	Lung	20–30
Eye (lens)	2–10	Kidney	20–30
Lung	7–10	Liver	35–40
Gastrointestinal	5–10	Skin	30–40
Colorectal	10–20	Thyroid	30–40
Kidney	10–20	Heart	40–50
Bone marrow	15–20	Lymphoid	40–50
Heart	18–20	Bone marrow	40–50
Liver	15–20	Gastrointestinal	45–50
Mucosa	5–20	Vasculoconnective tissue systems	50–60
Vasculoconnective tissue systems	10–20	Spinal cord	50–60
Skin	15–20	Peripheral nerve	65–77
Peripheral nerve	15–20	Mucosa	65–77
Spinal cord	15–20	Brain	60–70
Brain	15–25	Bone and cartilage	>70
Bone and cartilage	>30	Muscle	>70
Muscle	>30		

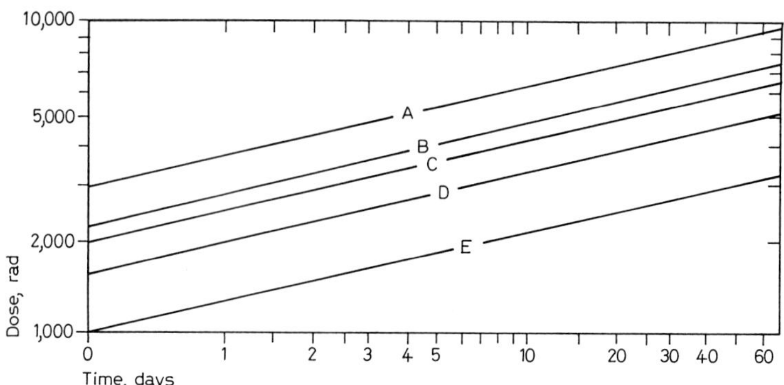

Fig. 3. Standqvist lines. The dose-time isoeffect line relates total dose delivered and total time indpendent of fractionation for different tissue and end points: A = skin necrosis; B = cure of skin carcinoma; C = moist desquamation of skin; D = dry desquamation of skin; E = skin erythema. [From ref. 7, with permission.]

could be found, yielding a favorable therapeutic ratio [24] (fig. 3). Although these lines were drawn parellel, it became apparent to many investigators that tumors may respond differently than normal tissues and that a divergence of the isoeffect slopes for normal tissue versus cancers exists. [29]. The importance of volume of the normal tissue [8] and dose-time factors needs to be stressed in considering tolerance or normal-tissue or organ effects (fig. 3). In revising and reexamining the tolerance doses for different vital and dose-limiting tissues and organs, the volume factor is even more relevant today in view of the increasing use of total body irradiation in which whole-organ systems are exposed. More time-concentrated schedules are in use which vary from single exposure to short intense fractionation schedules. Another new modality – intra-operative radiation therapy – has led to the use of large single doses to large tissue volumes and has provided new insights to the tolerance dose. Accordingly, a tabulation of the changing order is provided in table II, mainly based upon the dose, although the volume is also considered and will be discussed in another section.

Currently, the prescribed tolerance dose is at best a calculated estimate of the TD_5 and TD_{50} based upon recorded human and animal data [6, 7, 14]. The complication probability for either 5% (TD_5) and 50% (TD_{50}) assumes uniform irradiation of all or part of an organ, conventional fractionation schedules (1.8–2.0 Gy/fraction and five fractions/week), relatively normal organ function as a baseline, no adjuvant drugs or surgical manipulations, and normal age ranges. It is beyond the scope of this presentation to do more than provide a relative ordering of tissue/organ radiation sensitivity, since other speakers will address each organ site in more detail. In ordering the organ radiosensitivity according to dose level, a variety of factors were considered, including: the end point chosen (late more than acute), the use of single or fractionated regimens, and the volume of the organ. Since the literature is not always complete or precise [6,14], extrapolation is inevitably involved in using either clinical or experimental animal data, and the dose levels are rounded off rather than offering doses to one or two decimals as is occassionally reported. Such accuracy can be as misleading as the general estimates of tolerance doses offered.

Single Doses, Whole Organ

Two to Ten Gy (200–1,000 cGy)

At doses less than 10 Gy, the radiosensitive cells effected are the lymphoid tissue and lymphocytes, bone marrow, hematopoitic stem cells, lens epithlium, ovarian oocyte, testes spermatogonia, lung type II cells, and gastrointestinal epithilium and villi [4] (table III). Most of these are highly radiosensitive, rapidly dividing stem cells and are directly effected without injury to the microvasculature or connective tissue stroma.

Ten to Twenty Gy (1,000–2,000 cGy)

At doses between 10 and 20 Gy, the majority of other organ systems respond to irradiation and include upper aerodigestive mucosa, kidney, heart, liver, peripheral nerves, spinal cord, and brain. Skin probably would be effected as well. These are deliberately listed as organs with effects related to radiation damage to microcirculation and connective tissue interstitium as well as parenchymal cells. Due to the large single doses used, it is difficult to distinguish between the impact of indirect vascular injury as distinct from direct effects of irradiation on parenchymal cells that are often slow cycling.

Doses Greater than Twenty Gy (>2,000 cGy)

At doses greater than 20 Gy, there are a number of otherwise radioresistant structures which include bone and cartilage, muscle, endocrine organs such as pituitary and adrenals, reproductive organs such as uterus and prostate, and other organs such as pancreas and biliary system.

Table III. Tolerance doses

Target cell single dose/whole organ	Complication end point	TD_5–TD_{50} dose range, Gy
100–1,000 cGy		
Lymphoid and lymphocytes	lymphopenia	2–5
Bone marrow hematopoietic stem cells	aplasia	2–10
Lens epithelium	cataract	2–8
Ovarian oocytes	sterility	2–6
Testes spermatogonia	sterility	2–6
Lung type II cells	pneumonitis	7–10
Gastro intestinal epithelial cells	enteritis	5–10
1,000–2,000 cGy		
Colorectal epithelial cells	colitis	10–20
Upper Aerodigestive mucosa	mucositis	15–20
Kidney	nephritis	11–19
Heart	carditis	18–20
Liver	hepatitis	15–20
Peripheral nerve	neuropathy	15–20
Spinal cord	myelopathy	15–20
Brain	encephalopathy	15–20
Microcirculation	vasculitis	15–20
Connective tissue stroma	inflamation	15–20
>2,000 cGy		
Bone and cartilage	osteitis/fracture	>20
Muscle	myositis/myopathy	>20
Endocrines: pituitary/adrenals	hypopituitarism	>20
Pancereas	Addisonian pancreatitis/ diabetes	>20

Fractionated Doses, Whole and Partial Organ Volumes

The greatest clinical experience is with limited field irradiation to a part of an organ and has provided insights into tissue/organ radiation sensitivity. Many dose ranges have been avoided in human situations, and only animal data exist as a guide. Unfortunately, large fraction size and shorter time intervals are often exployed in experiments and are different from conventional clinical schedules, where 2 Gy daily and 10 Gy weekly are the standard. Despite these limitations, an ordering of radiation sensitivity according to fractionated regimens illustrates a shifting in relative position as compared to single exposures for these same tissues/organs [4, 14, 15] (table IV).

Table IV. Tolerance doses TD_5–TD_{50}

Target cell fractionated dose/whole or partial organ	Complication end point	TD_5–TD_{50} dose range, Gy
200–1,000 cGy		
Lymphocytes and lymphoid	lymphopenia	2–10
Testes spermatogonia	sterility	1–2
Ovarian oocytes	sterility	6–10
1,000–2,000 cGy		
Lens	cataract	6–12
Bone marrow stem cell	acute aplasia	15–20
2,000–3,000 cGy		
Kidney: renal glomeruli	arterionephrosclerosis	23–28
Lung: type II VCTS	pneumonitis/fibrosis	20–30
3,000–4,000 cGy		
Liver central veins	hepatopathy	35–40
Bone marrow	hypoplasia	25–35
4,000–5,000 cGy		
Heart/whole organ	pericarditis and pancarditis	43–50
Bone marrow microenvironments, sinusitis	permanent aplasia	45–50
5,000–6,000 cGy		
Gastrointestinal	infarction necrosis	50–55
Heart/partial organ	cardiomyopathy	55–65
Spinal cord	myelopathy	50–60
Brain	encephalopathy	50–60
>6,000–7,000 cGy		
Mucosa (UAD)	ulcer	65–75
Rectum	ulcer	65–75
Bladder	ulcer	65–75
Mature bones	fracture	65–70
Pancreas	pancreatitis	

UAD = Upper aerodigestive tract; VCTS = vasculoconnective tissue systems.

Two to Ten Gy (200–1,000 cGy)

With fractionated doses of less than 10 Gy, the testes spermatogonia, ovarian oogonia, and lens epithilium are injuried. The testes spermatogonia are very sensitive to smaller fractional doses are more efficiently destroyed than ovarian tissue. Lymphocytes and lymphoid tissues also will be suppressed with trivial doses.

Ten to Twenty Gy (1,000–2,000 cGy)

With fractionated doses of 10–20 Gy, the normal bone marrow hematopoietic stem cells will be depressed, but with limited volumes larger doses will be required to achieve suppression. In disease states unlike the normal state, small fractional doses, i.e., <10 Gy, may ablate the bone marrow. Growing cartilage and growing bone will also be arrested within this dose range.

Twenty to Thirty Gy (2,000–3,000 cGy)

Between 20 and 30 Gy, a number of vital organs reach their radiation threshold and decompensate despite fractionation. This is most apparent when an entire organ is so treated. The kidneys and lungs are both vulnerable to this dose level and reflect a combination of injury to the microvasculature and epithelial cell injury.

Thirty to Forty Gy (3,000–4,000 cGy)

The liver becomes vulnerable. For many organs, there are little data on whole-organ fractional therapy schedules, but skin and oropharyngeal mucosa can become acutely reactive. The liver displays a special veno-occlusive even secondary to platelet adhesion to central veins at or somewhat above this dose level.

Forty to Fifty Gy (4,000–5,000 cGy)

At this dose level, the heart and gastrointestinal organs are likely to experience severe and life-threatening injury, particularly with large or entire organ irradiation.

Fifty to Sixty Gy (5,000–6,000 cGy)

The majority of organs are vulnerable to fractionated schedules in the 50- to 60-Gy range. Gastrointestinal injury is significant, and the colorectal tissues become vulnerable. Spinal cord and brain may become demyelinated. The vascular connective tissue stroma is effected in this dose range and has a major effect even in partial organ irradiation as in lung, liver, kidney, and bone marrow, with long-term fibrosis occurring even if smaller volumes are irradiated

Sixty to Seventy Gy (6,000–7,000 cGy)

At this range, the brain is more likely to react to irradation by undergoing demyelination at the TD_{5-50} levels. Rectum and bladder become vulnerable to major injury at the TD_5 level. Mature bone and cartilage are able to withstand these levels as are pancreas, peripheral nerves, and muscle.

Changing Order of Radiosensitivity as a Function of Volume

The volume or an irradiated organ or tissue may be as important as the fractionation effect in determining the total dose prescribed [8] (table V). Paterson [12] first quantified the impact of volume on radiation response of normal skin showing an inverse relationship of dose and volume using similar fractionation schemas. Von Essen [29] indicated that increasing the volume of tumor and normal skin leads to as adverse therapeutic ratio, since the slopes for tumor curability and normal-tissue tolerance were different (fig. 4). Fractionation of dose resulted in favorable therapeutic ratios for skin tumors <3 cm^2 but was virtually impossible to achieve for large volumes exceeding 100 cm^2. A three-dimensional model relating dose, time, and volume indicated the balance required for an uncomplicated cure.

The concept of a 'tolerance volume' needs to be defined similar to a 'tolerance dose'. The volume is more critical to complication outcome and also serves as a clinical guide, since it is possible to obliterate or lose a certain volume of a vital organ with large doses, i.e., exceeding the $TD_{90\text{-}100}$ is akin to surgical resection. Loss of a certain volume does not effect organ survival, since the organ can offer compensate for loss of volume through regeneration or hypertrophy and remain within function tolerance for survival though impaired: (1) tolerance volume (TV)

Table V. Volume effects

	% ablated, compatible with detectable effect	% ablated incompatible with survival	Lethal event
Bone marrow	<25	>75–100	+
Ovary	50	100	0
Testes	50	100	0
Lens	<25	>75–100	0
Lung	25–50	>75–100	+
Gastrointestinal tract	>5	?	+
Kidney	50	76	+
Heart	25	>75–100	+
Liver	25–50	>75–100	+
Mucosa	25–50	>75–100	+
Peripheral nerve	>5	?	0
Spinal cord	>5	?	+
Brain	>5	>50–100	+
Bone/cartilage	>10	?	0

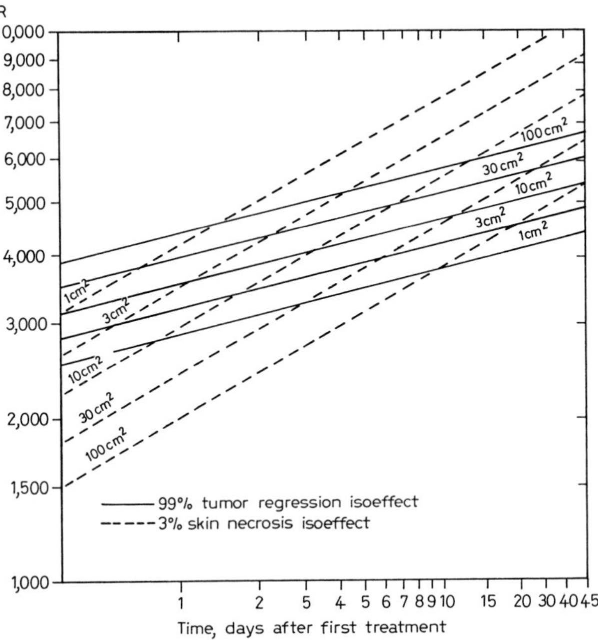

Fig. 4. Modification of the Strandqvist concept by volume factor. Isoeffect lines for tumor and skin (normal tissue) are no longer parallel. Despite increasing fractionation, it is not possible to achieve a favorable therapeutic ratio for larger skin cancers (100 cm^2) as compared to smaller ones (10 cm^2). R = Roentgen. [From ref. 29, with permission.]

5–25%: irradiation of 5–25% of the organ volume can result in a life-threatening or lethal complication; (2) tolerance volume (TV) 50–90%: irradiation of 50–90% of the organ volume can result in a life-threatening or lethal complication.

There are generally two levels of critical volumes for the dose-limiting or vital organs defined as class I – essential for life or survival. Only the gastrointestinal tract and the central nervous system can have disastrous outcomes after small volumes (TV 5–25%) are exposed to doses exceeding $TD_{5\text{-}50}$. It is also important to note that necrotic bowel can be resected, and on occasion necrotic foci can be successfully resected in brain. For the majority of organs often considered dose limiting, the bone marrow, the lung, the kidney, and in all probability the heart and the liver can tolerate higher doses to smaller volumes. Such organs may decompensate when more than 50% of the total volume (as applied to paired organs) is exceeded. When organ decompensation begins, clear-

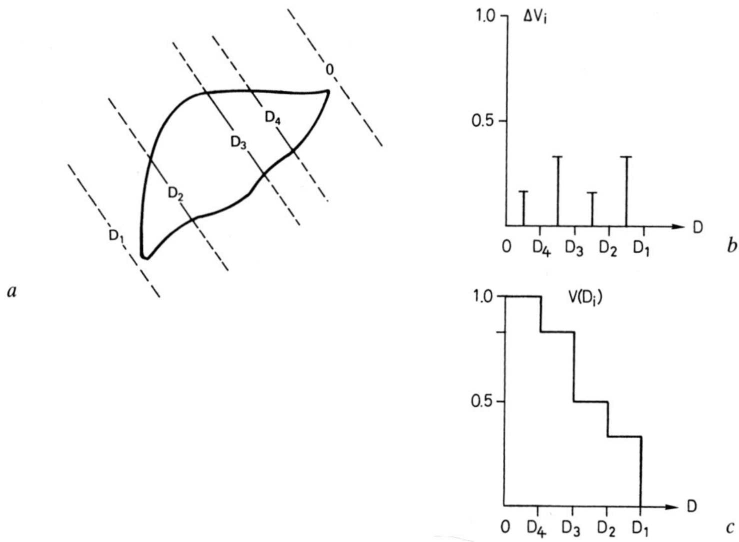

Fig. 5. Creation of a dose-volume histogram. Representation of the three-dimensional distribution of doses within a planar isodose map for the organ. The dashed lines in a show isodose lines outside the organ under consideration. Note the convention that the index i on D_i increases with decreasing dose. *b* Differential dose-volume histogram derived from a complete set of such maps. *c* The equivalent integral, or dose-cummulative volume, histogram. $V(D_i)$ refers to the fraction of the organ receiving dose D_i or more. [From ref. 9. with permission.]

ly depends upon the compensatory regnerative mechanisms that come into play when significant organ volume loss occurs. For example, there are numerous mechanisms that exist in the bone marrow when a certain percentage of the volume is ablated [4, 18, 19]. Paradoxically, there is in-field regeneration of bone marrow for 'ablative doses,' i.e., >3,000 cGy when more than 50% of its volume is irradiated. Thus, in Hodgkin's disease, irradiation of mantle fields (25% of the bone marrow organ volume) leads to permanent aplasia or hypoplasia of sternal marrow due to compensatory hyperplasia of the unirradiated bone marrow. However, with total nodal irradiation, which effects more than 50% of the bone marrow organ, compensating mechanisms lead to extension of bone marrow into the femoral shafts and humeri and a return of in-field vertebral bone marrow regeneration.

The dose-volume histogram is being adopted by numerous investigators to predict unfavorable outcomes as a result of volume loss in a critical structure [3] (fig. 5). Thus, the dose-response curves for an individual organ will change as a function of volume and dose. With computerized three-dimensional dosimetry programs, each patient's customized radiation therapy should be considered as a complete dose-response curve rather than as one point on a dose-response curve. The data in the clinical and experimental literature can be divided into four categories: (1) whole organ – single doses; (2) whole organ – fractionated doses; (3) partial organ – single doses, and (4) partial organ – fractionated doses.

From this type of analysis, it is possible to generate a modifying factor for dose and volume, but the data required are incomplete for many organ sites. Restated, the range of total doses used in the clinic varies with the volume and dose fractionation. Volume-modifying factors (VMF) and dose-modifying factors (DMF), therefore, can be approximated for different vital organs. Although it is beyond the scope of this presentation to present an accurate analysis of these data, hopefully it should be possible to reconstruct when the conference papers are published and retrospectively reviewed and analyzed. These modifying factors are defined:

$$\text{VMF} = \frac{\text{TD}_{5-50}\text{ for partial-organ irradiation}}{\text{TD}_{5-50}\text{ for whole-organ irradiation}} \qquad (1)$$

$$\text{DMF} = \frac{\text{TD}_{5-50}\text{ for fractionated irradiation}}{\text{TD}_{5-50}\text{ for single-dose irradiation}} \qquad (2)$$

Generally, the VMF for most organ systems allows for an increment in tolerance dose, as one decreases the volume from one to five times that utilized for whole-organ irradiation and more often is only two to three times. The DMF for most organ systems is similar, i.e., the tolerance dose increases by a factor of two to three times when the ratio of single doses is compared to conventional daily dose fractionation.

According to Lyman [8] and Lyman and Wolbarst [9], many authors have offered a simple model for dependence on irradiated volume of dose to achieve a specified complication, namely a power-law relationship of the form:

$$\text{TD(V)} = \text{TD(1)V}^{n} \qquad (3)$$

where TD = tolerance dose, V = the fraction of the volume (or the ratio of the size of irradiated tissue to some reference size), and n = a size-dependent parameter. Further Lyman [8] presented a three-parameter model which connects the three variables of interest: Complication probability (P), dose (D), and volume (V), expressed as follows:

$$P = \frac{1}{\sqrt{2\pi}} \int_{-\infty}^{t_{max}} e^{-t^2/2} dt \tag{4}$$

where $t = [D\text{-}TD_{50}(V)/(V)]$ and $(V) = m^*TD_{50}(V)$. Equation 3 is used to obtain $TD_{50}(V)$, and m is the third free parameter which is to be determined by the data. This formula is a combination of the power law dose-volume relationship (equation 3) and an error function representation of the complication-dose relationship and gives back these equations if complication probability or volume, respectively, are held constant.'

The three-dimensional display relating dose and volume with the probability of complications is important to this clinical concept [9] (fig. 6). The dose-response curve and its steepness varies as a function of volume, and organ tolerance should not be viewed or expressed simply as a function of dose. That is, there are a large number of dose-response curves to express organ tolerance according to the volume of the irradiated organ. The probability of a 5 or 50% complication rate is plotted in figure 7 and graphically demonstrates that as the volume decreases, the dose required to produce a complication increases [8].

Uniform Toxicity Scoring

To conclude on an important pragmatic note, there is a need to develop a uniform toxicity scoring for late effects [20, 21]. The introduction of mutlimodal management to cancer treatment has resulted in differences in reporting toxicity to treatment. The radiation oncologist is more concerned and aware of the importance of late effects once the acute phase of the reaction has been cared for in contrast to medical oncologists. However, chemotherapy produces late effects similar to irradiation, and these complications have been increasingly documented in the literature, but the focus still remains on relatively acute and subacute effects. As a result, two different scoring and grading systems for toxicity have emerged. The radiation scores have been oriented toward specific pathologic lesions, whereas chemotherapy grades usually reflect functional and physiologic changes. Toxicity reporting of multiagent chemotherapy combinations and/or their interaction with radiation effects has lad to national cooperative groups to form committees to mainly assess acute effects and develop scoring and grading systems for these toxicities. A

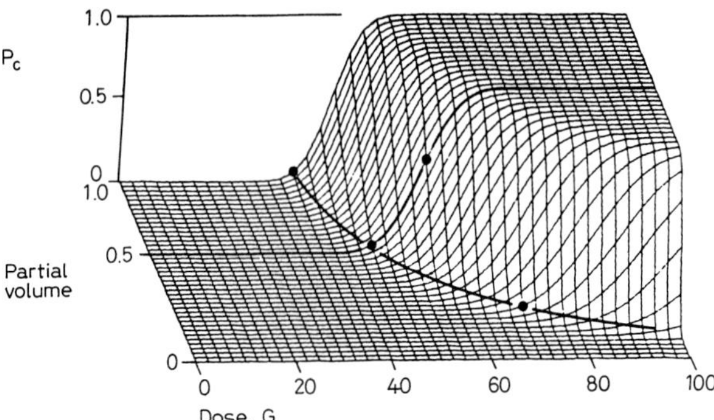

Fig. 6. Each organ has a spectrum of dose-response curves as a function of volume irradiated. A three-dimensional surface representation of the probability of complication (P_c) for the heart as a function of the dose and the partial volume which is uniformily irradiated. [From ref. 8, with permission.]

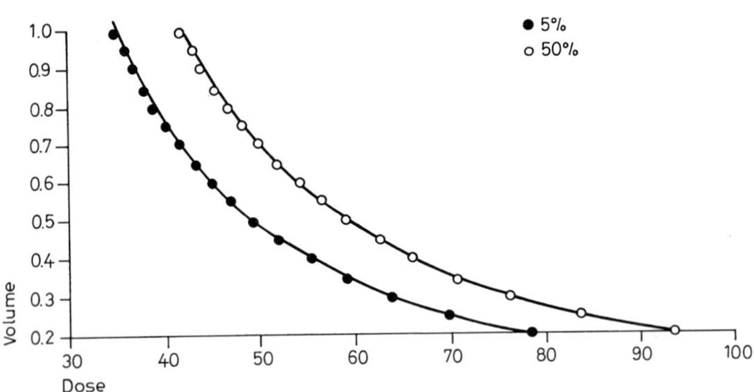

Fig. 7. Volume-dose relationship. As the volume of an organ irradiated decreases, the dose to produce 5 or 50% complications increases. This illustrates that there is no 'fixed' safe dose or tolerance dose TD_5 and TD_{50}, but it varies. [By courtesy of Lyman, unpubl. data.]

recommendation for a uniform system is the desired end product based upon 'consensus criteria'. In September 1985, a conference on toxicity was held in Baltimore, Md., USA. A subcommittee, comprised of representatives from several cooperative groups and the National Cancer Institute, was formed at this meeting with the aim of addressing the question

Table VI. Scale [from ref, 20, will permission]

Grade				
1 (mild)	2 (moderate)	3 (severe)	4 (life-threatening)	5 (fatal)
10% ↑ ↓	25% ↑ ↓	50% ↑ ↓	75% ↑ ↓	100% ↑ ↓
Range of Values, relative units				
1–3 (1.5 × NL)	3–5 (3 × NL)	5–8 (5 × NL)	8–10 (10 × NL)	>10 (> × NL)

NL = Normal.

of standardized toxic effects criteria. Conclusions and recommendations made by the committee are summarized below [20]:

(1) There is a need for uniform toxicity scoring, both for acute and late effects, but particularly with regard to late effects in vital organs.

(2) The toxicity scale should consists of five values including mild, moderate, severe, life-threatening, and fatal. The emphasis should be on grade 3, 4, and 5 levels with consideration for both peak grade and time in developing an appropriate index (table VI).

(3) In addition to the major modalities of radiation therapy and chemotherapy, which are known to produce such late effects, the effects of host cofactors, other modalities, and recurrent tumor need to be carefully considered.

(4) End points need to be clearly defined in terms of somatic, genetic, and second malignant tumors with appropriate time scales set, preferably more than 6 months following the introduction of treatment. There is a need for a working committee on late effects representing all major modalities including a radiation oncologist, a medical oncologist, and a surgical oncologist, depending upon the site.

(5) Protocols for longitudinal studies of key dose limiting normal tissues and organs in which the appropriate standard diagnostic laboratory and imaging tests are used need to be developed. These should include CT, MRI, and PET scans.

(6) Actuarial risk reporting and recall of long-term survivors should be done initially in select patient cohorts, namely survivors beyond 2 years. Although malignancies in which there are 50% survival have been considered most appropriate for such studies, this requirement may be too stringent, and instead the assessment of adverse effects should be done in all survivors beyond 2 years. This is particularly true for highly fatal cancers where intensive regimens of combined modalities are used.

(7) Publications should routinely present therapeutic ratios and use standard toxicity and late-effect scoring along with tumor response rates [20].

Further efforts were made at Williamsburg in 1987 to develop precise criteria for category I/II organ toxicity by defining the late-effect pathologic lesion, evaluative diagnostic tests, medical and surgical intervention, and whether the acute and late effects were different or similar by organ site (see table VII) [21]. Most recently, Wittes [30] has circulated a standardized system for acute toxicity scoring derived at a National Cancer Institute consensus meeting which was recommended by the national cooperative groups to all investigators involved in clinical trials (table VIII). A similar standardized late-effect classification needs to be more widely adopted and should be based upon the available RTOG-EORTC late-effect system (table IX). Protocols need to be developed prospectively to accurately document late effects in all long-term survivors, i.e., more than 2 years survival [21].

Predictive Assays for Late Effects

There is a need for predictive assays for late effects in vital normal tissues, as there is a need for predictive assays in tumors [22]. The ability to titrate the radiation dose would be ideal for radiation oncology practitioners prior to the completion of treatment to avoid later severe or life-threatening complications. A simple biochemical test that is accurate and reproducible would be ideal. Since there is no relationship between acute and late radiation effects in most vital organs, this is even more important for achieving a favorable therapeutic ratio. An illustration of this approach is the development of surfactant release as a measure or index of developing later fatal radiation pneumonitis [23]. In a number of different murine strains and different species, such as the rabbit, the detection of increased levels of alveolar surfactant and serum surfactant on day 7 after irradiation correlates with later lethality at 4 months [24]. [See also Lung Chapter; Rubin et al., this volume.] A similar assay has been developed for myelin basic protein released into the cerebrospinal fluid 1–2 months after radiation which correlates with late myelopathy [25]. Although these are laboratory models at present, protocols are available for human study. These are the first biochemical markers identified for later radiation effects and represent a line of study that would be extended to many other vital tissues and organs. The hypothesis is that unique antigens and other biochemical products and proteins are released into body fluids and sera during or at the conclusion of irradiation

Table VII. Class I/II organs: pathologic lesions, evaluative testing, and possible interventions for treatment-related injuries [form ref. 23, with permission]

Organ	Class	Pathologic lesion	Evaluative testing	Therapeutic intervention		Scoring/ grading
				medical	surgical	
Nervous system Peripheral	II	demyelinization hepatic necrosis	nerve conduction studies	anesthesia (e.g., nerve block)	surgery	A = L
Central Brain	I	demyelinization necrosis	CT/MRI, EEG, MBP in cerebrospinal fluid	steroids, antiepileptics, supportive	surgery	A = L
Spinal cord		demyelinization necrosis	myelogram, MRI, MBP	care, steroids, antiepileptics		A = L
Bone marrow	I	aplasia, fatty replacement	peripheral blood counts, bone marrow scanning MRI, bone marrow biopsy/aspiration	transfusion, antibiotics	bone marrow transplant	A = L
Lung	I	XRT: *acute:* pneumonitis, alveolar cell hyperplasia, intraalveolar hyaline membrane, thickened alveolar septum *chronic:* fibrosis chemo: *BNCU:* interstitial pneumonitis, pulmonary fibrosis *CTX:* proliferation of alveolar lining cells *Busulfan:* interstitial fibrosis	pulmonary function test (including exercise testing), CXR, CT: isotope scans, biochemical tests in serium or lung lavage (surfactant)	steroids O_2, assisted ventilation, surfasctant		A = L
Cardiac	I	XRT: pericarditis, endomyocarditis, pancarditis, vascular changes Chemo: anthracycline: myopathy	ECG, CXR, Echo, rest/exercise-gated nuclear angiography, endomyocardial biopsy, thallium scanning	medications	surgery (e.g., for tamponade)	A = L
Liver	I	hepatitis, veno-occlusive disease, cirrhosis	lab: SGOT, SGPT, alkaline phosphatase, bilirubin, nuclear scans, CT/MRI, ultrasound	medications	resection	A = L

(Table VII continued on next page)

Table VII. (continued)

Organ	Class	Pathologic lesion	Evaluative testing	Therapeutic intervention		Scoring/ grading
				medical	surgical	
Kidney	I	acute nephritis, chronic nephropathy, atrophy	Lab: serum: blood urea nitrogen, creatinine, albumin urine: protein, blood, blood presure, CT, nuclear scans, prostaglandin excretion	medications, dialysis	transplant	A = L
Skin	II	inflammation, ulceration, epilation, atrophy		Topical medications, wet/dry soaks, supportive care	surgery	A = L
Subcutaneous tissue	II	fibrosis, atrophy		supportive care (exercise, e.g., physical therapy)		A = L
Oral cavity Mucosa	II	Inflammation, ulceration, fibrosis		medications, supportive care		A = L
Bone		osteonecrosis	X-rays	supportive care	surgery	late only
Salivary glands		inflammation, fibrosis, atrophy	sialogram	supportive care, artificial saliva		A = L
Gastrointestinal						
Esophagus	I	inflammation, fibrosis, necrosis	radiography (plain films with contrast agents, barium swallow, fluoroscopy, CT, MRI), esophagoscopy	medications, supportive care	surgery	A = L
stomach	I	inflammation, ulceration, atrophy	radiography, endoscopy, barium swallow	medications, supportive care	surgery	A = L
UGI		inflammation, ulceration, fibrosis, necrosis	Radiography (plain films with contrast agents), endoscopy, stool guaiac	medications, diet	surgery	A = L

LGI		inflammation, ulceration, fibrosis, necrosis	radiography (plain films with contrast agents), endoscopy, stool guaiac	medications	surgery	A = L
Bladder	II	telangiectasia, fibrosis, necrosis	radiography (with contrast), cystoscopy, IVP, RUG	medications	surgery	A = L
Ears	II					
Hearing		Inflammation, serious otitis, scierosis	auditory testing	medication, mechanical device	surgery	A = L
Balance		labrynthitis	equilbrium testing	medication	surgery	A = L
Eye	II					
Retina		retinitis, vascular changes, detachment, fibrosis	ophthalmic exam, evoked responses	medication	surgery	A = L
Conjunctiva		Conjunctivitis, telangiectasia, ulceration	ophthalmic exam	medication		A = L
Cornea		keratitis, neovascularization	ophthalmic exam	medication		A = L
Angle of schlemm aqueous veins		glaucoma	ophthalmic exam, tonometry	medication	surgery	A = L
Lens		cataract	ophthalmic exam		surgery	late only
Cartilage	II					
Growing		growth arrest	sequential measurements, X-rays	mechanical lifts	epiphysectomy of contralateral epiphysis	Late
mature		chondritis, loss of vascularization, cellular dissarray, necrosis	X-rays including angiography		surgery	A = L
Bone	II	osteonecrosis	X-rays	supportive care, artificial saliva		A = L
Endocrine glands	II					
Hypothalmus/ pituitary		cellular changes (degranulation, vacuolation, necrosis), hemorrhage	baseline hormonal and stimulation testing	medication		A = L
Thyroid		atrophy	baseline hormonal and stimulation testing	medication		A = L

A = Acute toxic effects; L = late toxic effects; MBP = myelin basic protein; CT/MRI = computerized tomography/magnetic resonance imaging; XRT = radiation therapy; Chemo = chemotherapy; CXR = chest X-ray; Echo = echocardiogram; UGI = upper gastrointestinal series; LGI = lower gastrointestinal series; IVP = intravenous pyelogram; RUG = retrograde urogram.

Table VIII. Common toxicity criteria [from ref. 30, with permission]

Toxicity	Grade				
	0	1	2	3	4
Blood/bone marrow					
WBC	≥4.0	3.0 – 3.9	2.0–2.9	1.0–1.9	<1.0
PLT	WNL	75.0 – normal	50.0–74.9	25.0–49.9	<25.0
hemoglobin	WNL	10.0 – normal	8.0–10.0	6.5–7.9	<6.5
Granulocytes/ Bands	≥2.0	1.5 – 1.9	1.0–1.4	0.5–0.9	<0.5
Lymphocytes	≥2.0	1.5 – 1.9	1.0–1.4	0.5–0.9	<0.5
Hemorrhage (clinical)	none	mild, no transfusion	gross, 1–2 transfusion per episode	gross, 3–4 transfusion per episode	massive, >4 transfusion per apisode
infection	none	mild	moderate	severe	life-threatening
Gastrointestinal					
Nausea	none	able to eat reasonable intake	intake significantly decreased but can eat	no significant intake	—
Vomiting	none	1 episode in 24 hrs	2–5 episodes in 24 h	6–10 episodes in 24 h	>10 episodes in 24 h or requiring parenteral support
Diarrha	none	increase of 2–3 stools/day over pre-irradiation	increase of 4–6 stools/day or nocturna stools or moderate cramping	increase of 7–9 stools/day or incontinence or severe cramping	increase of ≥10 stools/day or groosly bloody diarrhea or need for parenteral support
Stomatitis	none	painless ulcers, erythema, or mild soreness	painful erythema, edema, or ulcers, but can eat	painful erythema, edema, or ulcers, cannot eat	requires parenteral or entaral support

Liver					
Bilirubin	WNL	—	<1.5 × N	1.5–3.0 × N	>3.0 × N
Transaminase (SGOT, SGPT)	WNL	≤2.5 × N	2.6 – 5.0 × N	5.1–20.0 × N	>20.0 × N
Alkaline phosphatase or 5′-nucleotidase	WNL	≤2.5 × N	2.6 – 5.0 × N	5.1–20.0 × N	>20.0 × N
Clinical	no change from baseline	—	—	precoma	hepatic coma
Kidney, bladder					
Creatinine	WNL	<1.5 × N	1.5–3.0 × N	3.1–6.0 × N	6.0 × N
Protainuria	no change	1 + or <0.3 g% or <3 g/1	2–3 = or 0.3–1.0 g% or 3–10 g/1	4+ or >1.0 g% or >10 g/1	nephrotic syndrome
Hemmaturia	negative	micro only	gross, no clots	gross, clots	requires transfusion
Alopecia	no loss	mild hair loss	pronounced or total hair loss	—	—
Pulmonary	none or no change	asymptomatic, with abnormality in PFTs	dyspnea on significant exertion	dyspnea at normal level of activity	dyspnea at rest
Heart					
Cardiac dys-rhythmias	none	asymptomatic, transient, requiring no therapy	recurrent or persistent, no therapy required	requires treatment	requires monitor-ing or (hypotension, or ventricular tachycardia, fibrillation)
Cardiac function	none	asymptomatic, decline of resting ejection fraction by less than 20% of baseline value	asymptomatic, decline of restion ejection fraction by less than 20% of baseline value	mild congestive heart failure, responsive to therapy	severe or refrac-tory congestive heart failure

(Table VIII continued on next page)

Table VIII. (continued)

Toxicity	Grade				
	0	1	2	3	4
Cardiac ischemia	none	nonspecific T wave flattening	asymptomatic, ST and T wave changes suggessting ischemia	angina without evidence for infarction	acute myocardial infarction
Cardiac-pericardial	none	asymptomatic effusion, no intervention required	pericarditis (rub, chest pain, ECG changes)	symptomatic effusion, drainage required	tamponada, drainage urgently re-quired
Blood pressure					
Hypertension	none or no change	asymptomatic, transient increase by greater than 20 mm Hg (diastolic) or to <150/100 if previously WNL; no treatment required	recurrent or per-sistent increase by greater than 20 mm Hg (diastolic) or to >150/100 if previously WNL; no treatment required	requires therapy	hypertensive crisis
Hypotension	none or no change	changes requiring no therapy (including transient orthostatic hypotension)	requires fluid replace-ment or other therapy, but not hospitalization	requires therapy and hos-pitalization: resolves within 48 h if stopping the agent	requires therapy and hospita-lization for <48 h after stopping the agent
Neurologic					
Sensory	none or no change	mild paresthesias. loss of deep tendon reflexes	mild or moderate objective sensory loss, moderate paresthesias	severe objective sensory loss or paresthesias that interfere with function	—
Motor	none or no change	subjective weakness, no objective findings	mild objective weakness without significant im-pairment of function	objective weakness with impairment of function	paralysis

Cortical	none	mild somnolence or agitation	moderate somnolence or agitation	severe somnolence, agitation, confusion, disorientation, or hallucinations	coma, seizures, toxic psychosis
Cerebellar	none	slight incoordination, dysdiadokinesis	intention tremor, dysmetria, slurred speech, nystagmus	locomotor ataxia	cerebellar necrosis
Mood	no change	mild anxiety or depression	moderate anxiety or depression	severe anxiety or depression	suicidal ideation
Headache	none	mild	moderate or severe, but transient	unrelenting and severe	—
Constipation	none or no change	mild	moderate	severe	ileus >96 hrs
Hearing	none or no change	asymptomatic, hearing loss on audiometry only	tinnitus	hearing loss interfering with function, but correctable with hearing aid	deafness not correctable
Vision	none or no change	—	—	symptomatic subtotal loss of vision	blindness
Skin	none or no change	scattered macular or papular eruption or erythema that is asymptomatic	scattered macular or papular eruption or erythema with pruritus or other associated symptoms	generalized symptomatic macular, papular, or vesicular eruption	exfoliative determatitis or ulcerating determatitis
Allergy	none	transient rash, drug fever <38 °C (100.4 °F)	urticaria, drug fever = 38 °C (100.4 °F), mild bronchospasm	serum sickness, bronchospasm, requiring parenteral medication	anaphylaxis
Fever in absence of infection	none	37.1–38.0 °C (98.7–100.4 °F)	38.1–40.0 °C (100.5–104.0 °F)	>40.0 °C (>104.0 °F) for less than 24 h	>40.0°C (104.0°F) for more than 24 h of fever accompanied by hypotension

(Table VIII continued on next page)

Table VIII. (continued)

Toxicity	Grade				
	0	1	2	3	4
Local	none	pain	pain and swelling with inflammation or phlebitis	ulceration	plastic surgery indicated
Weight gain/loss, %	<5.0	5.0–9.9	10.0–19.9	≥20.0	—
Metabolic					
Hyperglycemia	<116	116–160	161–250	251–500	—
Hypoglycemia	>64	55–64	40–54	30–39	<500 or keto-acidosis
Amylase	WNL	<1.5 × N	1.5–2.0 × N	2.1–5.0 × N	>30
Hypercalcemia	<10.6	10.6–11.5	11.6–12.5	12.6–13.5	<5.1 × N
Hypocalcemia	>8.4	8.4–7.8	7.7–7.0	6.9–6.1	≥13.5
Hypomagnesemia	>1.4	1.4–1.2	1.1–0.9	0.8–0.6	≤6.0
					≤0.5
Coagulation					
Fibrinogen	WNL	0.99–0.75 × N	0.74–0.50 × N	0.49–0.25 × N	≤0.24 × N
Prothrombin time	WNL	1.01–1.25 × N	1.26–1.50 × N	1.51–2.00 × N	>2.00 × N
					>3.00 × N
Partial thromboplastin time	WNL	1.01–1.66 × N	1.67–2.33 × N	2.34–3.00 × N	

WBC = White blood cell count; PLT = ; WNL = Normal value; N = ; PFT =

Table IX. RTOG/EORTC late radiation morbidity scoring scheme[1]

Organ/tissue	Grade				
	0	1	2	3	4
Skin	none	slight atrophy, pigmentation change some hair loss	patchy atrophy, moderate telangiectasia, total hair loss	marked atrophy, gross telangiectasia	ulceration
subcutaneous tissue	none	slight induration (fibrosis) and loss of subcutaneous fat	moderate fibrosis, but asymptomatic/slight field contracture/less than 10% linear reduction	severe induration and loss of subcutaneous tissue field contracture >10% linear measurement	necrosis
Mucous membranes	none	slight atrophy and dryness	moderate atrophy and telangiectasia/little mucous	marked atrophy with complete dryness/ severe telangiectasia	ulceration
Salivary glands	none	slight dryness or mouth/ good response on stimulation	moderate dryness of mouth/poor response on stimulation	complete dryness of mouth/no response on stimulation	fibrosis
Spinal cord	none	mild L'Hersitte syndrome	severe L'Hersitte syndrome	objective neurological findings at or below cord level treated	mono, para euadriplesis
Brain	none	mild headache/slight lethargy	moderate headache/great lethargy	severe headache, severe CNS dysfunction (partial less of power or dyskinesia)	seizures or paralysis/ coma
Eye	none	asymtomatic cataract, minor corneal ulceration or keratitis	symtomatic cataract, moderate corneal ulceration/minor retinopathy or glaucoas	severe keratitis, severe retinopathy or detachment/severe glaucoas	panophthalsitis, blindness
Larynx	none	noarseness/slight arytenoid edeas	moderate arytenoid edema/chondritis	severe edeas/severe chondritis	necrosis

(Table IX continued on next page)

Table IX. (continued)

Organ/tissue	Grade				
	0	1	2	3	4
Lung	none	asymptomatic or mild symptoms (dry cough), slight radiographic appearances	moderate symptomatic fibrosis or pneumonitis (severe cough), low-grade fever/patchy radiographic appearances	severe symptomatic fibrosis or pneumonitis, dnese radiographic changes	severe respiratory insufficiency/ continuous O_2/ assisted ventilation
Heart	none	asymptomatic or mild symptoms/transient T wave inversion and ST changes/sinus tachycardia >110 (at rest)	moderate angina on effort/mild pericarditis/ normal heart size/ persistent abnormality of T wave and ST changes/low QRS	severe angina/pericardial effusion/constrictive pericarditis/moderate heart failure/cardiac enlargement/ECG abnormalities	tasponde/severe heart failure, severe constrictive pericarditis
Esophagus	none	mild fibrosis/slight difficulty in swallowsing solids/no pain on swallowing	unable to take solid food normally/swallowing semisolid food dilatation may be indicated	severe fibrosis/able to swallow only liquids/ may have pain on swallowing, dilatation required	necrosis/perforation/ fistula
Small/large intestine	none	mild diarrhea/mild cramind/bowel movement 5 times daily/ slight rectal discharge or bleeding	moderate diarrhea and colic/bowel movement <5 times daily/ excessive rectal sucus or intermittent bleeding	obstruction or bleeding requiring surgery	necrosis/perforation/ fistula
Liver	none	mild lassitude/nausea dyspepsia/slightly abnormal liver function	moderate symptoms/ some abnormal liver function tests/serum albumin normal	disabling hapatic insufficiency/liver function tests grossly abnormal/low level edema or ascites	necrosis/hepatic coma or encephalopathy

Kidney	none	transient albuminuria, no hypertension/mild impairment of renal function/urea 25–35 mg%/creatinine 1.5–2.0 mg%/creatinine clearance >75%	persistent moderate albuminuria (2+)/mild hypertension/no related anesia/moderate impairment of the renal function/urea >36–60 mg%/creatinine 2.5–4.0 mg%/creatinine clearance 50–74%	severe albuminuria/severe hypertension/persistent anesia (<10 g%)/severe renal failure/urea >60 mg%/creatinine >4.0 mg%/creatinine clearance <50%	maligment hypertension/ureaic coma/urea >100%
Bladder	none	slight epithalial atrophy/minor telangiectasia (microscopic hematuria)	moderate frequency/generalized telangiectasia/intermittent macroscopic hematuria	severe frequency % dysuria/severe generalized telengiectasia (often with petechiae)/frequent hematuria/reduction in bladder capacity(<150 cm^3)	necrosis/contracted bladder (capacity <100 cm^3)/severe hemorrhasic cystitis
Bone	none	asymptomatic/no growth retardation/reduced bone density	moderate pain or tenderness/growth retardation/Irregular bone sclerosis	severe pain or tenderness/complete arrest of bone growth/dense bone sclerosis	necrosis/spontaneous fracture
Joint	none	mild joint stiffness/slight limitation of movement	moderate stiffness/intermittent or moderate joint pain/moderate limitation of movement	severe joint stiffness/pain with severe ligitation of movement	necrosis/complete fixation

[1] Grade 5 would indicate death directly related to radiation late effect.

that are measurable and useful as predictors. Furthermore, during the clinical latent period, when biochemical events are occurring but have not expressed themselves (i.e., cellular/tissue injury), corrective interventions can be applied. Bone marrow transplantation is widely used, and other tissue and organ transplant methods for restoration are under study. Radioprotectors (i.e., WR-2721 and others) have the potential to protect bone marrow, skin, mucosa, and salivary glands [27]. Dramatic results with avoidance of lung fibrosis have been demonstrated by Yu et al. [31].

Specific Organ $TD_{5\text{-}50}$: Conclusions

(1) There is a shifting of order in organ radiosensitivity, depending on different critical cell subpopulations in the organ, in addition to differences in repair, repopulation, and regeneration of the critical cell; (2) there is a wide range of radiosensitivity of organ failure, depending on volume and dose-time factors; (3) a thorough understanding of radiation pathophysiology of the multiple cell populations interacting is required to understand late effects in this multimodal era; (4) the tolerance doses $TD_{5/5}$–$TD_{50/5}$ for specific organs serve as a guide but are not 'safe doses' due to drugs and innovations; (5) volume is perhaps more critical as a clinical guide, i.e., a certain percentage of a critical volume is lost with high doses – akin to surgical resection –, but is within tolerance for survival; (6) VMFs need better definition and data similar to $TD_{5\text{-}50}$ such as tolerance volume 5–25 and 50–90; (7) tolerance scoring needs to be uniform both for acute and late effects and be adopted both by radiation and medical oncologists; (8) chemotherapy has altered concepts of 'early' and 'late' effects and produces late effects itself; (9) predictive assays using serum biochemical markers are possible, and (10) corrective and preventative maneuvers are possible to avoid late effects – late radiation damage should not be viewed as permanent and irreversible effects.

References

1 Bergonie, J.; Tribondeau, L.: Interprétation de quelques résultats de la radiothérapie et essai de fixation d'une technique rationelle. C. r. hebd. Séanc. Acad. Sci., Paris *143:* 938–985 (1906).
2 Casarett, G. W.: Radiation histopathology, vol. I and II (Chemical Rubber Press, Boca Raton, 1980).
3 Chen, G. T. Y.; Austin-Seymour, M.; Castro, J. C.; Collier, J. M.; Lyman, J. T.; Pitluck, S.; Saunders, W. M.; Zink, S. R.: Dose-volume histograms in treatment planning

evaluation of carcinoma of the pancreas. Proc. 8th Int. Conf. on Uses of Computers in Radiation Therapy, pp. 264–268 (Computer Society, Los Alamitos 1984).

4 Constine, L. S.; Rubin, P.: Total body irradiation: normal tissue effects; in Bleehen, Radiobiology in radiotherapy, pp. 95–121 (Springer, New York 1987).

5 Ellis, F.: Is NSD-TDF useful to radiotherapy? Int. J. Radiat. Oncol. Biol. Phys. *11:* 1685–1699 (1985).

6 Fajardo, L. F.: Pathology of radiation injury (Masson, New York 1982).

7 Hall, E. J.: Radiobiology for the radiologist (Harper & Row, New York 1978).

8 Lyman, J. T.: Complication probability as assessed from dose-volume histograms. Radiat. Res. *104:* suppl. 8, pp. 13–19 (1985).

9 Lyman, J. T.; Wolbarst, A. B.: Optimization of radiation therapy. III. A method of assessing complication probabilites from dose-volume histograms. Int. J. Radiat. Oncol. Biol. Phys. *14:* 103–109 (1988).

10 Orton, C. G.; Cohen, L.: A unified approach to dose-effect relationships in radiotherapy. I. Modified TDF and linear quadratic equations. Int. J. Radiat. Oncol. Biol. Phys. *14:* 549–557 (1988).

11 Orton, C. G.: A unified approach to dose-effect relationships in radiotherapy. II. Inhomogeneous dose distributions. Int. J. Radiat. Oncol. Biol. Phys. *14:* 561–565 (1988).

12 Paterson, R.: The treatment of malignancy by radium and X-rays. Being a practice of radiotherapy (Arnold, London 1947).

13 Rubin, P.: Radiation effect and tolerance, normal tissue; in Vaeth, Front. Radiat. Ther. Onc., vol. 6 (University Park Press, Baltimore 1972).

14 Rubin, P.; Casarett, G. W.: Clinical radiation pathology, vol. I and II (Saunders, Philadelphia 1968).

15 Rubin, P.; Siemann, D.: Principles of radiation oncology and cancer radiotherapy; in Rubin, Clinical oncology: a multidiciplinary approach; 6th ed., pp. 58–72 (American Cancer Society, New York 1983).

16 Rubin, P.; Van Houtte, P.; Constine, L. S.: Radiatioin sensitivity and organ tolerances in pediatric oncology: a new hypothesis. Front. Radiat. Ther. Onc., vol. 16, pp. 62–82 (Karger, Basel 1982).

17 Rubin, P.: The Franz Buschke Lecture: Late effects of chemotherapy and radiation therapy: a new hypothesis. Int. J. Radiat. Oncol. Biol. Phys. *10:* 5–34 (1984).

18 Rubin, P.; Landman, S.; Mayer, E., et al.: Bone marrow regeneration and extension after extended field irradiation in Hodgkin's disease. Cancer *32:* 699–711 (1973).

19 Rubin, P.; Constine, L. S.; Scarantino, C. W.: The paradoxes in patterns and mechanisms of bone marrow regeneration after irradiation. II. Total body irradiation. Radiother. Onc. *2:* 227–233 (1984).

20 Rubin, P.; Wasserman, T. H.: The late effects of toxicity scoring. Int. J. Radiat. Oncol. Biol. Phys. *14:* suppl. 1, pp. 29–38 (1988).

21 Rubin, P.; Constine, L. S.; Van Ess, J.: Lated effects of toxicity scoring. Natn. Cancer Inst. Monogr. *6:* 9–18 (1988).

22 Rubin, P.; Finkelstein, J. N.; Siemann, D. W.; Shapiro, D. L.; Van Houtte, P.; Penney, D. P.: Predictive biochemical assays for late radiation effects. Int. J. Radiat. Oncol. Biol. Phys. *12:* 469–476 (1986).

23 Rubin, P.; Shapiro, D.; Finkelstein, J. N.; Penney, D.: The early release of surfactant following lung irradiation of alveolar type II cells. Int. J. Radiat. Oncol. Biol. Phys. *6:* 75–77 (1980).

24 Rubin, P.; Siemann, D. W.; Shapiro, D.; Finkelstein, J.; Van Houtte, P.; Penney, D.:

Surfactant release as an early measure of radiation pneumonitis. Int. J. Radiat. Oncol. Biol. Phys. *9:* 1669–1673 (1983).

25 Rubin, P.; Whitaker, J. N.; Bryant, R. G.; Herman, P. K.; Ceckler, T. L.; Gregory, P. K.; Constine, L. S.; Baggs, R. B.: Myelin basic protein and magnetic resonance imaging for diagnosing radiation myelopathy. Preliminary report. Int. J. Radiat. Oncol. Biol. Phys. (in press, 1988).

26 Standqvist, M.: Studien über die kumulative Wirkung der Röntgenstrahlen bei Fraktionierung. Acta radiol. *55:* 1–300 (1944).

27 Takahashi, I.; Nagai, T.; Miyaishi, K.; Maehara, Y.; Niibe, H.: Clinical study of the radioprotective effects of amifostine (Ym-08310, WR-2721) on chronic radiation injury. Int. J. Radiat. Oncol. Biol. Phys. *12:* 935–939 (1986).

28 Thames, H. D.; Hendry, J. H.: Fractionation in radiotherapy (Taylor & Francis, London 1987).

29 Von Essen, C. F.: Roentgen therapy of skin and lip carcinoma: factors influencing success and failure. Am. J. Roentg. *83:* 556–570 (1960).

30 Wittes, R. E.: Personal commun. (1988).

31 Yu, S.; Yang, X. Y.; Zhan, Q. M.; Guo, R.; Liu, J. W.; Yang, C. Z.: The use of Chinese herb medicine in experimental radiotherapy. Int. J. Radiat. Oncol. Biol. Phys. (in press, 1989).

Philip Rubin, M. D., Department of Radiation Oncology, University of Rochester Cancer Center, 601 Elmwood Avenue, Rochester, NY 14642 (USA)

Vaeth JM, Meyer JL (eds): Radiation Tolerance of Normal Tissues.
Front Radiat Ther Oncol. Basel, Karger, 1989, vol 23, pp 41–59

Cell Depletion and Initial and Chronic Responses in Normal Tissues

Elizabeth L. Travis, Nicholas H. A. Terry

Department of Experimental Radiotherapy, University of Texas System Cancer Center, M. D. Anderson Hospital and Tumor Institute, Houston, Tex., USA

Introduction

It is current practice to divide all normal tissues into two categories based solely on the time after irradiation at which damage is observed, i.e., 'acute' or 'late' responding [1, 2]. This distinction is, however, potentially confusing as similar terms, acute and late responses (or effects), are used to refer primarily to *what* is observed, either clinically or pathologically, although a time component is implicit in these terms too. The classification based on when effects are observed does have a radiobiologic rationale. However, classifications based on either the time damage occurs or on what is observed may obscure rather than clarify the mechanisms involved. A concept which merges the time dependence of damage with the clinical and pathological expression of the injury would be useful.

It is likely that most, if not all, normal tissues exhibit two separable and distinct types of damage, both of which are due to cell depletion (fig. 1). The first type may occur soon after irradiation, as in 'acutely' responding normal tissues, or at longer intervals, as in 'late'-responding normal tissues, dependent on the turnover kinetics of the putative target cells of the tissue. However, regardless of the time after irradiation that this initial response occurs, the etiology is the same, i.e., depletion of parenchymal cells specific to the tissue. An example of the above would be the initial response in the esophagus – esophagitis – and in the lung – pneumonitis – an acutely responding and a late-responding normal tissue, respectively. Esophagitis appears within the 1st month after irradiation, whereas pneumonitis is not manifested until 3 months or longer after irra-

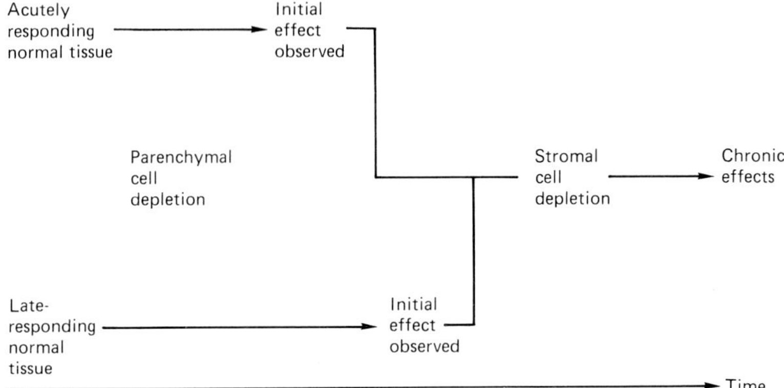

Fig. 1. Chronology of injury (i.e., initial and chronic phases) in 'acutely' and 'late'-responding normal tissues.

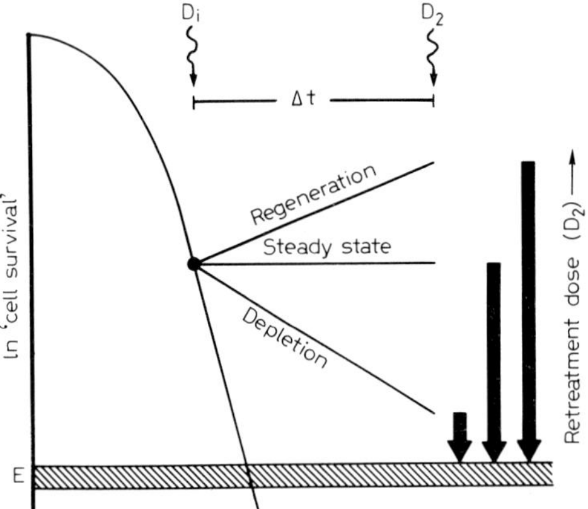

Fig. 2. Schematic showing the effect of target cell behavior on retreatment dose (D_2) after the same D_i for a given treatment interval.

diation. However, damage in both tissues is due to depletion of parenchymal cells, basal cells in the mucosa of the esophagus, and (most likely) type 2 pneumocytes of the alveolar epithelium. Subsequently, a later stromal response of nonparenchymal etiology occurs which is manifested as chronic tissue damage, i.e., fibrosis (as in the lung), obstruction, stenosis, or strictures (as in the esophagus). Thus, in the chronology of tissue damage the first observable (i.e. 'acute') response in an acutely and late-responding normal tissue represents the same type of injury with the same etiology, although it may occur at vastly different times. The chronic response occurring at longer times after irradiation refers to specific pathological changes and is to be distinguished from the late-responding normal tissue category which is purely time dependent.

Test of the Hypothesis

If it is assumed that (1) all damage (both initial and chronic) is due to depletion of putative target cells and (2) that any changes in target cell number in a tissue after irradiation will be reflected in changes in isoeffect dose, then one way to test this hypothesis is to quantify the 'remembered dose' (or residual damage) at various times after a range of first doses in 'acutely' responding normal tissues, 'late' responding normal tissues, and for chronic damage in both classes of tissues. Any changes in retreatment isoeffect dose compared to that for Elkind repair will indicate whether regeneration (increased isoeffect dose) or further depletion (decreased isoeffect dose) has occurred in the interval between the two doses. In such experiments the second dose acts simply as an indirect 'probe' of any relative changes in the number of putative target cells in the tissue at a given time after a first dose. A schematic of this concept is shown in figure 2 for a given first dose which reduces survival to a certain level. If regeneration of the target cells occurs in the time between this first and a second dose, thus repopulating the tissue, then the retreatment isoeffect dose will be larger than if continual cell death and loss depletes the tissue (which would result in a lower retreatment isoeffect dose). Clearly, if the tissue is in a steady state after the first dose, i.e., no further depletion but no regeneration either, or if the more likely situation exists where repopulation balances cell depletion, then the isoeffect for retreatment will be the same as that when full repair of sublethal damage occurs.

This concept has as variables both the size of initial dose and time, and the effects of each of these on retreatment dose are given in figures 3a and 3b, respectively, which assume that repopulation (primarily) occurs after the first dose. It is clear from figure 3a that after different-sized first doses, the retreatment dose at a fixed time will be inversely related to the size of the first dose (D_i), i.e., a larger D_i will require a smaller dose for isoeffect at any retreatment time. After a fixed first dose, the retreatment isoeffect dose will change as a function of time between the two doses, reflecting either regeneration (larger isoeffect dose) or continued depletion (smaller retreatment isoeffect dose; fig. 3b).

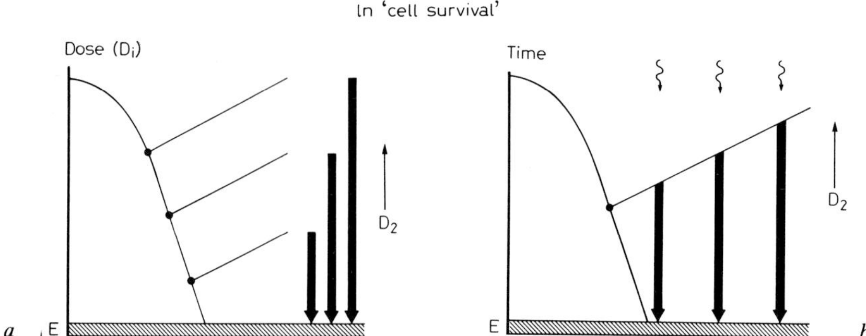

Fig. 3. Effect of dose (*a*) and increasing time (*b*) on retreatment isoeffect dose (D_2). E = observed isoeffect level.

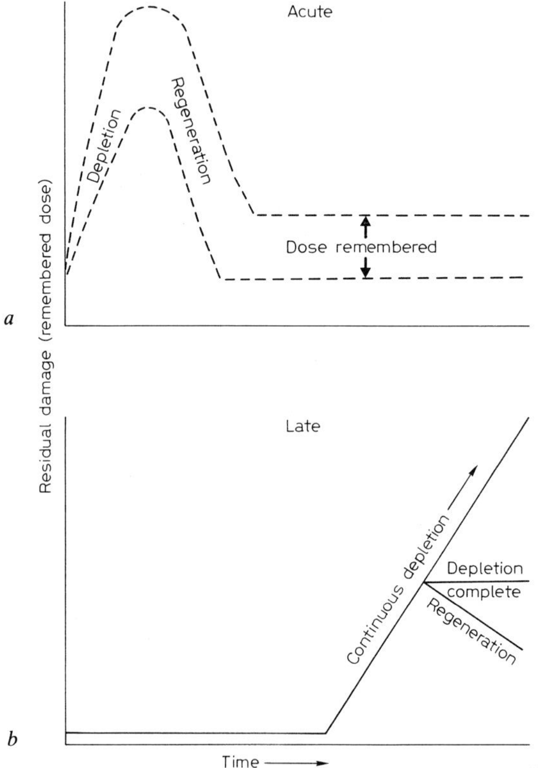

Fig. 4. Schematic representation of the hypothesis that the extent of residual damage measured should reflect the kinetics of depletion and regeneration of critical cells in acute-responding (*a*) and late-responding (*b*) normal tissues after irradiation (recovery curves).

If a series of experiments is conducted where a range of fixed first doses is given followed at various times by a range of second doses, the retreatment isoeffect dose can be obtained and plotted as a function of time between the two doses, allowing a time-dependent picture of relative cell depletion and repopulation to be constructed for each first dose given (i.e., a tissue recovery curve). If the original hypothesis is correct, that the initial response seen in all normal tissues, *irrespective of time of appearance*, is due to depletion of parenchymal cells specific to the tissue, then any memory of the first dose would be forgotten sooner and quickly in 'acute'-responding tissues but later and slowly in 'late'-responding normal tissues. Thus, there should be consistent differences in the recovery curves of these two classes of tissues. However, if the later chronic response is of nonparenchymal stromal origin with a common cellular etiology, then the decay of dose for this injury (e.g., contraction, fibrosis, stenosis) would be similar for all tissues, reflecting a common pathogenesis.

A schematic of this working hypothesis is given in figure 4 where the retreatment isoeffect dose is plotted as a function of time for acute- and late-responding normal tissues. This diagram represents the expected recovery curve for the initial injury in both classes of tissues. The shape of the recovery curve for the chronic response for both acute- and late-responding normal tissues would be similar to the form of that for the initial effect in the late-responding tissue (fig.4), except over a longer time scale.

It is important to point out that the data obtained from such experiments cannot be obtained from conventional split-dose experiments where two equal-sized doses are separated by increasing intervals. In the design of such experiments the total dose is deliberately increased with time (to account for any repopulation), and the initial dose then represents a sliding scale of initial target cell kill. Thus retreatment isoeffect doses at different intertreatment intervals are not comparable; such comparisons can only be made if a fixed first dose is given.

Although the two processes of target cell depletion and regeneration may occur independently of each other, the more likely situation in many tissues is that they occur simultaneously and that the change in retreatment dose reflects the dominant process. In addition, a third and equally important assumption not discussed previously is that the tissue does not overtly express injury until a critical level of depletion of the putative target cells is reached. Thus changes in retreatment dose reflecting target cell depletion may not always translate into observable damage, particularly if regeneration occurs simultaneously and maintains target cell numbers above this critical level.

Residual Damage Studies in Normal Tissues

Normal Tissues

Residual damage studies are important not only in understanding basic tissue responses to injury but have clinical implications for treatment of malignant tumors with radiation or drugs. However, there is a surprising lack of such studies in the literature. The data from these few normal tissues are described below.

'Acute'-Responding Normal Tissues

Skin Two well-defined types of damage occur in skin after irradiation, an 'acute' reaction consisting of erythema and desquamation which may be followed by subcutaneous fibrosis and telangiectasis. Skin is the one tissue for which a large body of retreatment data exists, allowing a detailed recovery curve to be constructed, as least for the acute reaction. Data from our laboratory are presented in figure 5b as retreatment dose as a function of time between the two doses [3]. The first doses given ranged from 15 to 37.5 Gy which on their own produced no observable reaction and near full effect, respectively. Isoeffect data were constructed from the dose-response relationships for all priming doses and retreatment intervals at an average skin reaction level of 1.1. The errors on the data points were derived from graphing envelopes of standard errors of the mean from the dose-response curves. The hatched area in figure 5b represents the isoeffect doses required to produce an average skin reaction of 1.1 for age-matched single-dose controls. Note that the retreatment doses (right-hand axis) are plotted as *decreasing* values *ascending* the y axis, i.e., the smaller the retreatment dose, the more damage (or dose) remaining. Thus, an ascending curve represents target cell depletion and increasing damage and a descending curve target cell regeneration and repopulation of the tissue. If repopulation is sufficient, then the tissue may return to its preirradiated state, and the retreatment isoeffect dose will be the same as that in a previously not irradiated tissue, i.e., the retreatment ED_{50} will lie in the hatched area of figure 5.

It is clear from figure 5 that if 2–6 months are allowed to elapse before retreatment, the skin, as far as acute epidermal response is concerned, behaves as if it had never experienced a first radiation exposure. Damage is 'remembered' after all first doses, however, if only 10 days or 1 month is allowed to pass before retreatment. The amount of damage 'remembered' in dose terms was dose dependent, 11 Gy after a first dose of 37.5 Gy and less after the lower first doses.

These data indicate that in acutely responding skin the 'memory' of the epidermis of previous irradiation has been forgotten by 2 months, and

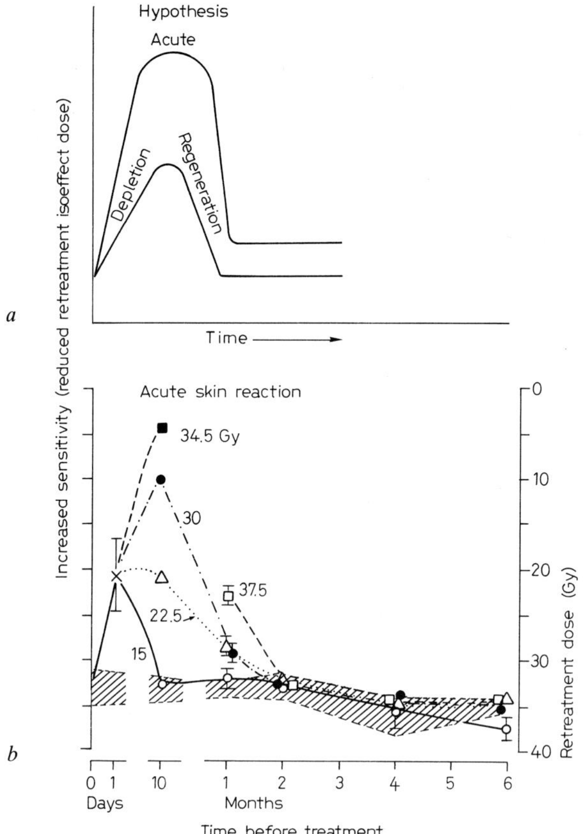

Fig. 5. a Schematic diagram showing that the extent of residual damage measured should reflect the kinetics of depletion and regeneration of critical cells in acute-responding tissues. *b* Skin retreatment data plotted in the above format, i.e., isoeffect data for an average skin reaction of 1.1 as a function of retreatment time. The hatched area represents the isoeffective doses for age-matched, single-dose control data. Damage was only 'remembered' over the 1st month – consistent with the hypothesis. Note the decreasing dose scale on the abscissa.

the tissue remains 'ignorant' of its previous history until at least 6 months after first treatment. Figure 5a shows the expected recovery curve for an 'acute'-responding normal tissue. It is clear that these data are in good agreement with the hypothesis which was based on cell depletion kinetic considerations.

As stated, the acutely reacting skin is one tissue for which a body of retreatment data do exist. These data are summarized in figure 6 where

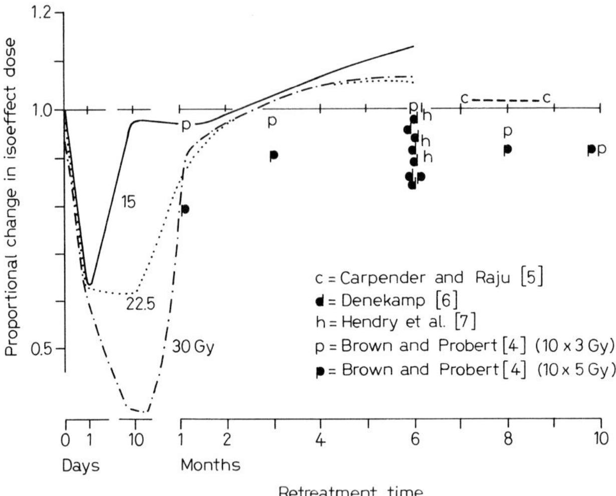

Fig. 6. Proportional change in retreatment isoeffective doses compared with controls (i.e., previously not irradiated skin) as a function of retreatment time for published data including data from Terry et al. [3].

they are plotted as the *proportional reduction* in retreatment dose for isoeffect after a variety of first radiation doses [4–7]. In this way data from several authors and systems can be compared. Our data after three priming doses (see figure 5) are shown, but the data points have been omitted for clarity. It is clear from all these data that skin fits the hypothesis, at least for the acute reaction.

'Late'-Responding Normal Tissues

Lung It has been suggested that the lung exhibits two waves of damage, firstly an initial pneumonitis, occurring between 3 and 7 months after irradiation, which is most likely due to depletion of type 2 epithelial cells [8]. A second chronic wave occurs from 9 months onward, but the etiology of this phase is controversial; is it merely a continuation of pneumonitis or rather a truly separable component of damage? A recent analysis by Bentzen et al. [9] suggests that it represents a truly separate and distinct component. If true, then this chronic damage is most likely due to depletion of a different cell in the lung.

The pneumonitis response in mouse lung is the one initial phase of damage in a late-responding normal tissue for which a detailed recovery curve exists for a range of initial doses [10]. The first doses used in that

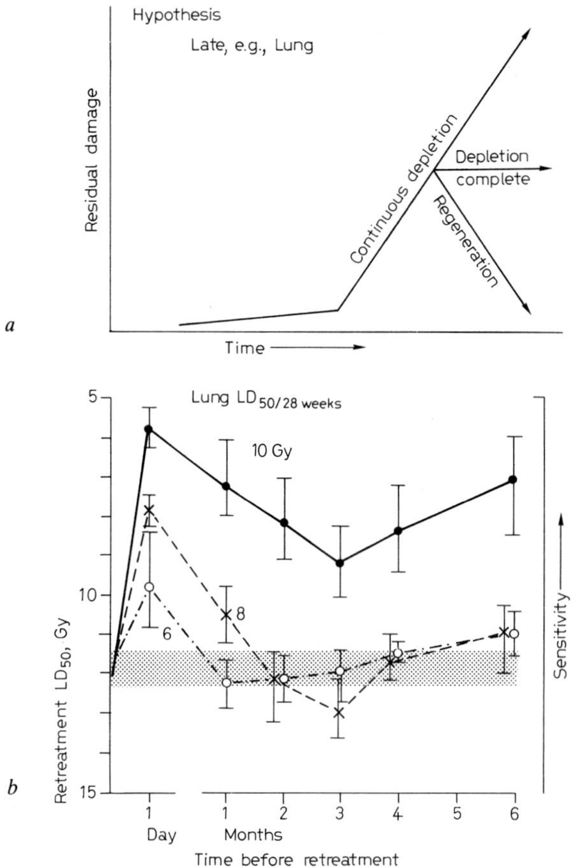

Fig. 7. *a* Schematic representation of the hypothesis that the extent of residual damage measured should reflect the kinetics of depletion and regeneration of critical cells in late-responding normal tissues. *b* $LD_{50/28}$ weeks retreatment doses for lung as a function of time before retreatment after the indicated first doses. The hatched area represents 95% confidence limits for single-dose controls. Errors on dose points are 95% confidence limits. Note the decreasing dose scale on the abscissa.

study (6, 8, and 10 Gy) were chosen to cover a range of injury and hence different levels of putative target cell depletion. Ten Gy, representing about 80% of the single-dose LD_{50}, was the highest dose that on its own produced neither changes in breathing rate nor deaths due to pneumonitis over the time of the study. The lowest dose (6 Gy) represented about 50% of the single-dose LD_{50}.

Retreatment isoeffect data were obtained at the LD_{50} level from logit fits to lethality data at 196 days, the end of the pneumonitis phase. These values are shown graphically in figure 7b as a function of retreatment interval. As in the plot of the skin data (see figure 5), the retreatment LD_{50} doses in figure 7 are plotted as decreasing values ascending the y axis. Hence, when cell depletion is the dominant process occurring between two doses, the ioseffect dose is smaller, and the converse is true when repopulation is the primary process occurring in the intertreatment interval. The hatched area of figure 7b represent the $LD_{50/196}$ for single-dose controls. The data show that at short-treatment intervals there was a considerable, first-dose-dependent, amount of dose remembered, and the lung was relatively radiosensitive (as indicated by a lower isoeffect dose). Furthermore, figure 7 clearly shows the influence of the time interval before retreatment. After the lower two doses, the lung returned to the sensitivity of control lungs by 2 months (i.e., the isoeffect doses in both groups were similar). Although lungs given a first dose of 10 Gy never returned to pretreatment sensitivity, the shape of the recovery curve was similar to that after the lower doses, i.e., after the contribution of Elkind recovery, there was most dose remembered at 1 month with some recovery over the next 2 months. After 3 months there was again an increase in the dose remembered by the lung, being greatest after 10 Gy.

These data show that the lung could not be retreated to the single-dose tolerance if only a 1-month interval elapsed after the higher first doses of 8 or 10 Gy. After the lower two first doses (6 and 8 Gy) recovery took place by 2 months. Lungs retreated at this time had returned to control levels of radiation sensitivity. Lungs given a first dose of 10 Gy never returned to pretreatment sensitivity, but some recovery did occur during the 3 months after the first treatment. The actual amounts of residual damage were very high, particularly on retreating at 1 month, and were dependent on the size of the first dose. After a first dose of 10 Gy, although some recovery occurred over the first 3 months, the amount of damage remembered never dropped below 25–35%

If these changes in retreatment isoeffect dose are due to cell depletion and subsequent regeneration, these data suggest then that, in the lung, depletion and subsequent regeneration of some cell type occurs quickly, within the first 3 months after irradiation. Recent data on the proliferation of type II pneumocytes after X-irradiation by Coggle [11] showed a significant increase in labeling index which peaked at 4 weeks after irradiation, returned to control values at 3–4 months, and then rose again significantly at 5 months (fig. 8).

These data, suggesting an early target cell depletion and regeneration, are not in agreement with the hypothesis described earlier and

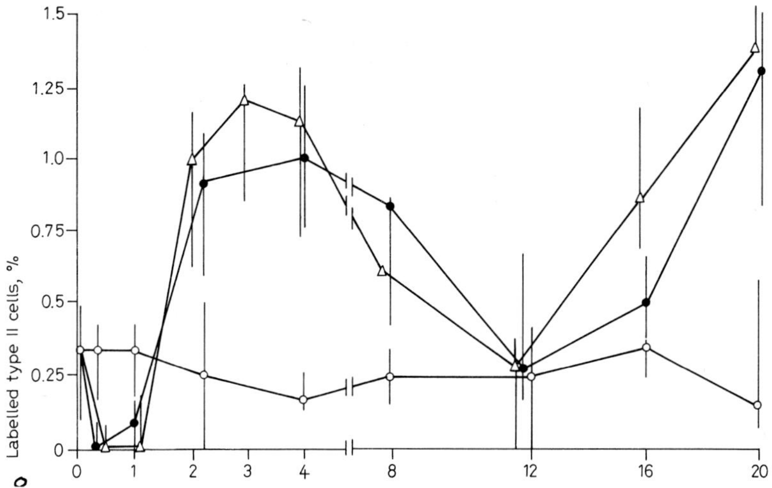

Fig. 8. DNA-labeling index of type 2 pneumocytes in mice after 10 Gy (•) and 12 Gy (△) thoracic irradiation compared with control mice (○). The points shown are median values. Units on the ordinate are weeks. [From ref. 11, reproduced with permission of Taylor and Francis, Ltd.]

shown schematically in figure 7a. It was expected that even for the initial response in late-responding tissues, such as lung, any damage remaining after a first treatment would be expressed late and develop slowly in keeping with the (assumed) slowly proliferating nature of the target cells and would appear more like the data after the 3-month retreatment interval (see figure 7). Before this time, however, the lung, in terms of retreatment sensitivity, acts more like skin, an acutely responding normal tissue.

Spinal Cord

Data in rat spinal cord imply that two distinct and separable types of damage occur after irradiation [12]. Based on the pathology, it has been suggested that these two waves have differing etiologies, although the clinical manifestation of the damage is the same, i.e., paralysis. The primary lesion of the initial phase at 7 months is white matter necrosis and is proposed to be due to glial cell depletion. The second, appearing at 18 months, has as its primary pathological component vascular lesions, and thus it is suggested that this 'chronic' response is of vascular etiology.

Although a detailed study of residual damage in spinal cord after a range of first doses has not been conducted, split-dose data of van der Kogel [13], using a fixed first dose of 15 Gy, fit the criteria for analysis.

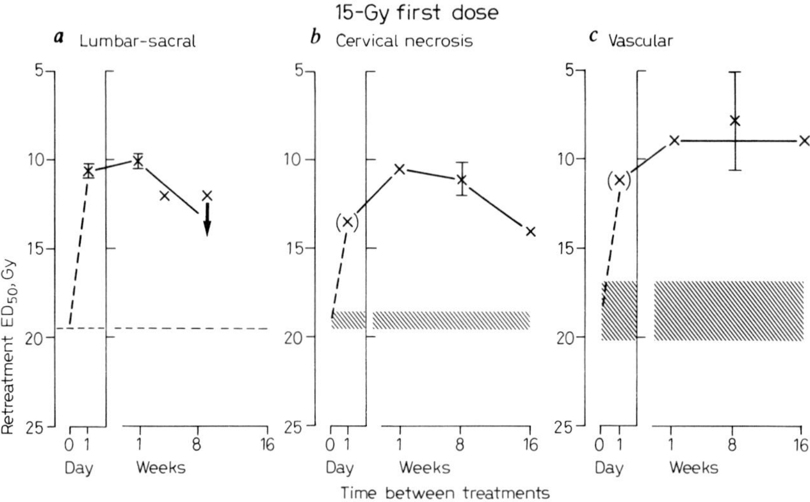

Fig. 9. Spinal cord data. Retreatment ED_{50} for paralysis after a first dose of 15 Gy as a function of time between treatments. (*a*) Paralysis at 7 months after depletion of Schwann cells in the lumbar sacral cord. Initial (*b*) and chronic (*c*) damage to the cervical cord (see text). Data drawn after van der Kogel [13].

Figure 9 show a plot of retreatment ED_{50} for paralysis as a function of time between two doses for the initial (7 months, fig. 9b) and chronic (18 months, fig. 9c) damage in the cervical spinal cord. Also shown in figure 9 are data after irradiation of the lumbar sacral cord in which paralysis again appears at 7 months, but the pathogenesis is suggested to be depletion of Schwann cells.

Figures 9a and b imply that there is some regeneration of the putative target cells for the initial response (paralysis at 7 months) between 8 and 16 weeks after irradiation of both the cervical and lumbar sacral cord. In fact, it appears that this recovery occurred even sooner in the lumbar sacral cord, between 1 and 4 weeks after irradiation. As in the lung, the suspected early regeneration of target cells in cervical cord is supported by the labeling studies of Hornsey et al. [14] which showed an increased labeling index in the neuroglial cells of the cervical cord as early as 15 and 40 days after a single dose of 20 Gy (fig. 10).

In this late responding tissue then, as in the lung, the data for the initial damage did not agree with the hypothesis of a late and slow depletion of the critical target cells. In contrast, the recovery curve for the 'chronic' vascular injury (fig. 10) are in agreement with the hypothesis.

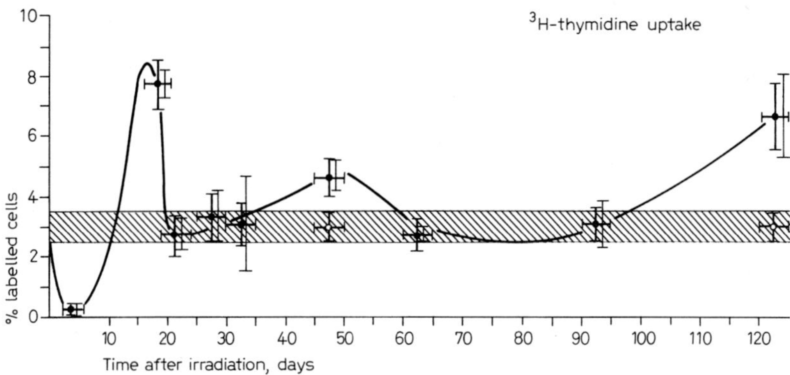

Fig. 10. Labeling of glial cells in the cervical spinal cord after a dose of 20 Gy as a function of time after irradiation. [From ref. 31, reproduced with permission of the British Institute of Radiology.]

Other Normal Tissues

Few retreatment data are available from experiments in other normal tissues which fit the design criteria of a fixed first dose. Those that do are given in table I where residual damage is expressed as a percentage change in retreatment isoeffect dose compared to previously not irradiated age-matched controls. The data in lung and spinal cord show that the retreatment dose is markedly dose dependent. Interestingly, only one tissue, intestine, required a higher dose for isoeffect at long retreatment times, but this was shown to be due to hypoxia rather than increased cell number [15].

It would be interesting if the surprising finding of a very early regenerative response in lung and spinal cord occurs for the initial response in other late-responding normal tissues, e.g., kidney or bladder. Although retreatment studies have not been performed in bladder, labeling data of Stewart et al. [16] suggest that such an early proliferation does not occur, but is observed 9 months after irradiation. It is important to note here again that the data from the radiation retreatment studies in lung and spinal cord, indicating regeneration of critical target cells between 1 and 2 months, were in agreement with the finding of increased labeling indices in type 2 cells in lung and glial cells of the spinal cord over this same time. Analysis of conventional split-dose studies in kidney indicate that some regeneration may occur after 25 days after irradiation, well before the injury becomes evident clinically [17].

Table I. Residual injury in different tissues [from ref. 25]

Tissue	Species	End point	Priming dose percentage of dose to give end point	Time between first and second doses	Dosage change	Reference
Haematopoietic	mouse	$LD_{50/30}$	10	3 weeks	−10	26
Haematopoietic	dog	$LD_{50/30}$	67	3 weeks	+13	27
Haematopoietic	sheep	$LD_{50/60}$	67	1 month	−22 to 29	28
Intestine[1]	mouse	10 surviving cells/jejunal circumference	78	2 months	+11	15
				6 months	+15	
				12 months	+7	
			100	2 months	+18	
				6 months	+24	
				12 months	+7	
Skin[2]	mouse	ND_{50}	70–90	6 weeks	−8–11	29
Lung	mouse	$LD_{50/80}$	76–85	4 weeks	−15 to 24	30
Spinal cord[1]	rat	white matter necrosis (ED_{50})	80	8 weeks	−42	13
				16 weeks	−26	
		vascular damage (ED_{50})	80	8 weeks	−58	
				16 weeks	−51	
Spinal cord	rat	$ED_{50/1year}$	25	14 weeks	−6	31
			50		−10	
			75		−29	
Skin[1]	mouse	Av reaction 1.1	45	10 days	−2	
					3	
				1 month	−4	
				2 months	−1	
				4 months	+7	
				6 months	+13	
			68	10 days	−37	
				1 month	−14	
				2 months	−2	
				4 months	+5	
				6 months	+4	

			90	10 days	−70	
				1 month	−11	
				2 months	−2	
				4 months	+2	
				6 months	+6	
			113	1 month	−32	
				2 months	−3	
				4 months	+3	
				6 months	+4	
Lung[1]	mouse	pneumonitis	50	1 month	+3	10
		(ED_{50})		2 months	+3	
				3 months	+1	
				4 months	−4	
				6 months	−7	
			67	1 month	−12	
				2 months	+2	
				3 months	+8	
				4 months	−3	
				6 months	−7	
			84	1 month	−39	
				2 months	−30	
				3 months	−22	
				4 months	−29	
				6 months	−39	

[1] Experiments which used a fixed first dose
[2] Many other values have been published for skin [reviewed in ref. 32].

Clearly more data are needed both for the initial response in late-responding normal tissues and especially for chronic tissue damage.

'Cell Depletion and Clinically Evident Injury'

The data in lung and spinal cord suggest an early dose-dependent depletion of cells and a regenerative response within 3 months, a surprising finding when it is considered that the actual overt expression of injury does not occur until at least 3 months in lung and 7 months in spinal cord, well after the end of this initial regeneration. Why this early cell depletion and regeneration in tissues does not result in an overt expression of damage at that time is unclear. One possibility is that any early proliferation offsets cell loss due to radiation-induced cell kill, and tissue function is maintained (because the critical level of depletion is not reached). At some point, however, doomed survivors incapable of unlimited proliferation begin to be lost from the tissue, offsetting any regeneration, and the critical level of cell depletion is now reached and the tissue overtly fails. Such an observation has been made after irradiation of bone marrow where defects in renewal ability of the stem cells were observed as a decrease in the number of progeny [18]. If true in lung and spinal cord, then both tissues should recognize and respond to the damage sooner after a higher first dose (because it is nearer to a critical threshold level of cell depletion), i.e., the latent period for the expression of damage should be shorter. Analysis of the latent time data in lung showed this to be true [10].

Another interpretation of the data shown in figure 7 for lung and figure 9 for spinal cord injury at 7 months is that the responses of two different target cells are being assessed. One population would be depleted quickly and would regenerate within the first 3 months after irradiation, whereas depletion in the second population becomes apparent only after 3 months. The extent of depletion and regeneration of this second population would be expected to be dependent on the level of injury (i.e., dose) sustained. At this time neither hypothesis can be excluded.

Clinical Implications

Retreatment studies have obvious implications for the radiotherapist when faced with treating a recurrence in a previously irradiated site. Although clinical studies are few, in general, those studies available indicate that the tolerance of a tissue to retreatment is remarkably similar to that of nonirradiated tissues, at least for 'acute' reactions even in late-responding normal tissues [19–22]. These clinical findings suggest then that those target cells responsible for the initial reactions do regenerate after treatment. This is further substantiated by the finding that retreatment tolerance increases as the interval between the two courses becomes longer.

Of equal importance, though perhaps less clear, is the implication of these experimental studies when chemotherapy is the retreatment modality or even when chemotherapy is given soon after completion of a full course of radiotherapy. Even fewer clinical data are available in this area, but, based on the available experimental data, one would predict that retreating the lung, or any other tissue for that matter, with a cycle-specific drug at a time when regeneration was occurring would elicit an unexpected and enhanced reaction. This would be particularly important in late-responding tissues where our data in lung indicate that regeneration occurs between 1 and 3 months after irradiation.

It is also possible that the mechanism of the so-called 'radiation recall' [23, 24] phenomenon, which occurs when drugs are given after irradiation, is simply that fewer cells remain in the tissue after irradiation. Thus, if the target cells for the drug are the same as those for radiation, then a response in the tissue will occur sooner (because it again is nearer to a critical level of depletion) and at a lower drug dose (because there are fewer target cells to kill). Since tissues have only a limited number of ways to respond to damage, drug-induced damage may look like radiation damage both clinically and pathological. Thus 'recall' of radiation damage by subsequent chemotherapy simply may be drug-induced damage.

Acknowledgements

The authors are grateful to Shelia A. Buckner for the preparation of this manuscript. This work was supported by grant CA-38106 from the National Cancer Institute.

References

1 Thames H. D., Withers H. R., Peters L. J., et al.: Changes in early and late radiation responses with altered dose fractionation: Implications for dose-survival relationships. Int J Radiat Oncol Biol. Phys 1982; *8:* 219–226.

2 Withers H. R., Thames H. D., Peters L. J.: Differences in the fractionation response of acutely and late-responding tissues; in Karcher K. H., et al. (eds): Progress in Radio-Oncology. New York, Raven Press, 1982, vol II, pp 287–296.

3 Terry N. H. A., Tucker S. L., Travis E. L.: Time course of loss of residual radiation damage in murine skin assessed by retreatment. Int. J. Radiat Biol, 1988 (in press).

4 Brown J. M., Probert J. C.: Early and late radiation changes following a second course of irradiation. Radiology 1975; *115:* 711–716.

5 Carpenter S. G., Raju M. R.: Residual radiation damage in the mouse foot after exposure to heavy particles. Radiology 1981; *138:* 483–485.

6 Denekamp J.: Residual radiation damage in mouse skin 5 to 8 months after irradiation. Radiology 1975; *115:* 191–195.

7 Hendry J. H., Rosenberg I., Greene D. S., et al.: Reirradiation of rat tails to necrosis at six months after a 'tolerance' dose of X-rays or neutrons. Br J Radiol 1977; *50:* 567–572.

8 Travis E. L., Down J. D., Holmes S. J., et al.: Radiation pneumonitis and fibrosis in mouse lung assayed by respiratory frequency and histology. Radiat Res 1980; *84:* 133–143.

9 Bentzen S. M., Thames H. D., Travis E. L., et al.: Direct estimation of latent times for radiation injury in late responding normal tissues using mixture models: Lung, spinal cord and gut. Int J Radiat Biol. Submitted 1988.

10 Terry N. H. A., Tucker S. L., Travis E. L.: Residual radiation damage in murine lung assessed by pneumonitis. Int J Radiat Oncol Biol Phys 1988; *14:* 929–938.

11 Coggle J. E.: Proliferation of type II pneumocytes after X-irradiation. Int J Radiat Biol 1987; *51:* 393–399.

12 van der Kogel A. J.: Radiation-induced damage in the central nervous system: An interpretation of target cell responses. Br J Cancer 1986; *53:* 207–217.

13 van der Kogel A. J.: Late effects of radiation on the spinal cord; PhD thesis University of Amsterdam, 1979.

14 Hornsey S., Myers R., Coultas P. G., et al: Turnover of proliferative cells in the spinal cord after X-irradiation and its relation to time dependent repair of radiation damage. Br J Radiol 1981; *54:* 1081–1085.

15 Reynaud A., Travis E. L.: Late effects of irradiation in mouse jejunum. Int J Radiat Biol. 1984; *46:* 125–134.

16 Stewart F. A., Denekamp J., Hirst D. G.: Proliferation kinetics of the mouse bladder after irradiation. Cell Tissue Kinet 1979; *13:* 75–84.

17 Williams M. V., Denekamp J.: Radiation induced renal damage in mice: Influence of fraction size. Int J Radiat Oncol Biol. Phys 1984; *10:* 885–893.

18 Hendry J. H., Xu C. X., Testa N. G.: A cellular analysis of residual hemopoietic deficienies in mice after 4 repeated doses of 4.5 gray X-rays. Int J Radiat Oncol Biol Phys 1983; *9:* 1641–1646.

19 Hunter R. D., Stewart J. G.: The tolerance to re-irradiation of heavily irradiated skin. Br J Radiol 1977; *50:* 573–575.

20 McNeese M. D., Fletcher G. H.: Retreatment of recurrent nasopharyngeal carcinoma. Radiology 1981; *138:* 191–193.

21 Fu K. K., Newman H., Phillips T. L.: Treatment of locally recurrent carcinoma of the nasopharynx. Radiology 1975; *117:* 425–431.

22 Langlois D., Eschwege F., Kramar A., et al.: Reirradiation of head and neck cancers. Radiother Oncol 1985; *3:* 27–33.

23 Hill A. B., Tattersall S. F.: Recall of radiation pneumonitis after intrapleural administration of doxorubicin. Med J Aust 1983; *i:* 39–40.

24 Stein R. S.: Radiation-recall enteritis after actinomycin D and adriamycin therapy. South Med J 1978; *71:* 960–961.

25 Thames H. D., Hendry J. H.: Fractionation in Radiotherapy. London, Taylor and Francis, 1987, pp 130–136.

26 Porteous D. D., Lajtha L. G.: on stem cell recovery after irradiation. Br J Haematol 1966; *12:* 177–188.

27 Ainsworth E. J., Leong G. F.: Recovery from radiation injury in dogs as evaluated by the split-dose technique. Radiat Res 1966; *29:* 131–142.

28 Hanks G. E., Page N. P., Ainsworth E. J., et al.: Acute mortality and recovery studies in sheep irradiated with cobalt-60 gamma rays or 1-MV X-rays. Radiat Res 1966; *27:* 397–405.

29 Hendry J. H.: The tolerance of mouse tails to necrosis after repeated irradiation with X-rays. Br J Radiol 1978; *51:* 808–813.

30 Field S. B., Hornsey S., Kutsutani Y.: Effects of fractionated irradiation on mouse lung and a phenomenon of slow repair. Br J Radiol 1976; *69:* 700–707.

31 Hornsey S., Myers R., Warren P.: Residual injury in the spinal cord after treatment with X-rays or neutrons. Br J Radiol 1982; *55:* 516–519.

32 Chen F. D.: A cellular analysis of residual injury in skin; PhD thesis University of Manchester, 1986.

Elizabeth L. Travis, PhD, Department of Experimental Radiotherapy, Box 66,
M. D. Anderson Hospital, 1515 Holcombe Boulevard, Houston, TX 77030 (USA)

Vaeth JM, Meyer JL (eds): Radiation Tolerance of Normal Tissues.
Front Radiat Ther Oncol. Basel, Karger, 1989, vol 23, pp 60–74

Repair of 'Sublethal Damage': Key Factor in Normal Tissue Tolerance to Fractionated and Low Dose Rate Irradiation

Emmanuel van der Schueren, Willy Landuyt, Pierre Scalliet

Department of Experimental Radiotherapy, Division of Oncology,
Universitair Ziekenhuis St. Rafaël, Leuven, Belgium

Introduction

After an irradation, apparent repair takes place of what has been called 'sublethal damage'. Such repair occurs repeatedly when irradiation is given with increasing fractionation, leading to a much higher tolerance of tissues to fractionated irradiation as to single-dose irradiations. The relationship between isoeffect doses and number of fractions (or inversely the fraction size) over which the irradiation is given can be translated in isoeffect curves, the slope of which is an expression of the capacity of a tissue to repair sublethal damage. While initially it was assumed that this repair capacity was the same in all tissues, it has gradually become evident that there are wide divergencies between different tissues [25, 35, 36]. The consequence of this being that increasing fractionation will spare some tissues to a larger extent than others. Conversely, it implies that loss of tolerance will occur to a larger extent in some tissues than in others when large fraction sizes are used. This evolution in concepts is illustrated by the transition from the use of the Ellis formula [11] with a standard factor for fractionation for all tissues to the application of the linear-quadratic model in which a range of different parameters are applied for the definition of the fractionation effect, depending on the type of tissue investigated [7, 26].

These data on differential repair capacities for a variety of normal tissues have led to the activation of clinical studies on fractionation with f.i. and to the use of large fraction sizes for melanomas and of small fraction sizes in head and neck tumors and brain tumors.

While an important part of the radiation damage can indeed be repaired, a certain fraction of it is irreversible. The relationship between repairable and irrepairable damage will be expressed in the previously described limits of the repair process. At a certain, relatively small, fraction size, all repairable damage will effectively be repaired, and further fractionation will not give corresponding increases in tolerance. This point has been operationally described as flexure dose [12, 30, 35]. As a working definition, it has been proposed to use a dose ten times lower than the dose at which contributions from repairable and irrepairable damage are equal. At this dose, contribution to cell kill by repairable damage will be negligible. It is important to realize that this is not a biologically well-defined point, as there is a gradual transition with progressive fading out of the role of sublethal damage, the detection of which will then be limited by the resolution of the biological system. This phenomenon of 'flexure dose' determines the limit to clinical usefulness of fractionation, and exact information on it is vital for the planning of fractionation schedules with small fraction sizes.

The use of a certain fraction size is thus linked to a 'tolerance dose' for a specific tissue. Application of different fraction sizes within one radiotherapy treatment has led to questions on the relative impact of the different fractionation modalities. Experimental studies have confirmed the validity of the concept of 'partial tolerance', using half the tolerance in a single top-up dose [1, 3]. In this concept, it is possible to add up the biological effect of several series of irradiations given with different fraction sizes, by converting each series with a specific fraction size to the percentage of tolerance 'used up' in this way. This has proven to be a very useful clinical concept. It has to be kept in mind, however, that experimental data also have indicated the limits of application of such a concept, especially with the use of fraction sizes, whereby significantly more than half of the tolerance is exhausted [unpubl. data].

Finally, a very important aspect of the repair of sublethal damage is the rate at which it is occurring. Indeed, the kinetics of this process will determine the minimum time necessary for a complete repair or 'fading away' of the damage before a subsequent irradiation can be given. If this is not taken into account, a cumulative effect would develop by the combination of unrepaired radiation damage, remaining from the previous irradiation, and the damage induced by the next irradiation. This phenomenon could become especially important in situations where series of irradiations are applied within very short intervals. This was already hinted at in a few clinical studies where accelerated treatment [34] or hyperfractionated treatments [19] were investigated. Indeed, such treatments necessitate an increase in the number of fractions per day to more than one with either a reduction in the total number of treatment days (accelerated) or an increase in the number of fractions for the same overall treatment time (hyperfractionation). Until now, common practice was to give the irradiations within an interval of at least 24 h which seems to be sufficient for completion of repair. During the 'normal' working day of a radiotherapy department, the overall time would be limited to 10–12 h, thus bringing intervals down to 6 or even 4 h, depending on the number of fractions given per day (two or three).

Again, evidence has been emerging in recent years as to the very different kinetics of repair for different tissues. Slowly proliferating tissues, which have usually a larger capacity of repair as compared with rapidly proliferating tissues, also require longer times to finish this repair [2, 4; for a review see ref. 28]. It is not yet clear to which extent these two factors of larger repair capacity and longer time needed for full repair are interrelated. The consequence, however, seems to be that there may be different needs for time intervals for tissues with early or late side effects which suggests that long-term follow-up is necessary to assess the effects of reduced time intervals between irradiations.

Both the extent and the kinetics of repair will also have important consequences for the repercussions of the dose rate at which the radiation is delivered. Indeed, when the dose rate is lowered significantly, the rate at which lesions are inflicted slows down, and more time is offered for repair of sublethal lesions before they can combine with other sublethal lesions to irrepairable damage. The increasing tolerance of a number of tissues in function of a decreasing dose rate has been described before [15, 16, 18, 20, 22, 23]. The indication that large differences existed in the repair capacities of different tissues led to the hope that decreasing dose rates would differentially spare slowly proliferating tissues, thus diminishing the critical late side effects. However, in a situation where the lesions have to be repaired during irradiation, kinetics of the repair process become extremely critical. The capacity of repair, as assessed during fractionated irradiation, is always based on the possibility of the tissue to finish repair of all induced lesions within intervals of 6–24 h. This is certainly not the case during a decreased dose rate irradiation, which means that clinical application of low dose rate irradiation can only be planned based on predicted tolerance which takes into account capacity as well as kinetics of repair.

Capacity of Repair

In our experimental group, two tissue types were extensively investigated as to their repair capacity, namely mouse lip mucosa and rat spinal cord. They were selected as models for a rapidly and a slowly proliferating tissue in view of the suggestions at that time that repair capacity could

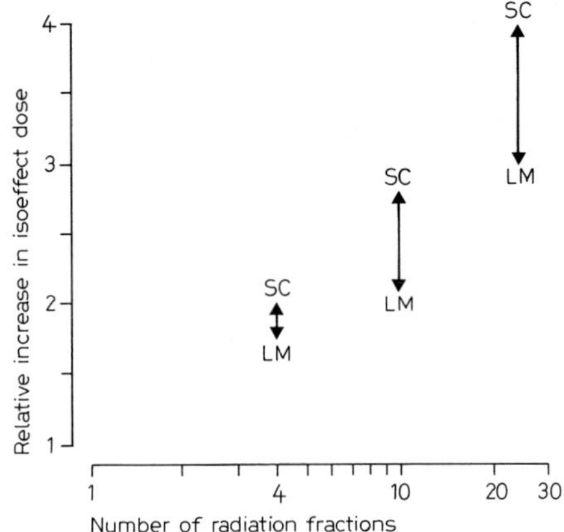

Fig. 1. Illustration of the difference in relative raise (size of arrows) in isoeffective dose (normalized to single-dose irradiation) with increasing number of fractions between mouse lip mucosa (LM) and rat cervical spinal cord (SC). For references of data see text.

be correlated to a certain extent to the proliferation characteristics of the target cells.

The central nervous system is a tissue in which already previously a great capacity for repair of sublethal damage was demonstrated [3, 31, 32]. Isoeffect curves were at that time obtained, having an exponent of 0.43–0.45 for the influence of the number of fractions. This was drastically different from the exponent used before in the Ellis formula which had been calculated on the basis of a different target tissue [11]. It is good to remind that the limitations for application of the Ellis formula were clearly expressed at the time it was proposed and that it was the indiscriminate application of the formula to a number of other situations that has led to problems with its clinical application.

The investigation of the repair capacity of mouse lip mucosa yielded an isoeffect curve with a slope of 0.32–0.35 in function of the number of fractions [1, 38]. This did confirm the significant difference in capacity of repair between tissues with slow and rapid proliferation kinetics [36]. When applying the linear-quadratic model to these data, an α/β value of 6–8 Gy was found for the lip mucosa [1] and of 1.7–2 Gy for the spinal cord [5]. The direct consequence is that the differential effect of fractionated irradiation on these two tissues can be drastically increased by further fractionation. This is illustrated in figure 1 where the size of the arrows is proportional to the difference in raise in tolerance with progressive

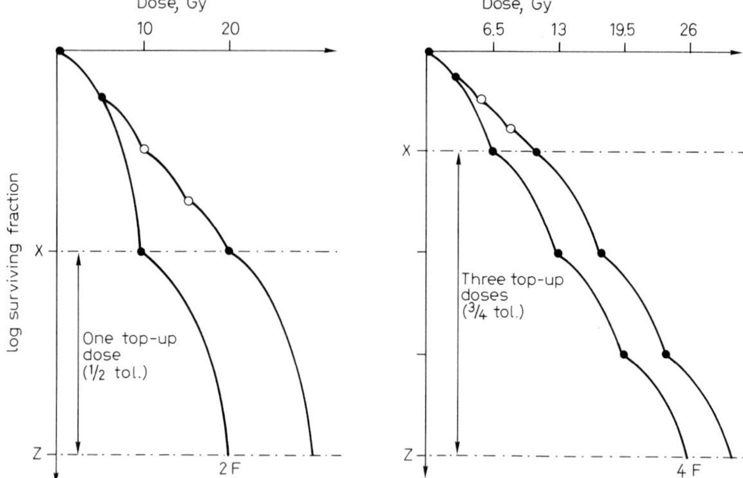

Fig. 2. Schematic presentation of the concept of partial tolerance, using hypothetical survival curves for the involved target cells (assuming equal effect per fraction, F). The left panel shows the application of a fixed '$^1/_2$ of the tolerance' single top-up dose. This single top-up dose represents the fraction size of a two-fraction regimen. The right panel demonstrates the use of fixed '$^3/_4$ of the tolerance' top-up doses. The three top-up doses each correspond with the fraction size of a four-fraction regimen.

fractionation for mouse lip mucosa and rat spinal cord. This is the biological basis of the unforeseen spinal cord lesions which did develop after the application of clinical fractionation schedules with large fraction sizes to treat bronchial cancer. Indeed, the correction in total dose was then based on the assessment of acute side effects.

Partial Tolerance

The mixture of irradiations with different fraction sizes occurs sometimes in clinical practice and leads to problems in estimating the total biological effect of such treatments. Also, in experimental work, it is sometimes necessary to use a concept of 'top-up' dose in order to obtain certain biological damage levels when applying very small fraction sizes. These two situations have led to the necessity of investigating the concept of 'partial tolerance'. In this, part of the treatment is given in a single large fraction or in a limited number (up to 3) of fractions (fig. 2). The extrapolation to total tolerance, when 'wiping out' 50 or 75% of the tolerance of the treated tissue by such 'top-up' irradiation, was investigated.

For a number of situations, it was proven that this was well feasible. Indeed, for the lip mucosa [1] as well as for the spinal cord [3], a single top-up dose corresponding to the fraction size of a two-fraction regimen could be given in combination with fractionated series of irradiations over a wide range of fraction sizes without affecting the slope of the isoeffect curve. This means that about half of the tolerance could be given in a single irradiation without affecting the repair characteristics of the tissue to a series of small-fraction sizes.

In the lip mucosa model, the top-up dose could even be increased to 75% of the tolerance dose, using three irradiations with a fraction size corresponding to the tolerance dose given in a four-fraction regimen [1]. Even under these circumstances, the slope of the isoeffect curve of fractionated regimens given in combination with the three top-up fractions was still 0.35, in very good concordance with the slope obtained after straightforward fractionation regimens without top-up dose (fig. 3) [1, 38].

However, in the rat spinal cord model, the use of fraction sizes covering significantly more than half of the tolerance led to increasing scatter in the data when combinations were carried out with fractionated irradiations. As a result, no clear isoeffect curves could be obtained [unpubl. data]. This was the case when a single top-up dose of 20 Gy was used (comparing to 22 Gy of isoeffect dose to obtain 50% of paralysis after single irradiation) as well as when three fractions of about 10 Gy were given (comparing to the 50% paralysis level obtained with four fractions of 10 Gy). These results suggest a certain limitation to the use of the 'top-up' practice in experimental situations. This finding also implies a limit to the straightforward application of the concept in clinical practice, especially when doses close to tolerance have been used in one of the considered treatment regimens.

Flexure Dose

With increasing fractionation, there will be a limit to the possibility of further increase in tolerance dose as all repairable damage is repaired. The point at which no further increase in tolerance can be obtained is to be considered the flexure dose. The flexure dose is a theoretical concept, of which the definition will be limited by the resolution of the models investigated. As a working tool, it has been defined as the dose which is ten times lower than the dose at which cell kill occurs with equal efficiency by directly lethal and by sublethal damage [12, 30, 35]. It can thus either be theoretically calculated from the isoeffect curve or one can attempt to

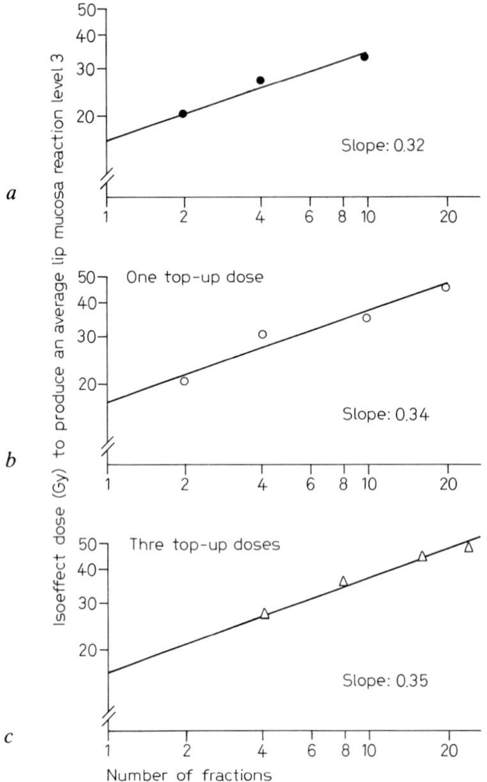

Fig. 3. Isoeffect curves for the different series of experiments in mouse lip mucosa involving fractionated irradiation, either without *(a)* or with one top-up dose (1/2 of the tolerance) *(b)* or three top-up doses ($^3/_4$ of the tolerance) *(c)*. The number of fractions indicated on the figure and corresponding with the isoeffect doses consists of the number of fractions of the fractionated part multiplied by a factor of 2 *(b)* or by a factor of 4 *(c)* with regard to the tolerance concept involved. [From ref. 1, with permission.]

experimentally define it. The experimental definition is extremely important in order to correlate the theoretical concepts with biological facts, but it is also limited by the inevitable scatter occurring in the experimental (or clinical) observation methods.

In lip mucosa, no further sparing could be demonstrated by reduction of the fraction sizes below 2 Gy, since the isoeffect doses for fraction sizes of 2, 1.5, and 1.2 Gy remained at the same level [1]. The same type of

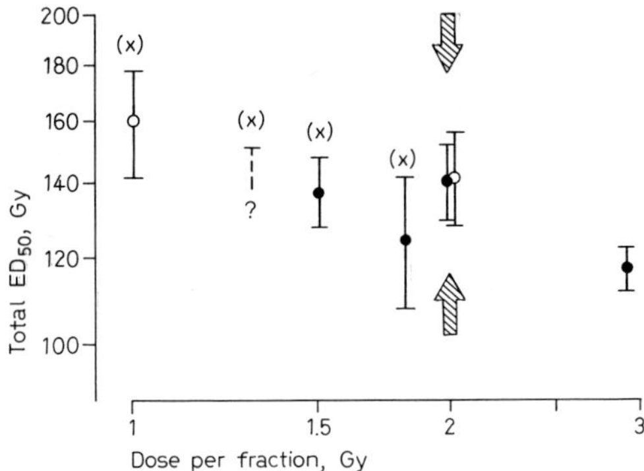

Fig. 4. Isoeffect doses for induction of paralysis in rats (due to white-matter necrosis) after cervical spinal cord irradiation, plotted as a function of the fraction size (range between 1 and 3 Gy). Calculated values (based on the application of the linear-quadratic model) are indicated (×) for comparison. For further details see text. [From ref. 33, with permission.]

experiments was carried out for the rat spinal cord where more extensive repair was still expected at fraction sizes below 2 Gy. In a first series of experiments, no additional repair could be demonstrated when comparing fraction sizes of 2 and 1.8 Gy to 1.3 Gy [5,6]. In a second series of experiments, the investigation was extended down to fraction sizes of 1 Gy (fig. 4) [33]. Here, an increase in radiation tolerance of about 15% (increase of isoeffect dose from 140 to 159 Gy) was detected. However, there is an overlap of the 95% confidence limits between the two isoeffect dose points. This suggests that there is still some gain in tolerance, but, in view of the scatter of the experimental data, it will be extremely difficult to confirm or negate the possibility.

A very important point in these studies on flexure dose, carried out with very small fraction sizes, is the correlation between the values for increase in tolerance with decreasing fraction size (calculated with the linear-quadratic model) and the experimental data. Both in the lip mucosa model and in the spinal cord, the experimental data remain well below the calculated (namely extrapolated) data. In the spinal cord, e.g., with an α/β ratio of 1.7, an increase in tolerance would still be expected from 140 Gy at 2 Gy per fraction to 192 Gy for a fraction size of 1 Gy [33]. This stresses the fact that one should be very careful in extrapolating data outside the range which is experimentally confirmed.

Kinetics of Repair

In addition to the large amount of information on the differential aspects of repair capacity for the various types of tissues, increasing data are now also becoming available, pointing to the diverging rates in the kinetics of repair.

Indeed, it has been shown both for fractionated [4, 26, 37] and continuous low dose rate irradiation [10, 15, 18, 20] that repair halftimes differ to a similar extent between early- and late-reacting normal tissues as do their respective repair capacities. The results of fractionated irradiations, delivered with variable intervals between the successive fractions, suggest a monoexponential time course for repair. About half of the possible amount of repair seems to be finished within 60 min for early-reacting tissues, whereas about 90 min are necessary to complete 50% of the repair for slowly proliferating tissues. In our experience in mouse lip mucosa [6] and rat spinal cord [4] the calculated halftimes were exactly within these ranges. When the percentage of the potential repair per fraction (comparison made with repair occurring during an interval of 24 h) is plotted against the time interval between fractions (fig. 5), this difference in rate of repair between lip mucosa and spinal cord is easily recognized. From these data it appears that repair after relatively small fraction sizes is essentially complete within 2 h in the lip mucosa, while up to 15% of potential repair for similar fraction sizes is still uncompleted in the spinal cord after time intervals of up to 4 h. The fact that repair kinetics are closely related to the proliferation rate of a given tissue was nicely documented by Withers et al. [37], using the hair follicle as the biological system. These studies show the smaller α/β value and the longer halftime of repair for hair follicles in the telogen phase, whilst the reverse was found for the hair follicles in the anagen phase. The different ranges of halftime values are not to be taken as absolute values or a unified approach of the problem, since there are indications that the rate of repair might be related to the size of the dose per fraction in both types of tissue effects [4, 6, 39]. This latter observation, however, can be obscured by the differences in experimental approach and in mathematical models used for the analysis of the data. This has been pointed out by Ang et al. [2] for rat spinal cord following calculations of halftime of repair with either the 'F_R' method [13] or the 'incomplete repair' method [27].

Furthermore, several in vitro as well as in vivo experimental data demonstrated the possible existence of two components of repair, i.e., a fast component with a halftime of 10–20 min and a much slower component of the order of 1.5–2 h [9, 17]. Although the existence of these different values seems to be confirmed, until now a reasonable approach

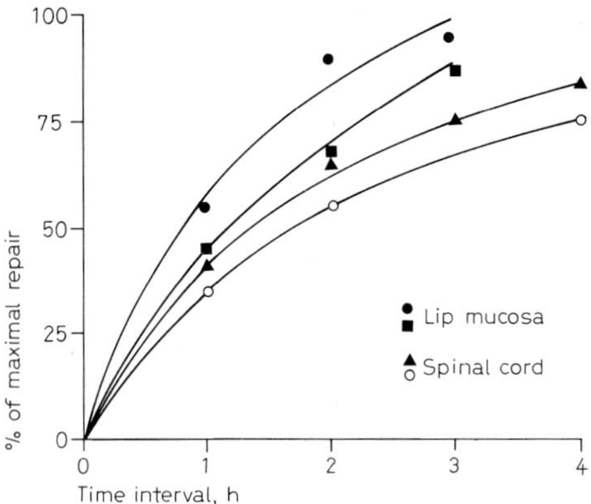

Fig. 5. Difference in the kinetics of repair between mouse lip mucosa and rat spinal cord. Comparison of the percentage of maximal repair (24-hour interval) at different time intervals is done with similar fraction size. Two fractions: lip mucosa (■) and spinal cord (○); two and five fractions: lip mucosa (●); four fractions: spinal cord (▲).

of repair rate can be obtained with the acceptance of a monoexponential function of damage repair and time.

Another important factor, determining the biological effectiveness of radiation and related to repair kinetics, is the dose rate effect. Already decades ago, a number of studies demonstrated a sparing effect when irradiation was delivered at lower dose rates. This was interpreted as repair of sublethal damage occurring during treatment. Several reviews have considered the extent of repair during a decreased dose rate irradiation for different types of biological systems [14, 24]. Analyzing this dose rate effect necessitates not only quantitative information on the extent of repair, but also on the rate at which this repair takes place during continuous radiation exposure. Our group [20] has investigated the effect of decreasing radiation dose rates using the mouse lip mucosa model. Applying a mathematical method developed by Dale [8] made it possible to easily derive the halftime of repair, based on the comparison of tolerance increases for decreasing dose rates during continuous irradiation and for increasing fractionation with high dose rate treatments in the same biological system (fig. 6). It was found that the halftime of repair during continuous irradiation did not differ from the value of 47 min obtained with experiments using the fractionated irradiations with fraction sizes of 5 Gy and less, given with different time intervals. Furthermore there seemed no dependency of the repair kinetics on the radiation quality,

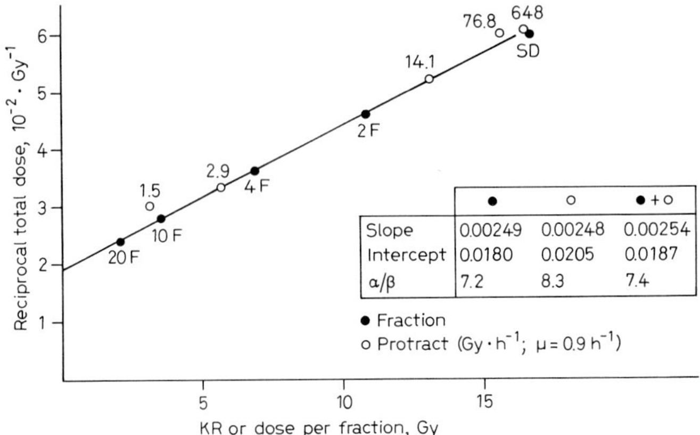

Fig. 6. Derivation of a value for halftime of repair using the method of Dale [8] on mouse lip mucosa data. The reciprocal total isoeffective dose is plotted against KR (low-dose irradiation) and against the dose per fraction(fractionated irradiation). The obtained value was 47 min, with an α/β ratio of 7.4 Gy. (From ref. 20, with permission.]

comparing radiation experiments with ^{60}Co gamma rays and d(50) + Be neutrons [23].

Similarly, in the rat cervical spinal cord, values for halftime of repair were very close, whether the calculations were based on fractionated irradiation or on different dose rates [22]. Data obtained for the lung also indicated a similarity between kinetics of repair derived from either fractionated irradiation [28, 29] or continuous low dose rate treatment [10].

This implies that the rate at which irradiations are delivered mainly influences the extent of repair, but not the speed of this process. The realization of the impact of repair kinetics on the sparing effect of low dose rate irradiations affects the concepts of tolerance in relation to, e.g., overall treatment times in brachytherapy. Using a theoretical approach, it was attempted to quantify the different aspects involved in the total amount of repair under such conditions. The results of these calculations are displayed in figure 7 [21]. From these theoretical isoeffect curves it is evident that in the considered overall treatment times of 3–7 days repair kinetics would play a less important role in determining the biological effect of irradiation on slowly proliferating tissues, as compared with acutely reacting tissues. This observation thus contrasts with the impact of repair kinetics during fractionated radiation treatments. Indeed, the benefit of using a large number of small dose fractions (2 to 1 Gy) given several times per day (interval times of 4 hours or less) could be limited

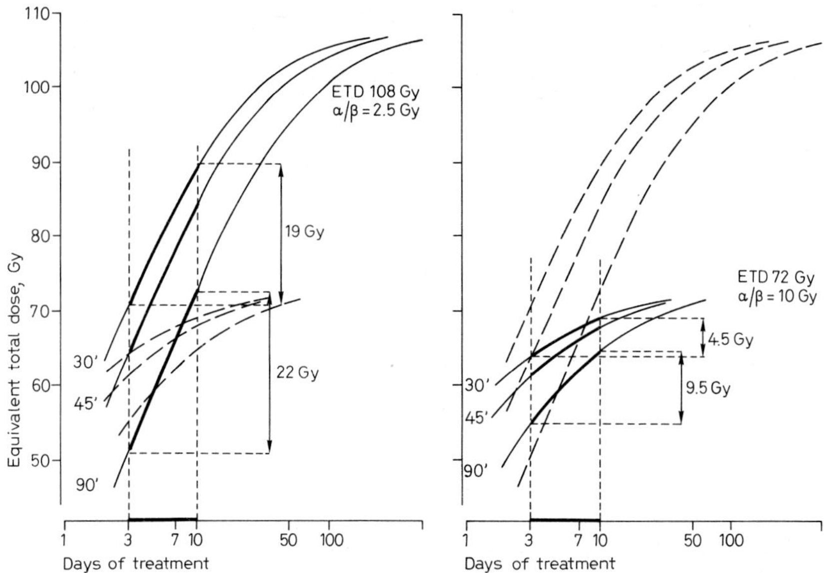

Fig. 7. Theoretical isoeffect curves for the equivalent total dose to be delivered in function of the treatment time (i.e., the dose rate) in brachytherapy. The ETD values have been derived from an equivalent dose of 60 Gy delivered in 30 fractions of 2 Gy. Three different halftimes have been used for the construction of the curves (30, 45, and 90 min), using the mathematical model of Dale [8]. For a large α/β (right), the variation of the equivalent total dose is small between 3 and 10 days of treatment and is dependent on the repair kinetics (4.5 Gy for $t_{1/2} = 30$ min vs. 9.5 Gy for $t_{1/2} = 90$ min). For a small α/β (left), the variation of the equivalent total dose is large within the same range of time, but is only slightly influenced by the kinetics of repair (22 Gy for $t_{1/2} = 90$ min vs. 19 Gy for $t_{1/2} = 30$ min). [From ref. 21, with permission.]

by the lower rate of repair of the late-reacting normal tissues inbetween the subsequent irradiations.

Conclusion

Repair of sublethal damage, although only representing a limited part of the total recovery processes taking place after irradiation, is the most important factor playing a role in defining the biological effect of fractionated irradiations on tissues. The wide divergencies in the capacities of different tissues to effect this process, but also the differences in rates at which it takes place, are the basis of differential effects observed in a number of clinical situations. Further refining of our insights and knowledge, with especially quantitative data, on this process will lead to a better control of the side effects of clinical radiotherapy and to improvements in the therapeutic ratio. One of the next vital steps to take is gaining similar information on the repair characteristics of human tumors in order to tailor individual treatment schedules to specific clinical situations.

References

1 Ang, K. K.; Landuyt, W.; Xu, F. X.; Vanuytsel, L.; Schueren, E. van der: The effect of small radiation doses per fraction on mouse lip mucosa assessed using the concept of partial tolerance. Radiother. Oncol. *8:* 79–86 (1987).

2 Ang, K. K.; Thames, H. D.; Kogel, A. J. van der; Schueren, E. van der: Is the rate of repair of radiation-induced sublethal damage in rat spinal cord dependent on the size of dose per fraction? Int. J. Radiat. Oncol. Biol. Phys. *13:* 557–563 (1987).

3 Ang, K. K.; Kogel, A. J. van der; Schueren, E. van der: The effect of small radiation doses on the rat spinal cord: the concept of partial tolerance. Int. J. Radiat. Oncol. Biol. Phys. *9:* 1487–1491 (1983).

4 Ang, K. K.; Kogel, A. J. van der; Schueren, E. van der: The kinetics of repair of sublethal damage in the rat spinal cord during fractionated irradiations. Radiother. Oncol. *1:* 247–253 (1984).

5 Ang, K. K.; Kogel, A. J. van der; Schueren, E. van der: Lack of evidence for increased tolerance of rat spinal cord with decreasing fraction doses below 2 Gy. Int. J. Radiat. Oncol. Biol. Phys. *11:* 105–110 (1985).

6 Ang, K. K.; Xu, F. X.; Landuyt, W.; Schueren, E. van der: The kinetics and capacity of repair of sublethal damage in mouse lip mucosa during fractionated irradiations. Int. J. Radiat. Oncol. Biol. Phys. *11:* 1977–1983 (1985).

7 Barendsen, G. W.: Dose fractionation, dose rate and isoeffect relationships for normal tissue responses. Int. J. Radiat. Oncol. Biol. Phys. *8:* 1981–1997 (1982).

8 Dale, R. G.: The application of linear-quadratic dose effect equation to fractionated and protracted radiotherapy. Br. J. Radiol. *58:* 515–528 (1985).

9 Dikomey, E.; Franzke, J.: DNA repair kinetics after exposure to X-irradiation and to internal beta-rays in CHO cells. Radiat. environ. Biophys. *25:* 189–194 (1986).

10 Down, J. D.; Easton, D. F.; Steel, G. G.: Repair in mouse lung during low dose-rate irradiation. Radiather. Oncol. *6:* 29–42 (1986).

11 Ellis, F.: The relationship of biological effect to dose-time fractionation factors in radiotherapy. Curr. Top. Radiat. Res. Q. *4:* 357–397 (1968).

12 Fowler, J. F.; Joiner, M. C.; Williams, M. V.: Low doses per fraction in radiotherapy: a definition for 'flexure dose'. Br. J. Radiol. *56:* 599–601 (1983).

13 Fowler, J. F.; Denekamp, J.; Thames, H. D.; Travis, E. L.: Repair factors for multifraction irradiations. Radiother. Oncol. *1:* 281–286 (1984).

14 Hall, E. J.: Radiation dose-rate: a factor of importance in radiobiology and radiotherapy. Br. J. Radiol. *45:* 81–97 (1972).

15 Henkelman, R. M.; Lam, G. K. Y.; Kornelsen, R. O.; Eaves, C. J.: Explanation of dose rate and split dose effect on mouse foot reactions using the same time factor. Radiat. Res. *84:* 274–289 (1980).

16 Hill, R. P.: Response of mouse lung to irradiation at different dose rates. Int. J. Radiat. Oncol. Biol. Phys. *9:* 1043–1047 (1983).

17 Hopewell, J. W.; Aardweg, G. J. M. J. van der: Current concepts of dose-fractionation in radiotherapy normal tissue tolerance. Br. J. Radiol. (in press, 1988).

18 Huczkowski, J.; Trott, K. R.: Dose fractionation effect in low dose rate irradiation of jejunal crypt stem cells. Int. J. Radiat. Biol. *46:* 293–298 (1984).

19 Nguyen, T. D.; Panis, X.; Froissart, D.; Legros, M.; Coninx, P.; Loirette, M: Analysis of late complications after rapid hyperfractionated radiotherapy in advanced head and neck cancers. Int. J. Radiat. Oncol. Biol. Phys. *14:* 23–25 (1988).

20 Scalliet, P.; Landuyt, W.; Schueren, E. van der: Effect of decreasing the dose rate of irradiation on the mouse lip mucosa. Comparison with fractionated irradiations. Radiother. Oncol. *10:* 39–47 (1987).

21 Scalliet, P.; Landuyt, W.; Schueren, E. van der: Kinetics of repair: its influence in low dose rate irradiations. Radiother. Oncol. *11:* 249–251 (1988).

22 Scalliet, P.; Landuyt, W.; Schueren, E. van der: Importance of repair kinetics for determining the tolerance of central nervous system during low dose rate irradiation. Radiother. Oncol. 1988.

23 Scalliet, P.; Landuyt, W.; Vynckier, S.; Schueren, E. van der; Wambersie , A.: Kinetics of sublethal damage recovery in mouse lip mucosa comparing low and high LET radiation. Strahlentherapie 1988.

24 Steel, G. G.; Down, J. D.; Peacock, J. H.; Stephens, T. C.: Dose-rate effects and the reapir of radiation damage. Radiother. Oncol. *5:* 321–331 (1986).

25 Thames, H. D.; Withers, H. R.; Peters, L. J.; Fletcher, G. H.: Changes in early and late radiation responses with altered dose fractionation: implications for dose-survival relationships. Int. J. Radiat. Oncol. Biol. Phys. *8:* 219–226 (1982).

26 Thames, H. D.; Withers, H. R.; Peters, L. J.: Tissue repair capacity and repair kinetics deduced from multifractionated or continuous irradiation regimens with incomplete repair. Br. J. Cancer *49*: suppl VI, pp. 263–269 (1984).

27 Thames, H. D.: An 'incomplete repair' model for survival after fractionated and continuous irradiations. Int. J. Radiat. Biol. *47:* 319–339 (1985).

28 Thames, H. D.; Hendry, J. H.: Fractionation in radiotherapy, (Taylor and Francis, London 1987).

29 Travis, E. L.; Thames, H. D.; Helbing, S. J.; Kiss, I.; Watkins, T. L.: Kinetics of repair in mouse lung after fractionated radiation. Int. J. Radiat. Biol. (submitted, 1987).

30 Tucker, S. L.; Thames, H. D.: Flexure dose: the low-dose limit of effective fractionation. Int. J. Radiat. Oncol. Biol. Phys. *9:* 1373–1383 (1983).

31 Kogel, A. J. van der: Radiation tolerance of the rat spinal cord: time-dose relationship. Radiology *122:* 505–509 (1977).

32 Kogel, A. J. van der: Late effects of radiation on the spinal cord. Dose-effect relationships and pathogenesis (Radiobiological Institute TNO, Rijswijk 1979).

33 Schueren, E. van der; Landuyt, W.; Ang, K. K.; Kogel, A. J. van der: From 2 Gy to 1 Gy per fraction: sparing effect in rat spinal cord. Int. J. Radiat. Oncol. Biol. Phys. *14:* 297–300 (1988).

34 Vanuytsel, L.; Ang, K. K.; Vandenbussche, L.; Vereecken, R.; Schueren, E. van der: Radiotherapy in multiple fractions per day for prostatic carcinoma: late complications. Int. J. Radiat. Oncol. Biol. Phys. *12:* 1589–1595 (1986).

35 Withers, H. R.: Responses of tissues to multiple small dose fractions. Radiat. Res. *71:* 23–33 (1977).

36 Withers, H. R.; Thames, H. D.; Peters, L. J.: Differences in the fractionation response

of acute and late responding tissues; in Karcher, Kogelnik, Reinartz, Progress in radiooncology, vol. 2, pp. 257–296 Raven Press, New York 1982).

37 Withers, H. R.; Hunter, N.; Tucker, S. L.; Thames, H. D.: Response of resting and proliferating hair follicle cells in the mouse to multi-fraction X-rays. Int. J. Radiat. Biol. (in press, 1988).

38 Xu, F. X.; Schueren, E. van der; Ang, K. K.: Acute reactions of the lip mucosa of mice to fractionated irradiations. Radiother. Oncol. *1:* 369–374 (1984).

39 Gray Laboratery Annual Report (1986).

Emanuel van der Schueren, MD, Department of Experimental Radiotherapy, Divison of Oncology, Academisch Ziekenhuis St. Rafaël, Capucijnenvoer 35, B-3000 Leuven (Belgium)

Vaeth JM, Meyer JL (eds): Radiation Tolerance of Normal Tissues.
Front Radiat Ther Oncol. Basel, Karger, 1989, vol 23, pp 75–84

Morphologic Patterns of Radiation Injury[1]

Luis F. Fajardo

Stanford University School of Medicine and Veterans Administration Medical Center, Palo Alto, Calif., USA

The conventional descriptions of radiation pathology are organized according to organ systems [1, 2] or to the chronology of the injury (i.e., acute vs. chronic) [3] or to the extent of the radiation exposure (e.g., local vs. total body) [3–5].

In this article I will present a system of organization based not on the above variables, but on the morphologic patterns (mainly histologic patterns) produced in mammalian tissues by ionizing radiation. The purpose of this organization is twofold: (1) It is easier to remember the patterns that are common to many tissues, and then to learn the exceptions, than to retain in one's memory the lesions of each organ. Hence this is simple. (2) This classification emphasizes the pathways (the morphogenesis) of radiation damage for both radiation therapists and pathologists.

Therefore, here we group the radiation lesions into those that occur in *epithelia* (and parenchymatous cells of various organs), *blood vessels*, and *stroma*. Since not all lesions fit into the general patterns, the exceptions are described as *characteristic lesions of some organs*.

Unless specified otherwise, the following descriptions refer to the effects of ionizing electromagnetic radiations (i.e., X-rays and gamma rays) as used in humans for localized, fractionated, clinical radiation therapy.

It is important to remember that *there are no pathognomonic features of radiation injury*. Nevertheless, although not specific individually, combined radiation lesions are characteristic enough to be recognized. This review does not contain photographs. The readers interested in examples of the lesions described here are referred to the publications cited in the bibliography [1–10, 14, 16, 21, 22].

Epithelial and Parenchymal Lesions

Atrophy is one of the most consistent delayed effects of therapeutic irradiation. It occurs in all lining epithelia (skin, alimentary, respiratory, and urinary tracts) as well as in all glands (e.g., salivary, pancreatic, mannary, cutaneous, etc.). Atrophy also affects parenchymatous tissues such as kidney, lung, or gonads. It is clear, however, that some epithelia or parenchymas suffer more often or more severely than others. Qualitatively such tissues may be separated into three groups: (1) severe atrophy is seen in epidermis, sebaceous glands (perhaps the most affected in the skin), alimentary epithelium (especially intestine), urothelium, salivary glands, and germinal cells of the testis; (2) moderate atrophy occurs in the epithelia of the upper respiratory and alimentary tracts, lung, mammary glands, prostate, and kidney, and (3) atrophy is less common or less severe in sweat glands, liver, and endocrine glands. In fact the latter are rarely affected by external electromagnetic radiations, but, of course, are seriously altered by internally administered radionuclides (thyroid) or by heavy particle beams (pituitary). Atrophy is characteristically focal and random. It is not uncommon to observe relatively intact minor salivary glands adjacent to totally atrophic ones, all within the same radiation field.

Necrosis occurs in many epithelial and parenchymal cells during the *acute* phase of radiation injury, but, with exception of the skin and mucosas, such early lesions are seldom seen in humans. Delayed necrosis generally results from ischemia. It causes interruption(s) of the lining epithelia (i.e., *ulcers* of variable depth and chronicity) in the skin, upper alimentary and respiratory tracts, intestine, urinary tract, and genitalia. One of the most characteristic sites for delayed necrosis is the central nervous system, particularly the white matter of the cerebral hemispheres.

Atypia of epithelial cells is not only a striking, usually delayed, alteration, but also a source of confusion and error. It may affect either nucleus or cytoplasm or both. Most often there is enlargement of both nucleus and cytoplasm of individual cells. The nuclei may appear hyperchromatic, but the chromatin is 'smudged', i.e., chromatin granules are not distinct. Nucleoli are often prominent. Generally, only some of the cells of a given structure (duct, gland, epithelial surface) show atypia, and architecturally there is no suggestion of neoplasia. Thus, with experience, a differential diagnosis can be made between radiation-induced atypia of nonneoplastic epithelium and residual or recurrent tumor. We have observed atypia in epidermis, squamous mucosas (mouth, larynx, vagina, cervix, etc.), bronchi and pulmonary alveoli, stomach, minor salivary glands, endometrium, urothelium, mammary gland, and prostate. In the last three sites this atypia has caused considerable diagnostic difficulty even to experienced pathologists.

Dysplasia induced by irradiation of epithelia is not uncommon in epidermis and squamous mucosas and is rare in nonsquamous epthelia. It is a late lesion (usually several years after exposure) characterized by nuclear atypia with hyperchromatism, lack of polarity (directional, organized maturation), involvement of large clones of cells, and architectural alterations. Dysplasia implies genetic damage, and abnormal ploidy can be documented. It should be distinguished from the benign atypia described above and should be considered premalignant, although not all cases evolve necessarily into neoplasms.

Neoplasia of epithelia and parenchymatous organs resulting from irradiation is well documented for a number of tissues and organs (see separate articles on the subject of radiation oncogenesis in this volume) [23]. Neoplasia often follows dysplasia in skin and squamous mucosas, years after exposure. However, not all radiation-induced neoplasms of these tissues are preceded by dysplasia.

Hypermaturation and the converse, *dedifferentiation* of cells as the result of radiation, have been observed in carcinomas and could possibly occur in nonneoplastic epithelia, but we have not encountered such cases. However, *metaplasia* (especially squamous metaplasia) is not uncommon in tissues like prostate and urothelium.

Stromal Lesions

Of all the lesions described here, those of the stroma are the ones best recognized by pathologists as radiation induced or radiation associated. The most typical combinations of the features described below occur in the submucosa and in the deep soft tissues of mouth, pharynx, larynx, and genitalia. Typical stromal lesions can be seen also in skin and lower urinary tract. Some of the features occur in the alimentary tube. Although fibrosis is a characteristic feature of delayed radiation injury in parenchymatous organs (e.g., lung and kidney), the other stromal features, such as atypical fibroblasts, are rarely observed in such organs.

Fibrosis is one of the commonest delayed manifestations. It occurs in practically all tissues and organs, but extent and severity vary from site to site. Fibrosis is very much time and dose dependent, and, of course, it has been used to measure both of these variables. The typical radiation-induced fibrosis is inhomogeneous: some areas have very dense, acellular collagen, while next to them other areas have only a few fibrous bands.

The fibrous areas are within the irradiated field, but do not fill it entirely. It is easiest to appreciate this alteration in adipose tissue, skeletal or cardiac muscle, or parenchymatous organs.

It will be more practical to list the sites where fibrosis does not occur, or is rare, than to list the many tissues where it is often found. Fibrosis does *not* occur in the lens or in the central nervous system (even gliosis, the CNS counterpart of fibrosis, is not a prominent result of irradiation). In the hemopoietic bone marrow replacement by adipose tissue is the result of high doses; fibrosis does not occur *unless* a neoplasm or an inflammatory lesion had been present prior to the irradiation, in which case the stroma of such a lesion persists in the marrow space. Radiation injury to the bone itself leads, after high doses, to necrosis rather than fibrosis. The delayed hepatic injury shows surprisingly little fibrosis, except in the areas that contained tumor prior to exposure. The same can be said of lymph nodes: when high doses result in lymphocyte depletion, the skeleton of the node remains, with little additional connective tissue, except in the areas that harbored tumor.

Fibrosis is much more than a mark of radiation damage; it is damaging in itself. Crippling or deforming skin retraction and esophageal, intestinal, or urinary stenosis with obstruction, myocardial failure, pericardial restrictive disease, and reduction in pulmonary function are some examples of its effects.

A very characteristic feature is the presence of *fibrin in the stroma*. Probably it occurs in most irradiated mesenchymal tissues, but it is only detectable by light microscopy in some soft tissues. Fibrinous exudate appears as a delicate network of acidophilic fibrils in the midst of collagen and fibroblasts. It is not seen throughout the entire area of fibrosis, but rater occurs in widely separate foci. Special stains, such as phosphotungstic acid-hematoxylin or the Fraser-Lendrum techniques, facilitate the recognition of fibrin. This finding is valuable in the differential diagnosis of delayed radiation fibrosis, but only in sites that do not have other causes for active inflammatory exudate (particularly ulcers); fibrin is a well-known component of the inflammatory exudate, and, therefore, it is expected to be present wherever there is inflammation.

Fibrinous exudate is found months to many years after exposure, in sequential biopsies of a given site, suggesting its persistence in the stroma due to decreased fibrinolysis or to repeated formation of fibrin or, more likely, both mechanisms.

Atypical fibroblasts (so-called 'radiation fibroblasts') are very characteristic of delayed radiation injury. These are large, bizarre cells, usually basophilic, with angulated and elongated cytoplasm. Triangular or even star shapes are observed, and a common configuration is reminiscent of a 'swallow tail'. The nuclei are almost invariably hyperchromatic (probably polyploid) and 'smudged', but mitotic figures are practically never seen.

Atypical fibroblasts are found in delayed lesions, predominantly of the submucosa of the upper respiratory tract, the entire alimentary tract, the lower urinary tract, and genitalia. They are less common in the nonulcerated skin and in the deep soft tissues. Atypical fibroblasts are practically never seen in deep organs such as lungs, heart, liver or brain. Maximow [6] who recognized them many years ago observed that atypical fibroblasts only occur in sites subject to inflammation, and this is still generally, but not absolutely, true. We have noted that they are more common in the presence of infection [1]. Cells almost identical to atypical fibroblasts are seen occasionally in nonirradiated chronically inflammed tissues, particularly at the base of chronic pressure ulcers (decubitus ulcers).

Necrosis of stromal elements is uncommon in the absence of ulceration, superimposed infection, or tumor. When it occurs, it is not necessarily helpful in the diagnosis, but it may suggest severe ischemia, perhaps as the result of the vascular lesions described separately. Fat necrosis is also rare. It has been described in the irradiated breast [7], and in such a location it may present as a mass mimicking clinically a recurrent tumor [7]. Most instances of necrosis in irradiated tissues are associated with radiation-induced ulcers. The beds of such chronic ulcers have the usual elements: necrotic debris, granulation tissue, fibrosis, etc. In contrast to the ulcers of other etiologies, cellular (leukocytic) exudate seems to be less prominent, and 'fibrinoid' necrosis of small arteries is more common. Although not specific, these ulcers are typical because of their chronicity. Aside from bleeding, the inflammatory events that occur in the beds of these ulcers contribute eventually to fibrosis, deformities, stenosis, etc.

Vascular lesions are very prominent morphologically and very important in the pathogenesis of delayed radiation injury. Although these could be considered also as stromal, the vascular changes are described separately.

A consistent feature of *delayed* radiation injury in mammalian tissues is the *lack or paucity of cellular inflammatory response*. With rare exceptions (such as ulcers) the stromal reactions described above are devoid of granulocytes and contain only a few lymphocytes or macrophages. This is best seen in deep tissues such as myocardium, pericardium, renal parenchyma, etc., but to a certain degree it is true of practically all tissues, as long as there is no ulceration or superimposed infection. This absence of cellular inflammatory response is helpful in the differential diagnosis of radiation pathology. Furthermore, it supports the concept that radiation injury is not mediated through an immune mechanism.

Vascular Lesions

Alterations of the blood vessels were recognized by radiation workers as early as 1899 [8]. Since then pathologists have become familiar with the most commonly detected changes of the vasculature, i.e., those in arterioles and capillaries [9]. For the purpose of this presentation the blood vessels are described in decreasing order of radiation sensitivity.

Blood capillaries and sinusoids: The narrowest and most ubiquitous elements of the vasculature appear to be also the most radiosensitive. This, of course, is related to the sensitivity of endothelial cells which constitute the most important part of their wall. Only some lesions of these vessels are appreciated by light microscopy: dilatation is common, and, when superficially located, it can be detected clinically as telangiectasia of skin or mucous membranes; asymmetry with irregularity of the wall; focally prominent endothelial cells; and, rarely, thrombosis. Electron microscopy [1, 9] allows detection of earlier and more subtle alterations. These are best observed in sequential experimental studies of various mammalian tissues — kidney [1], heart [10], lung [11], etc. — and include irregularity of cytoplasm with formation of pseudopodia or 'fronds', 'swelling' or 'blebs' of cytoplasm (often obstructing the lumen) detachment of endothelial cells from the basal lamina, cell pyknosis, rupture of plasma membrane, thrombosis, rupture of capillary wall, loss of entire capillary segments, and, in some organs, regrowth of the lost vessels, [1, 10, 11]. The above changes probably occur in many tissues, perhaps in all, but have been documented only in a few [1, 9–11].

Neither light microscopic studies of human tissues nor electron microscopy reveal the most important result of the above-mentioned acute damage: a reduction in the microvascular network which ultimately results in ischemia. This has been well documented in some tissues such as myocardium, central nervous system, and skin, [10, 12, 13].

Small-sized arteries (measuring up to 100 μm in external diameter) have a muscular wall which, although thin, gives some protection from rupture. These segments may develop necrosis, soon after irradiation or in the delayed phase (e.g., 'fibrinoid' necrosis of arterioles in the brain), but this is not observed often. More common are subendothelial or adventitial fibrosis, 'hyalinization' of the media (dense, acellular, acidophillic, collagenous material), and accumulation of lipid-laden macrophages in the intima (see below). Thrombosis may occur with any of the above.

Medium-sized arteries (100–500 μm) develop late lesions often recognized by pathologists. The most common is intimal fibrosis, characterized by deposition of collagen and fibroblasts (myofibroblasts). Lipid-containing macrophages (foam cells) may accumulate in the intima, in variable numbers, sometimes causing narrowing or complete obstruction. Fibrin may be present among the foam cells, and there may be occlusive thrombosis. Spontaneous atherosclerosis often produces these foam cell plaques in arteries of large size, but rarely in medium- and small-sized vessels. Therefore, although not specific, foam cell plaques in medium and small arteries are highly suggestive of irradiation. These tend to occur more often in the wall of the intestine and in the ovaries [1, 9, 14].

Vasculitis may occur as a rare, delayed lesion. It is an exception to the general rule (see Stromal Lesions) that cellular inflammatory exudate is absent or minimal in delayed radiation pathology. We have found examples of active arteritis in the wall of the intestine, in the pelvic adipose tissue, and in the breast [9]. The infiltrate is generally lymphocytic, moderate to heavy, and localized in media, adventitia, or, less commonly, in the intima. If the latter, there may be thrombosis. We can recognize scars in these vessels (of presumed vasculitis) [9], and in the acute cases that we have been able to follow no generalized vasculitis has developed. Thus we feel that these radiation-associated vasculitis are self-limited and heal without therapy [9, 15]. Hence these should not be confused with ominous systemic vasculitis.

Large arteries (>500 μm) are clearly less often affected than the smaller vessels, perhaps because their ample lumen and thick wall, made of relatively radioresistant cells, protect them [9, 15]. Nevertheless, lesions can occur and are well documented by publications because of their dramatic effects: myointimal proliferation, with or without lipid deposits (which may be greater in irradiated sites than in the rest of the body), thrombosis, mural or occlusive, and, finally, rupture of large arteries. The latter is an often fatal complication that tends to occur in the carotid or the femoral arteries or in the aorta. [9, 16]. It may not result necessarily from irradiation alone, and, in fact, many of such ruptures are clearly caused by other factors such as infections, exposure to digestive enzymes (e.g. saliva), or exposure to air [16]. However, recent experimental evidence indicates that some arterial perforations may result solely from high-dose irradiation [17].

Small veins (having only a few layers of muscle) are affected, overall, less often than their arterial counterparts. Nevertheless, in the wall of the intestine one finds intimal or medial fibrosis, or even thrombosis, of the veins as often or more often than similar arterial lesions [9, 14]. In the liver, of course, irradiation produces a venous lesion (see below) and not an arterial one.

Large veins (≥500 μm) seem to be the least affected of the blood vessels by irradiation, while they are quite often damaged by tumor invasion. Thus, in irradiated tissues, the veins showing transmural scars are often in fact vessels that contained neoplasms prior to irradiation [1, 9].

Some Characteristic Organ Lesions

Although the above-described patterns are found in the immense majority of delayed radiation lesions, it is obvious that a number of them do not fit into these patterns. Examples of such exceptions are: congenital malformations, growth delay, bone deformities, rapid cell depletion of hemopoietic or lymphopoietic organs, acute sialoadenitis, and lens opacities (posterior cataracts). Some of these exceptional tissue lesions deserve a brief description.

Permanent *bone marrow hypoplasia or aplasia* is common. It occurs as *focal,* sharply circumscribed lesions several months after FR doses in excess of 4,000 rad (2nd wave of aplasia) [18]. In this case the hemopoietic cells are decreased in number or absent [18]. Plasma cells and lymphocytes may be the only remaining cells. But these normal elements are not replaced by fibrous tissue as in other organs. They are replaced by adipocytes. Furthermore, there is no fibrinous exudate, and fibroblasts (atypical or otherwise) are not seen [1]. The only areas where collagen is found are those that existed prior to irradiation: the stroma of preexisting tumor nodules or inflammatory foci will remain, even if the neoplastic cells or the inflammatory exudate have dissapeared [1]. Deposition of thorium dioxide, however, does result in delayed fibrosis, but this is very rarely encountered today [1].

Acute radiation pneumonitis has a constellation of typical changes [1, 19]: enlargement and atypia of type II pneumocytes, edema of alveolar walls, variable number of alveolar macrophages, and, most prominently, hyaline membranes (mainly made of fibrin) lining alveolar ducts and alveoli. These are, of course, the features of 'acute, diffuse alveolar injury' or 'adult respiratory distress syndrome', a condition that may result from many etiologies besides radiation: shock, toxic substances (systemic or inhaled), various drugs, infections, etc. [1, 19]. However, the morphology of acute radiation pneumonitis, 7–16 weeks after initiation of therapy, is characteristic enough to distinguish it sometimes from even the adult respiratory distress syndrome produced by antineoplastic compounds which closely mimick it.

Colitis cystica profunda (CSP) is an uncommon condition that occurs chiefly in the distal colon and particularly in the rectum. Most of the reported cases, which by now probably are more than 200, are *not* associated with irradiation. The ordinary CSP is characterized by the penetration of nonneoplastic colonic epithelium (lining as well as glandular) through the muscularis mucosa and into the submucosa, replacing focally the submucosal stroma. The invaginated glands often form mucus-filled cysts. CSP is viewed as an inflammatory disease, often very symptomatic and sometimes rather difficult to treat. Its pathogenesis is unknown, and it does not appear to be related to a consistent group of disease entities.

The association of CSP with delayed irradiation effects in the colon was noted some time ago [14, 20]. We have now seen, or read of, 4 cases. What sets apart the radiation-associated CSP from the rest of the CSP is its morphology: in radiation CSP, the glands not only penetrate into the submucosa, but also into the main muscularis; also there is very little or no cellular inflammatory infiltrate around these glands. Thus, there is a remarkable growth of benign-looking glands in the midst of the muscular coat. Inexperienced observers may confuse these features with those of a well-differentiated adenocarcinoma. Additionally, radiation-associated CSP may occur in the (irradiated) right colon, an uncommon location for nonradiation CSP.

Veno-occlusive liver disease usually appears within 90 days of initiation of therapy. The lesion occurs in the centrilobular veins and in the terminal portion of their afferent sinusoids, as well as in some sublobular veins [1, 21]. Probably due to endothelial injury, delicate fibrin strands are formed in the lumina [21]. This is followed by collagen deposition producing a network that obstructs the lumina and traps erythocytes [1, 21]. Acute centrilobular congestion with subsequent necrosis ensues, causing most of the clinical manifestations, if the affected area is large enough, and even leading to death [21]. However, most cases subside and heal, leaving only minimal scars [22]. It is remarkable that the liver arterioles show no evidence of damage. The veins (including some portal venules) [21] seem to bear the brunt of the injury.

Acknowledgements

This work was supported in part by Veterans Administration Research Funds (Grant No. MRIS 2735-01). I appreciate the assistance of Donna L. Buckley.

References

1 Fajardo L. F.: Pathology of Radiation Injury. New York, Masson, 1982.
2 Rubin P, Casarett G. W.: Clinical Radiation Pathology. Philadelphia, Saunders, 1968.
3 White D. C.: An Atlas of Radiation Histopathology. Technical Information Center

Publication T/D-26676. Washington, US Energy Research and Development Administration, 1975.

4 Warren S.: The Pathology of Ionizing Radiation. Springfield, Thomas, 1961.

5 Liebow A. A., Warren S, DeCoursey E.: Pathology of atomic bomb casualties. Am. J. Pathol 1949; *25:* 21–26.

6 Maximow A. A.: Studies on the changes produced by roentgen rays in inflamed connective tissue. J. Exp. Med. 1923; *37:* 319–340.

7 Clarke D., Curtis J. L., Martinez A., et. al.: Fat necrosis of the breast stimulating recurrent carcinoma after primary radiotherapy in the management of early stage breast carcinoma. Cancer 1983; *52:* 442–445.

8 Gassmann A.: Zur Histologie der Roentgenulcer. Fortschr Geb Roentgenstr. 1899; *2:* 199–211.

9 Fajardo L. F., Bethrong M.: Vascular lesions following radiation. Pathol. Annu. 1988; *23:* 297–330.

10 Fajardo L. F., Stewart J. R.: Pathogenesis of radiation-induced myocardial fibrosis. Lab. Invest. 1973; *29:* 244–257.

11 Phillips T. L.: An ultrastructural study of the development of radiation injury in the lung. Radiology 1966; *87:* 49–54.

12 Hopewell J. W., Campling D., Calvo W., et. al.: Vascular radiation damage: Its cellular basis and likely consequences. Br. J. Cancer 1986; *53(suppl. VII):* 181–191.

13 Archambeau J., Ines A., Fajardo L. F., et. al.: Response of swine skin microvasculature to acute single exposures of X-rays: Quantification of endothelial changes. Radiat Res 1984; *98:* 37–51.

14 Berthrong M., Fajardo L. F.: Radiation injury in surgical pathology. Part II. Am. J. Surg. Pathol. 1981; *5:* 152–178.

15 Reinhold H. S., Fajardo L. F., Hopewell J. W.: The vascular system; in Altman K. I. (ed.): Relative Radiosensitivities of Human Organ Systems. Academic Press, vol. II, 1989.

16 Fajardo L. F., Lee A.: Rupture of major vessels after radiation. Cancer 1975; *36:* 904–913.

17 Fee W. E. Jr., Goffinet D. R., Fajardo L. F., et. al.: Safety of ^{125}I and ^{192}Ir implants to the canine carotid artery: Preliminary report. Laryngoscope 1985; *95:* 317–320.

18 Sykes M. P., Chu F. C. H., Wilkerson W. G.: Local bone marrow changes secondary to therapeutic irradiation. Radiology 1960; *75:* 919–924.

19 Gross N. J.: Pulmonary effects of radiation therapy. Ann. Intern. Med. 1977; *86:* 81–92.

20 Gardiner G. W., McAuliffe N., Murray D.: Colitis cystica profunda occurring in a radiation-induced colonic stricture. Hum. Pathol. 1984; *15:* 295–298.

21 Fajardo L. F., Colby T. V.: Pathogenesis of veno-occlusive liver disease following radiation. Arch. Pathol. Lab. Med. 1980; *104:* 584–588.

22 Lewin K., Millis R. R.: Human radiation hepatitis. A morphologic study with emphasis on the late change. Arch. Pathol. 1973; *96:* 21–26.

23 Fajardo L. F.: Ionizing radiation and neoplasia (chapter 5). In Fenoglio C., Weinstein R. S. (eds): New concepts in neoplasia as applied to diagnostic pathology. Williams & Wilkins 1986: 97–125.

Luis F. Fajardo, M.D., Stanford University School of Medicine and Veterans Administration Medical Center, Palo Alto, CA 94304 (USA)

Vaeth JM, Meyer JL (eds): Radiation Tolerance of Normal Tissues.
Front Radiat Ther Oncol. Basel, Karger, 1989, vol 23, pp 85–95

Effects of Radiation on the Microvasculature

Implications for Normal-Tissue Damage

J. W. Hopewell[a], *W. Calvo*[b], *D. Campling*[a], *H. S. Reinhold*[c], *M. Rezvani*[a], *T. K. Yeung*[a]

[a]CRC Normal Tissue Radiobiology Research Group, Research Institute, University of Oxford, Churchill Hopsital, Oxford, UK;
[b]Department of Clinical Physiology and Occupational Medicine, University of Ulm, FRG;
[c]Erasmus University, Rotterdam, and TNO Radiobiological Institute, Rijswijk, The Netherlands

Introduction

Irradiation with therapeutic doses of X-rays may result in the development of early and/or late effects in normal tissues. These range in severity from relatively insignificant changes to life-threatening complications. Although the underlying mechanisms responsible for the development of acute effects are relatively well understood and can largely be predicted on the basis of the hierarchical organization of the appropriate target cell population [16], the pathophysiological changes involved in the development of late effects are not as clearly defined. In patients that develop late radiation-induced sequelae, pathological lesions in the walls of blood vessels are a frequent finding, and this has been largely responsible for the evolution of the hypothesis that vascular damage is the predominant factor leading to the development of late effects in irradiated normal tissues.

Extensive experimental studies have shown a clearly defined association between vascular damage and the development of late radiation effects; however, the exact role played by vascular lesions remains uncertain [13]. In order to 'sift' definitive evidence in support of a vascular hypothesis from the large amount of speculation, two key questions need to be answered: (1) What are the time- and dose-related changes in the number of potential target cells within the walls of blood vessels, and (2) what are the vessel types at risk?

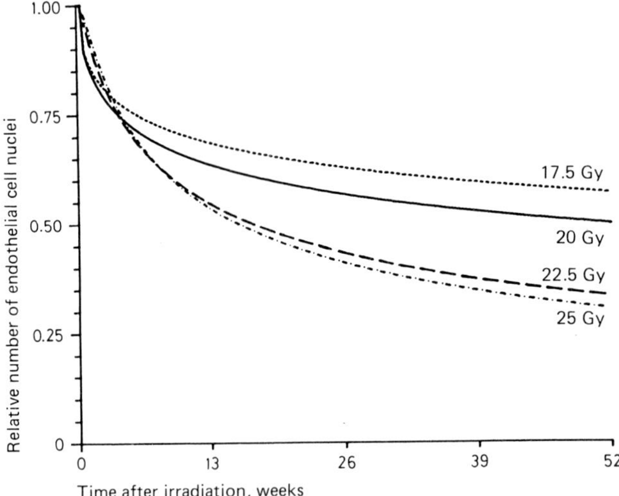

Fig. 1. Time-related changes in the relative number of endothelial cell nuclei (per unit length of basement membrane) in the vasculature of the choroid plexus of the rat brain after single doses of 17.5–25 Gy of X-rays. Data fitted by the Weibull regression method. [Redrawn from ref. 13.]

In an attempt to answer these basic questions, relatively simple tissue systems have been used, namely the choroid plexus of the rate brain and the hamster cheek pouch. The results obtained with these systems have been used to help in the understanding of more complex effects seen in irradiated pig skin and in the white matter of the rat brain after irradiation. These studies were largely carried out as part of the Collaborative Research Programme of the European Late Effects Project Group (EULEP).

Radiation Effects on Potential Target Cells

The choroid plexus, in the lateral ventricle of the rat brain, was used to examine the time- and dose-related changes in two potential target cells. In this system endothelial cells and smooth muscle cells in the wall of the blood vessels can easily be identified [3, 4].

The numbers of endothelial cell nuclei were reduced within 1 week of irradiation [14], and the rate of the initial decline in their number appeared to be independent of the size of the radiation dose (fig. 1). By 8

weeks, this reduction in the number of endothelial cell nuclei was highly significant ($p<0.001$), and between 26 and 52 weeks the reduction was dose-related, ranging from ~40% after 17.5 Gy to ~65% after 22.5 and 25 Gy. Associated with this loss of endothelial cell nuclei was evidence for reactive and/or regenerative changes. These included the appearence of grossly enlarged endothelial cell nuclei and the presence of the occasional mitotic figure. Further evidence in support of repopulation was provided by the presence of pairs or groups of endothelial cell nuclei at specific 'sites' in the walls of blood vessels otherwise depleted of cells.
These 'sites' represented ~15% of all endothelial cell nuclear positions 26 weeks after irradiation with 17.5 and 20 Gy and 25–30% of all 'sites' after 22.5 and 25 Gy [4]. Sometimes these groups of nuclei appeared to totally occlude the lumen of blood vessels. Although these changes have been reported in many normal tissues after irradiation [11], this represents the first occasion on which their frequency has been quantified.

The choroid plexus contains very few arterioles, and hence rather than count smooth muscle cells in the tunica media of only a limited number of vessels after irradiation, the histological sections from each animal were simply scored so as to assess the presence or absence of smooth muscle atrophy in these vessels. The resulting quantal data were analyzed by probit analysis to establish the latency associated with a 50% incidence (LP_{50}) of the effect (fig. 2). This latency was dose dependent, ranging from 29.8 ± 3.77 weeks after 25 Gy to an extrapolated value of 57.0 ± 4.2 weeks when the data for 17.5 and 20 Gy were combined.

Blood Vessel Types at Risk after Irradiation

The time- and dose-related changes in the density of blood vessels of differing calibre have been assessed in vivo in the hamster cheek pouch [2]. The time-related changes in the relative number of all blood vessels and of vessels in three broad subgroups were determined after irradiation with a single dose of 25 Gy. These findings are shown in figure 3. The first significant change, 1 month after irradiation, was an ~23% reduction ($p<0.005$) in vessels of 7–16 μm in diameter. Focal occlusive changes have been reported previously in small arterioles of this experimental model from approximately this time after irradiation [11]. A significant reduction ($p<0.005$) in the number of capillaries, i.e., vessels <7μm in diameter, was not seen until 3 months after irradiation. A maximum reduction of ~50% in vessels <7μm in diameter was seen after 5 months. A consistent reduction in the number of larger vessels, i.e., >16μm in diameter, was seen only at ≧7 months after irradiation. At these later times

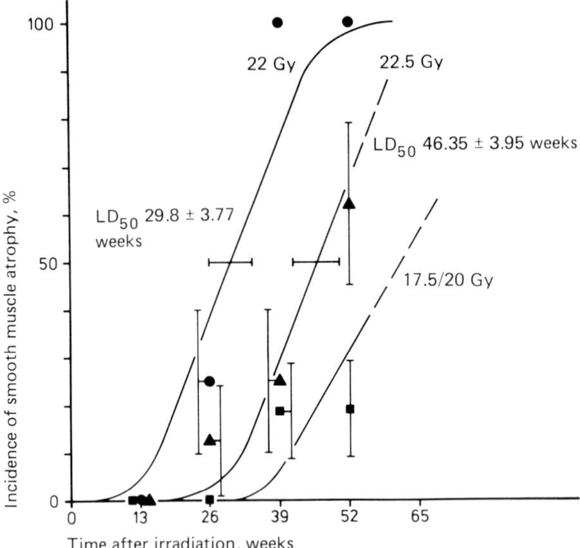

Fig. 2. Time-related changes in the percent incidence of smooth muscle atrophy in the tunica media of arterioles in the choroid plexus of the rat brain after single doses of 17.5/20 (combined data), 22.5, and 25 Gy.

the reduction in the density of vessels <7 and 7–16 μm in diameter was dose-dependent for doses between 15 and 25 Gy. A significant reduction in the number of blood vessels >16μm in diameter was seen only after 25 Gy.

Role of Vascular Changes in Normal Tissue Damage

Pig Skin

Atrophy of the dermis and subcutaneous tissues is a frequently reported complication after radiotherapy. It is often referred to clinically as subcutaneous induration or fibrosis [6]. Recently the time course for the development of late dermal atrophy has been established in pig skin after single doses of ^{90}Sr β-irradiation [14] or 250-kV X-rays [7]. The time-related changes in dermal thickness were measured 'in vivo' using pulsed ultrasound [7]. During the first 12 weeks after β-irradiation, there was no significant change in the relative thickness of the dermis. Then atrophy developed rapidly between 12 and 18 weeks (fig. 4), the rate of develop-

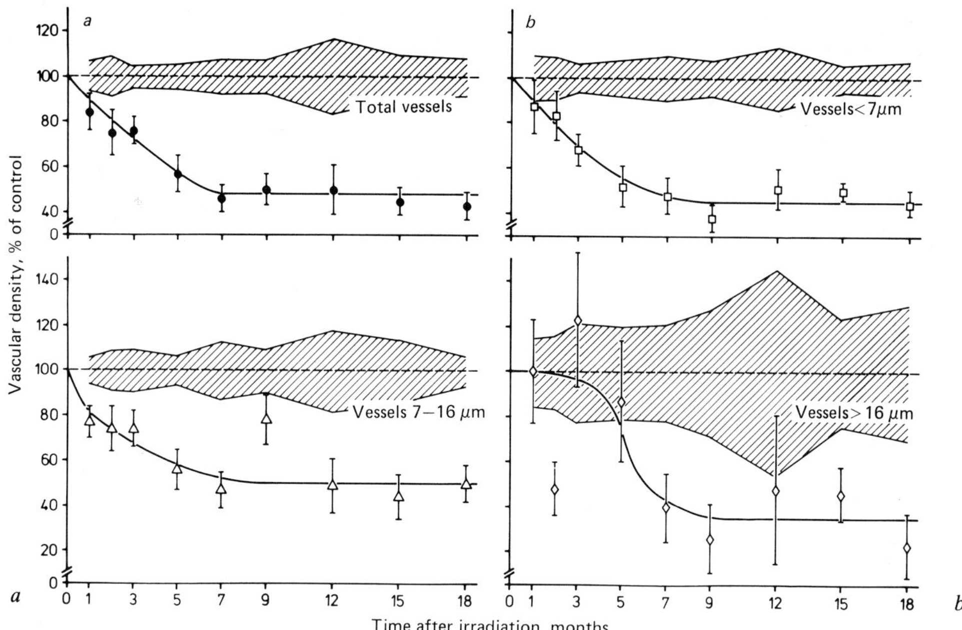

Fig. 3. Time-related changes in the total number (±SE) of blood vessels and of blood vessels in three subgroups in the irradiated hamster cheek pouch as compared with that in an unirradiated pouch in the same group of animals, after irradiation with a single dose of 25 Gy. The hatched areas represent ±SE of unirradiated control values.

ment being independent of the radiation dose. The values for the changes in relative dermal thickness, which plateaued between 20 and 50 weeks, were dose related, i.e., <10% after 10 Gy, rising to ~20% after 27 Gy of ^{90}Sr β-rays. A single dose of 18 Gy of 250-kV X-rays produced ~20% dermal thinning over this time period. A second wave of dermal thinning developed between 50 and 64 weeks after irradiation, and here again, although the severity was dose dependent, the rate of development of damage was independent of the irradiation dose.

The first wave of dermal thinning was preceded by a sequence of changes in the vasculature. These included a general reduction in both the number of endothelial cells and in the density of blood vessels [1]. After large single doses of X-rays (>20 Gy), these vascular changes were so severe that ischaemic dermal necrosis developed. A reduction in dermal blood flow has also been shown to precede the development of dermal necrosis or atrophy in pig skin [17]. A comparison of the radiation

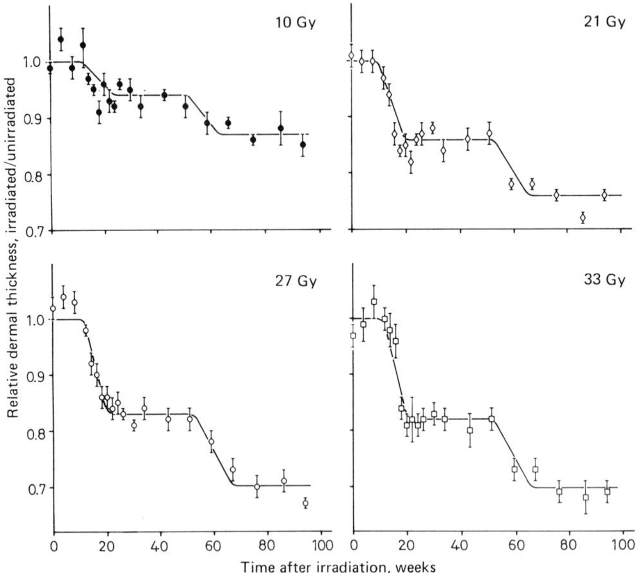

Fig. 4. Time-related changes in the relative thickness (±SE) of the dermis of pig skin after irradiation with single doses from 22-mm ^{90}Sr plaques.

reaction of skin to β-emitters of varying energies has also suggested that the arterioles in the deep dermal plexus are an important target in the development of late radiation injury [12]. This is an area where vessels that are occluded by groups of endothelial cell nuclei are to be found [11].

Preliminary observations would suggest that the second wave of dermal thinning was associated with a diffuse degeneration of the blood vessel walls. The tunica media of arterioles appeared to become vacuolated or was replaced by hyaline material. There was also histological evidence for the development of telangiectasis in the capillaries of the papillary dermis and for the extravasation of red blood cells, with the presence of focal parenchymal degeneration.

Rat Brain

Delayed radiation-induced lesions may develop from several months up to many years after the therapeutic irradiation of the brain. Although all regions of the brain have been reported to be affected, damage tends to be most severe in the white matter. This has been confirmed by the

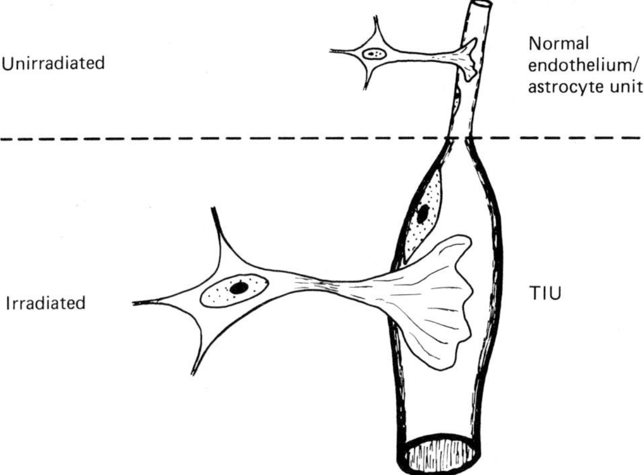

Fig. 5. Diagrammatic representation of a TIU seen in the white matter of the irradiated rat brain prior to the development of necrosis. The TIU was characterized by a dilation of the blood vessel lumen, a thickening of the blood vessel wall, an enlargement of endothelial cell nuclei, and a hypertrophy of the adjacent astrocytes when compared with an endothelial/astrocyte unit in the unirradiated brain.

results of numerous experimental studies [10]. In a recent investigation in the rat brain [5], necrosis of the white matter was seen only at intervals of ≧39 weeks after single doses of ≧22.5 Gy. However, of the various regions of white matter examined in histological sections of animals killed at regular time intervals after irradiation, the fimbria of the hippocampus appeared to be the most radioresponsive. For example, in the fimbria the LP_{50} associated with the use of a single does of 25 Gy was 35.9 ± 2.6 weeks. This can be compared with 48.9 ± 2.8 and 47.2 ± 2.7 weeks in the corpus callosum and in the internal capsule, respectively.

Necrosis of the white matter was preceded by changes in the vasculature. These changes, in common with necrosis, appeared to be both time and dose related. The vascular changes were characterized by the dilation of blood vessels, the enlargement of endothelial cell nuclei, the thickening of the blood vessel wall, and a reactive hypertrophy of the adjacent astrocytes. These four parameters were highly correlated with each other and collectively, as illustrated diagrammatically in figure 5, appeared to represent a tissue injury unit (TIU). Incidence and severity of damage to this vascular/glial unit appeared to increase with time after irradiation until necrosis developed. The relationship between the LP_{50} for the TIU and necrosis of the fimbria is shown in figure 6a. The LP_{50} times for the TIU were 11–13 weeks shorter than those for necrosis after single doses of 22.5 and 25 Gy.

After a single dose of 20 Gy, selective necrosis of the white matter was not seen within the natural life span of these rats. The late change developing in the brain after this dose was telangiectasia. This was found in regions of grey and white matter [5, 18]. Similar lesions were seen after higher doses, but after a shorter latent period (fig. 6b). Although the underlying mechanisms responsible for the development of telangiectasia are uncertain, it is perhaps significant that the LP_{50} times for smooth muscle atrophy in the arterioles of the choroid plexus were 15–17 weeks shorter than those for telangiectasia. The effects of radiations on arterioles in other regions of the brain will have to be examined before any general conclusions can be reached.

Discussion and Conclusions

In the choroid plexus of the rat brain, which has a relatively simple vascular system, it has been shown that endothelial cells are lost fairly soon after irradiation. This is consistent with the proposal that cell death occurs only in a small proportion of endothelial cells which have a short cell cycle time [8]. The initial rate of loss of endothelial cells from the choroid plexus was independent of the irradiation dose. This finding, like that of an early loss of cells, is not consistent with the concept of an 'F-type' or flexible target cell population in a late responding normal tissue [16].

The loss of smooth muscle cells from the arterioles in the choroid plexus occurred later, and in this instance the latency time was dose related, with the suggestion of a threshold dose higher than that for the loss of endothelial cells. A higher threshold dose and a longer latency were also associated with loss of larger vessels ($>16\,\mu m$ diameter) from the hamster cheek pouch. The initial loss of small arterioles and later of capillaries in the cheek pouch was associated with microscopic evidence of occlusive vascular changes which were consistent with the effects attributed to regeneration in the endothelial cells of the choroid plexus.

In the two more complex normal tissues, pig skin and white matter of the rat brain, two distinct waves of development of late damage were seen. After a threshold dose the initial reaction developing in the brain and skin was necrosis. Atrophy of the skin was also reported after lower doses. These effects were preceded by vascular changes in both tissues. A TIU was identified in the brain, its presence preceded the development of

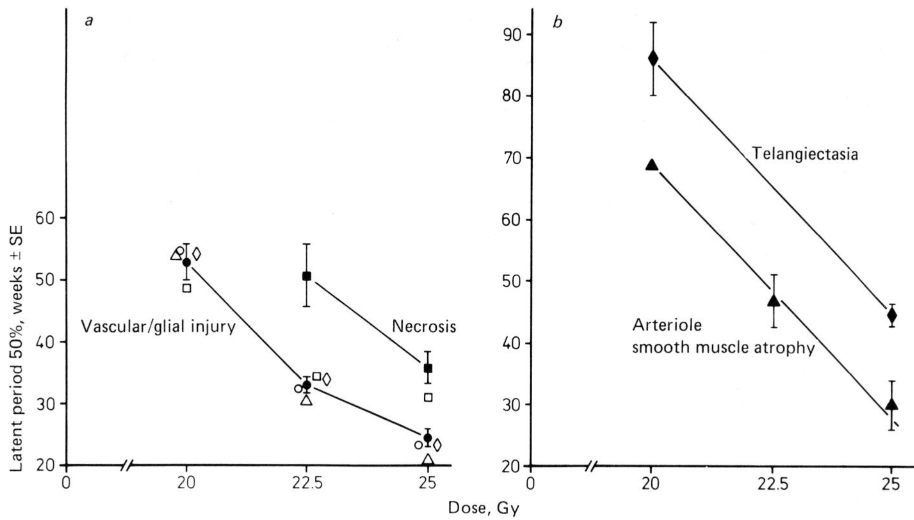

Fig. 6. Dose-related changes in the latency (±SE) for an LP_{50} of specific pathological lesions in the rat brain after irradiation: *a* Latency for the appearance of damage to a vascular/glial unit (TIU; ●) compared with that for necrosis in the fimbria (■). ○ = Blood vessel dilation; △ = endothelial cell enlargement; □ = wall thickening; ◇ = astrocyte hypertrophy. For further explanation see the text and figure 5. *b* Latency for the development of atrophy in the smooth muscle cells of arterioles in the choroid plexus (▲) compared with that for telangiectasia in grey and white matter in the rat brain (◆).

necrosis by several weeks. The histological characteristics of the TIU were thought to represent a series of reactive changes apparently in response to an earlier reduction in the capillary density [5]. A similar phenomenon preceded the development of necrosis and/or atrophy in pig skin [1].

The second later phase of development of damage in pig skin and in the rat brain was telangiectasia. Foci of necrosis and a general atrophy were also identified in pig skin at these later times. Such changes were associated with the degeneration of smooth muscle cells in arterioles with their replacement by hyaline material. Such changes have also been reported at these later times after irradiation in mesenteric blood vessels [9] and in the brain [11]. The loss of smooth muscle cells could result in a reduction in the control of capillary pressure; the consequence of which would be the appearance of grossly dilated, telangiectatic capillaries.

Although in general terms similarities exist between effects seen in pig skin and in the rat brain, there are also important differences. In the brain, the time of development of the relatively early necrotic changes in the white matter and the later telangiectatic effects were both dose related. However, the development of the two waves of atrophy in the skin and of necrosis in the initial phase after higher doses [15] was independent of the size of the radiation dose. This may simply reflect species differences or the different end points used for the analysis. The times of development of telangiectasia in human skin have been found to be dose dependent [19]. This suggests the need for additional investigations, including some in other normal tissues, before the now indisputable role of vascular damage in the development of late effects can be fully explained.

Acknowledgements

This work formed part of the Collaboration Programme of the European Late Effects Project Group (EULEP) and was partly supported by the Radiation Protection Programme of the Commission of European Communities (Contract No B16-099-D). The Research Institute, Churchill Hospital, is supported by the Cancer Research Campaign.

References

1 Archambeau, J. O.; Ines, A.; Fajardo, L. F.: Response of the swine skin microcirculation to acute single exposure of X-rays: quantification of endothelial changes. Radiat. Res. *98:* 37–51 (1984).
2 Campling, D.; Hopewell, J. W.: Time- and dose-related changes in the vasculature of the hamster cheek pouch after X-irradiation. Int. J. Radiat. Biol. *52:* 484 (1987).
3 Calvo, W.; Hopewell, J. W.; Reinhold, H. S.; Yeung, T. K.: Radiation-induced damage in the choroid plexus of the rat brain. An histological evaluation. Neuropath. appl. Neurobiol. *12:* 47–61 (1986).
4 Calvo, W.; Hopewell, J. W.; Reinhold, H. S.; Berg, A. P. van der; Yeung, T. K.: Dose-dependent and time-dependent changes in the choroid plexus of the irradiated rat brain. Br. J. Radiol. *60:* 1109–1117 (1987).
5 Calvo, W.; Hopewell, J. W.; Reinhold, H. S.; Yeung, T. K.: Time- and dose-related changes in the white matter of the rat brain after single doses of X rays. Br. J. Radiol. (November 1988).
6 Gauwerky, F.; Langheim, F.: Der Zeitfaktor bei der strahleninduzierten subkutanen Fibrose. Strahlentherapie *154:* 608–616 (1978).
7 Hamlet, R.; Rezvani, M.; Hopewell, J. W.: Ultrasound measurement of atrophy in pig skin following X- or β-irradiation. Bioeng. Skin *2:* 49–57 (1986).
8 Hirst, D. G.; Denekamp, J.; Hobson, B.: Proliferation studies of the endothelial and smooth muscle cells of the mouse mesentery after irradiation. Cell Tiss. Kinet. *13:* 91–104 (1980).
9 Hirst, D. G.; Denekamp, J.; Travis, E. L.: The response of mesenteric blood vessels to irradiation. Radiat. Res. *77:* 259–275 (1979).

10 Hopewell, J. W.: Late radiation damage to the central nervous system. A radiobiological interpretation. Neuropath. appl. Neurobiol. *5:* 329–343 (1979).
11 Hopewell, J. W.: Radiation effects on vascular tissue; in Potten, Hendry, Cytotoxic insult to tissue: effects on cell lineage, pp. 228–257 (Churchill Livingstone, Edinburgh 1983).
12 Hopewell, J. W.: Mechanisms of action of radiation on skin and underlying tissues. Br. J. Radiol., suppl. *19*, pp. 39–47 (1986).
13 Hopewell, J. W.; Campling, D.; Calvo, W.; Reinhold, H. S.; Wilkinson, J. H.; Yeung, T. K.: Vascular irradiation damage; its cellular basis and likely consequences. Br. J. Cancer *53:* suppl. VII, pp. 181–191 (1986).
14 Hopewell, J. W.; Calvo, W.; Campling, D.; Lauk, S.; Reinhold, H. S.; Reyners, H.; Rezvani, M.; Yeung, T. K.: The role of the vasculature in normal tissue responses; in Fielden, Fowler, Hendry, Scott, 8th Int. Congr. of Radiation Research, Edinburgh 1987; vol. 2: radiation research, pp. 789–794 (Taylor & Francis, London 1987).
15 Hopewell, J. W.; Young, C. M. A.: The effects of field size on the reaction of pig skin to single doses of X rays. Br. J. Radiol. *55:* 356–361 (1982).
16 Michalowski, A.: Effects of radiation on normal tissues: hypothetical mechanisms and limitations of in situ assays of clonogenicity. Radiat. environ. Biophys. *19:* 157–172 (1981).
17 Moustafa, H. F.; Hopewell, J. W.: Blood flow clearance changes in pig skin after single doses of X rays. Br. J. Radiol. *53:* 693–696 (1980).
18 Reinhold, H. S.; Hopewell, J. W.: Late changes in the architecture of blood vessels of the rat brain after irradiation. Br. J. Radiol. *53:* 693–696 (1980).
19 Turesson, I.; Notter, G.: The predictive value of skin telangiectasia for late radiation effects in different normal tissues. Int. J. Radiat. Oncol. Biol. Phys. *12:* 603–609 (1986).

J. W. Hopewell, PhD, CRC Normal Tissue Radiobiology Research Group,
Research Institute, University of Oxford, Churchill Hospital, Oxford OX3 7LJ (UK)

Vaeth JM, Meyer JL (eds): Radiation Tolerance of Normal Tissues.
Front Radiat Ther Oncol. Basel, Karger, 1989, vol 23, pp 96–112

The Unique Physiology of Endothelial Cells and Its Implications in Radiobiology

Luis F. Fajardo

Stanford University School of Medicine and Veterans Administration Medical Center, Palo Alto, Calif., USA

Introduction

Much has been learned about endothelial cells (EC) since the classical ultrastructural work on cell transport and permeability of the 1960s [1, 2]. Studies such as those on platelet-endothelial interactions [3, 4] were made possible by key developments. These included the design of continuous EC cultures [5, 6], new angiogenesis systems [7, 8], as well as the identification of angiogenic factors [9–11]. The effects of cytokines on EC are being defined [12–14], and currently the 'communications' between EC and adjacent smooth myocytes are the subject of intensive research.

This brief review of the functions peculiar to EC is limited to the salient facts and does not have a complete bibliography. It is focused mainly – but not exclusively – on aspects relevant to radiation biology. Those readers desiring additional information are referred to more extensive reviews [10, 14, 15]. Only the endothelium of the cardiovascular system will be considered here, since the lymphatic vessel endothelium has not been well studied.

Endothelial Functions

The EC functions concerning this review are those related to coagulation, inflammation, immune response, angiogenesis (including synthesis of stromal elements), and special metabolic activities. These functions are diagrammatically indicated in figure 1 and described in the paragraphs that follow.

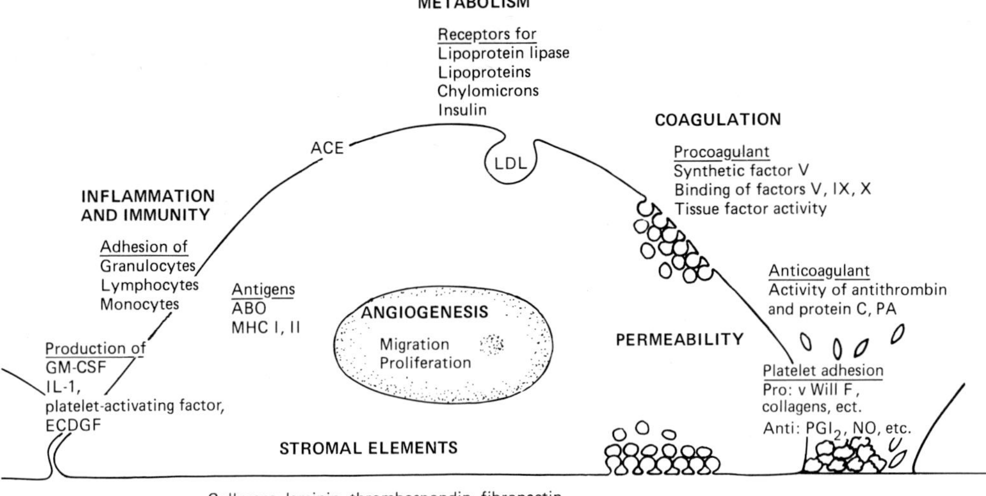

Fig. 1. Diagram representing a perpendicular section of an endothelial cell attached to its basal lamina (bottom) and to an adjacent cell (left), but leaving a gap of denuded basal lamina to the right which is partially filled by aggregating platelets. The main functions of the EC described in this review are indicated in bold capital letters, with examples of such functions in small case letters. ABO = ABO antigens; ECDGF = EC derived growth factor; GM-CSF = granulocyte monocyte colony-stimulating factor; LDL = low-density lipoproteins; MHC I-II = major histocompatibility complexes I and II; NO = nitric oxide. For explanation of the other abbreviations see text. See also figure 2.

Endothelium and Coagulation

The roles of the EC in the soluble coagulation process can be separated into two groups: procoagulant and anticoagulant. The same applies in relation to the contribution of EC in platelet aggregation: agonist and antagonist effects.

The procoagulant effects include the synthesis and release of factor V [16] (which is also produced by hepatocytes). In addition EC bind factors V, IX_a, and X_a and enzymatically activate factor XII. EC activated by endotoxin, thrombin, interleukin 1 (IL-1), tumor necrosis factor (TNF-α), or lymphotoxin (LT; TNF-β) markedly increase the – otherwise minimal – activity of tissue factor (thromboplastin, etc.). Leukocytes and platelets also stimulate such activity. Tissue factor reacts with factor VII and calcium, thus accelerating the activation of factor X [15].

The anticoagulant effects are also varied. Thrombomodulin and protein S (produced by EC) enhance the ability of thrombin to activate protein C, a liver-synthesized substance that suppresses factors V and VIII by proteolysis [15]. Heparin sulfate – and probably other similar molecules on the EC membrance – accelerates the inactivation of thrombin by plasma antithrombin III [15]. Probably through a similar mechanism EC may support the inactivation of factors IX_a, X_a, and XII_a by antithrombin III [15].

EC secrete both plasminogen activators (PA; urokinase and tissue type) *and* an inhibitor of PA (tissue type) [15]. IL-1 and TNF-α enhance the production of such an inhibitor [17]. These cytokines in addition decrease surface thrombomodulin [14, 15].

Platelets adhere to the basal lamina, at the sites where it is denuded of EC, or to the stroma surrounding a ruptured basal lamina. This adhesion to the basal lamina is dependent upon the interaction of von Willebrand factor (v Will F; factor VIII associated antigen) with collagens I, III, IV, and V, particularly the latter two. EC synthesize and secrete v Will F. The release of v Will F is induced by thrombin [15].

Adherent platelets proceed to aggregate and degranulate in succeeding waves, releasing multiple substances which include adenosine di- and triphosphate, platelet factor 4, thromboxane A_2, platelet-derived growth factor, etc. [15].

Unstimulated ('resting') platelets do not adhere to EC [15] because of an endothelium-derived relaxing factor on the surface of EC which has been identified as nitric oxide [18]. Even stimulated platelets do not adhere to normal EC, and in this instance such a property appears to be mediated by prostacyclin (PGI_2), a potent vasodilator and inhibitor of platelet adhesion. EC synthesize and secrete PGI_2 in response to the stimulus of numerous substances which include thrombin, histamine, bradykinin, lipoproteins (especially high-density lipoproteins), adenine nucleotides, cytokines (IL-1, TNF-α), trypsin, etc. [15]. Also cellular events such as shear stress and activation of neutrophils stimulate PGI_2 secretion [15]. Ectoenzymes of EC also limit platelet aggregation by metabolizing adenosine di- and triphosphate with the production of adenosine, a strong inhibitor of platelet function [15].

Role of Endothelium in Inflammation and Immune Response

Leukocyte adhesion to the endothelium, an important step in inflammation, is modulated (aside from physical characteristics) by the presence of specific receptors on the cell membranes.

Adhesion of granulocytes, monocytes-macrophages, and lymphocytes is enhanced by the action of cytokines, most prominently IL-1 and TNF-α. Certain molecules serve as receptors for leukocytes on the surface of EC [14]. ICAM-1, a molecule found in fibroblasts, lymphocytes, and normal EC, probably serves as a receptor for lymphocytes [14].

ELAM-1, another molecule, is expressed by *activated* EC and appears to serve as a receptor for granulocytes *in vitro* [14]. Certain proteins on the leukocyte surface, probably LFA_1 in lymphocytes, and MAC_1 in macrophages and granulocytes may be the ligands that interact with the EC receptors (ICAM-1 in lymphocytes and perhaps ELAM-1 in neutrophils). The in vivo interaction of leukocytes with EC is likely far more complex than what has been shown in vitro [Butcher, personal communi., 1988].

The mechanisms that regulate the selective exit of circulating lymphocytes into specific organs such as intestine, skin, lung, and lymphatic tissues are of current interest. Jalkanen et al. [19] and Streeter et al. [20] have found in lymphocytes a family of ~90-kD glycoproteins that seem to act as recognition molecules and have named them 'homing receptors'. These homing receptors recognize specific molecules on the membrane of the EC which probably vary from tissue to tissue. Because of their function the latter molecules have been named 'addressins' [Butcher, personal communi., 1988, 20].

In addition to IL-1 and TNF-α, other cytokines are involved in the EC response to inflammation [21]: lymphotoxin (LT; TNF-β) and gamma interferon (γ-IFN) are important. These cytokines and other circulating compounds such as thrombin and endotoxin (lipopolysaccharide) induce the synthesis and/or release, by the EC, of various substances involved in the immune response. Such substances include: PGI_2, granulocyte-monocyte colony stimulating factor, platelet-activating factor, endothelial cell derived growth factor, and a substance similar to platelet-derived growth factor. IL-1 can be produced by EC upon induction by endotoxin, thrombin, TNF-α, LT, and probably by IL-1 itself [14].

The role of the endothelium in immunity is closely linked with its antigenic makeup. EC, as other cells, contain the antigens of the ABO system. In addition they have major histocompatibility complex antigens I and II. The surface expression of the major histocompatibility complex can be induced by cytokines: α-, β-, and γ-IFN, TNF-α, and LT induce class I (HLA-A and B); γ-IFN induces class II (HLA-DR, DP, DQ). Resting EC cells express rarely class II (Ia) antigens, while EC stimulated by activated T lymphocytes or γ-IFN consistently express Ia [15]. It is apparent that EC are phagocytic under appropriate conditions. Furthermore, there is evidence that EC can act as antigen-presenting cells [15].

Angiogenesis and the Endothelium

The most dynamic functions of the endothelium are accomplished during the process of angiogenesis which is defined here as the formation of new microvessels in the fully developed vertebrate. A similar process also occurs, of course, in the embryo, leading to the formation of the cardiovascular system.

Angiogenesis occurs physiologically, e.g., in the proliferative endometrium and in wound repair. It also occurs as part of pathological processes, particularly in neoplasms and inflammatory disease. Since the former is beneficial and the latter often deleterious, the control of angiogenesis by external means is highly desirable. Thus, there is extensive research in this field [7, 8, 10, 22–24].

From in vivo models the major steps of the angiogenic process are generally known: in response to an angiogenic stimulus, EC in a 'mother' vessel separate from each other, leaving uncovered segments of the basement membrane which are rapidly digested. Through the gaps so formed EC migrate. Other EC divide. Migrating and proliferating cells form loops and then tubes. New basement membrane is secreted, and the lumen of these tubes communicates with that of the mother vessel. The process continues until the needed microvascular network is formed [23]. Then the neovessels are remodeled, or (if the stimulus ceases) the vessels stop growing, regress, and eventually may disappear.

The above process is modulated by agonists and antagonists of angiogenesis [7, 9, 10, 23]. Several normal tissues have angiogenic activity, best demonstrated in brain (especially hypothalamus), pituitary, retina, ovary, testis, salivary gland, synovium, and liver. Individual cells such as adipocytes, epidermal cells, macrophages, and T lymphocytes also show angiogenic activity. A number of angiogenic factors have been isolated from such mammalian normal tissues [9, 10, 25]. Best known are: epidermal growth factor from mouse submaxillary gland, acidic fibroblast growth factor from bovine hypothalamus, and basic fibroblast growth factor from bovine pituitary [10, 27].

Since neoplasms need their own microvascular network, it can be assumed that they have angiogenic activity. In fact, multiple tumor-derived factors have been isolated, and some have been purified [7, 8, 10, 11, 26, 27]. Some have been obtained from nonhuman tumors (rat chondrosarcoma, Walker 256 rat carcinoma, rat ascites tumor); others from cells of human tumors (melanoma, hepatoma, etc.). From human tumors a substance named transforming growth factor alpha has been isolated [27].

Angiogenic factors often stimulate both migration and proliferation of EC. It has been postulated that some substances – especially heparin – promote only EC migration. The morphologic characteristics of the microvessels depend considerably on the characteristics of the supporting stroma [28]. The formation of tubes, for instance, requires a matrix composed of the basement membrane collagens IV and V and laminin [28] (see 'Synthesis of Connective Tissue,' below).

As indicated above, there are also angiogenic inhibitors. These include corticosteroids (especially hydrocortisone), γ-IFN, and transforming growth factor beta (from human platelets). Protamine and the protein kinase C activators (PDBu) are also important antagonists [29]. TNF-α inhibits angiogenesis in vitro, but may actually stimulate it in vivo.

Special Metabolic Functions

Aside from the characteristic transport of molecules – e.g., within pinocytotic vesicles – across their cytoplasm (and all their basic cellular functions), certain metabolic activities, peculiar to endothelial cells, have been recognized.

EC produce and express on their surface angiotensin-converting enzyme (ACE) which converts angiotensin I to the active vasococonstrictor angiotensin II [15, 30]. In addition ACE inactivates bradykinin. Angiotensinases A and C, which inactivate angiotensin II, also are present in EC [15].

Human arterial EC bind 2.5 times more insulin than do venous EC [31]. In the retinal (but not in the aortic) endothelium, insulin increases glucose incorporation into glycogen and thymidine incorporation into DNA [15, 32]. EC have receptors for lipoproteins (high-density, beta low-density, acetyl low-density) and chylomicrons, and activated EC internalize low-density lipoproteins [15]. Lipoprotein lipase binds with high affinity to heparan sulfate and related molecules on the surface of EC.

Synthesis of Connective Tissue

The endothelium secretes the components of its own basement membrane, especially collagens IV and V and laminin [15, 28]. Also EC secrete other stromal constituents in vitro (and presumably in vivo), including collagens I and III, thrombospondin, fibronectin, elastin (from tropoelastin), and the mucopolysaccharides heparan, dermatan, and chondroitin sulfate [15, 28]. The types of stromal constituents secreted by cultured EC vary with the animal and the site from which such EC have been obtained [33], and this is further proof of EC heterogeneity. The stimulated EC contain and/or release collagenases capable of digesting collagens I, II, III, IV, and V [15]. These are important in the process of angiogenesis (remodeling phase) described above.

Heterogeneity of EC

To most careful observers of vessel morphology and function, EC are not a homogeneous population. There is now clear evidence of important differences in EC not just between species, but, more importantly, among EC from different sites of the same animal.

Examples of such differences are presented in table I. Some of the data are described in greater detail in the preceding or following sections of this review.

Effects of Radiation on the Endothelium

Unquestionably one of the most important targets of irradiation in mammalian tissues – at the therapeutic dose levels – is the microvasculature and within it the endothelium. This is not to say that EC are more important radiation targets than parenchymal cells (e.g. epithelia) or that EC are the only targets in the mesenchyma. We do feel that many of the delayed radiation effects in mammals are mediated through vascular injury, but we are aware of the opinions of respected investigators who do not agree with this point of view [34]. In fact, the delayed effects probably result from damage to multiple cell systems, the microvasculature being the one most consistently affected. Figure 2 shows diagrammatically some of the EC functions known to be affected by ionizing radiation.

There is not enough space here to list all of the numerous studies that have probed the radiation sensitivity of EC in vivo and in vitro. It should be sufficient to say that in the majority of the mammalian tissues observed [35–39] and in the majority of cultured systems assayed [40–46], a dose-dependent injury of endothelial cells has been demonstrated.

Some of the initial studies, using human umbilical vein EC, showed a 37% growth inhibition by 160 rad and complete inhibition by 750 rad [40]. Dose-dependent growth inhibition and decrease in attachment efficiency was sknown in bovine aortic EC exposed to single doses (SD) of 250–2,000 rad [41]. These effects were significantly greater than those in smooth myocytes also from bovine aortas, cultured under comparable conditions [41]. Intimal cells explanted from aortas of rabbits or monkeys showed a 50% reduction in outgrowth from a dose of 200 rad and a 99% reduction from 750 rad [47]. These cells were also more radiosensitive than medial cells (presumably smooth myocytes) and adventitial cells (presumably fibroblasts) from the same vessels [47].

When clonogenic assays for EC became available, these were, of course, used to determine more precisely the ability of radiation to inhibit EC replication. For instance, cultured rabbit aortic EC showed a D_0 of 120 rad and an extrapolation (n) number of 7 [43]. Porcine EC have shown a D_0 value of 157 rad for aortic cells (n 1.21) and 147 rad for brain capillary cells (n 1.74) [44]. Bovine aortic EC showed a D_0 of 101 rad (n

Table I. Evidence of endothelial cell heterogeneity

		Reference
Morphology		
Variations in size and shape		
Continuous cytoplasm: myocardial capillaries, etc.		83
Fenestrated cytoplasm: glomerular capillaries		
Special organelles		
Weibel-Palade bodies, common in primates and rats, rare in other mammals		84, 91
Antigen expression		
HLA-DR+ in most arterioles, capillaries, venules, and sinusoids, but not in umbilical vein		85
v Will F + in arterioles, capillaries, venules, but not in glomerular capillaries or spleen sinusoids		85
Addressins (for homing receptors) are organ specific		20
Insulin effects		
Insulin increases incorporation of glucose into glycogen and of thymidine into DNA in retinal, but not in aortic endothelium		32
Arterial EC bind 2.5 times more insulin than venous EC		31
Prostaglandin secretion		
Most EC from large vessels secrete mainly PGI_2		86
EC from human foreskin capillaries secrete PGE_2, $PGF_{2\alpha}$		
Collagen secretion		
Type of collagen (I, II, III, IV, V) secreted by EC and site of release in vitro (medium or matrix) vary with the tissue of origin of EC, the size of the vessel, and the animal species		15, 33
Some valvular EC are deficient in fibronectin synthesis		87
Cell kinetics		
% of EC in S phase		
Rabbit capillaries	0.6	79
Rabbit mid-size arteries and veins	0.1–1.1	
Rabbit aorta	0.003–0.08	
Cycle time		
Retina of adult mouse	≥3 years	81
Various adult-mouse organs	≥ 2 months	80
Various murine neoplasms	2.4–13 days	82
Radiation response in vitro		
Bovine aortic clones	D_0 101 rad n 1.9	46
Rabbit aortic clones	D_0 120 rad n 7	43
Porcine aortic clones	D_0 157 rad n 1.21	44
Radiation response in vivo		
Lung and myocardial capillaries: early evidence of damage (hours to days)		52, 90
Renal glomerular capillaries: late evidence of damage (weeks to months)		54
Endocardium of mice: mural thrombosis (≥2,000 rad SD)		88
Endocardium of man and rabbit: no damage (up to 8,000 rad SD)		89, 90

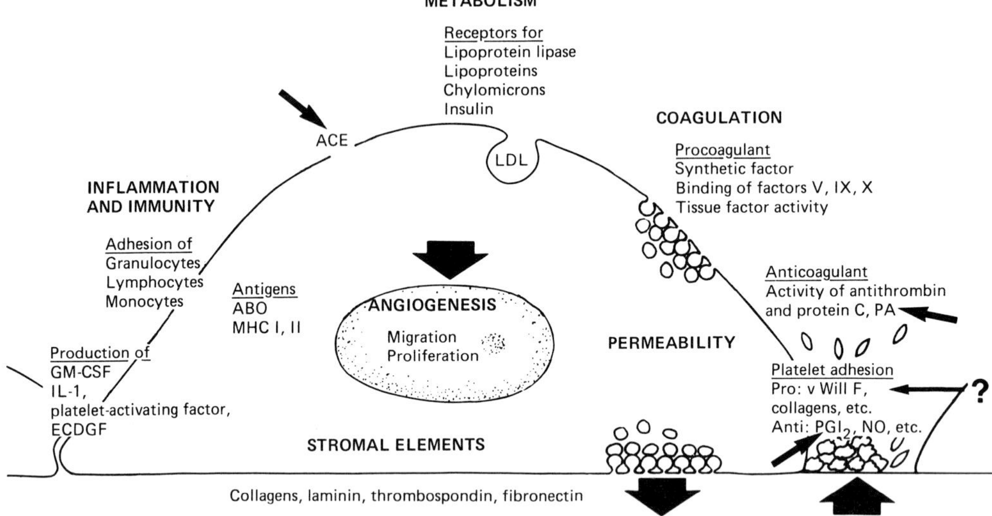

Fig. 2. Diagram of an endothelial cell similar to that shown in figure 1. The best-documented sublethal radiation effects (as described in the text) are indicated by arrows: inhibition of proliferation and angiogenesis, early increase in permeability, platelet aggregation (from denudation of basal lamina following EC loss), decrease in prostacyclin (early), PA, and ACE. There is increased release of v Will F, although this has not been proven in vivo. Cell death occurs, of course, following high doses of irradiation (see text). For explanation of abbreviations see figure 1 legend.

1.9) [46]. The effect in these cells was not only dose dependent, but also dose rate dependent [46].

The morphologic alterations of EC resulting from lethal or from sublethal doses have been described in detail either in cultures [41] or in samples of irradiated mammalian tissues [36, 42, 48–50].

In general, sequential sample studies have shown progressive degenerative changes of EC, best seen by some electron microscopy observations of capillaries [36, 51, 52]. Formation of 'blebs' or of cytoplasmic pseudopods is, in some cells, followed by severe swelling of the cytoplasm, with narrowing or occlusion of capillaries. Other cells show increased cytoplasmic density with concomitant decrease in size, then pyknosis, and, finally, detachment from the basement membrane and sloughing. Platelet aggregation occurs then, and the resulting platelet-fibrin thrombus also obstructs the capillary. Some capillaries are then permanently lost and replaced by a fibrous scar, e.g., in the myocardium

[36]. Others are obliterated temporarily and eventually are recanalized, e.g., in the lung [52], although their function may be impaired.

Morphologically the time of expression of this injury and its chronological progression vary from organ to organ: in the lung it appears as early as 1 day after a SD of 2,000 rad to the rat hemithorax [52] and may be seen even within a few hours in mice [53]. Complete loss of endothelial lining occurs 3–6 months later, and, following a period of prominent mast cell infiltration and collagen deposition, new capillaries are formed in many, but not all, of the affected alveolar septa [52]. In mice receiving total-body irradiation of 650 or 1,000 rad SD, a compensatory increase in pulmonary endothelial DNA synthesis occurs between 2 and 8 weeks after exposure [51].

In the myocardium of rabbits exposed to local SD of 2,000 rad, some endothelial abnormalities are detected almost immediately (3 min), but become generalized only at 20 days and reach maximum severity by 40 days [36]. Unlike in the lung, the capillaries that are destroyed by 70 days do not become recanalized: a compensatory EC proliferation (detectable by increased endothelial cell DNA synthesis) between 20 and 70 days does not result in sufficient repair of the capillary network, and ischemia with diffuse fibrosis occurs beyond 100 days [36].

In the renal parenchyma, on the other hand, the endothelial lesions appear to occur later. Mouse kidneys irradiated in situ with total doses of fractioned irradiation of 3,000–5,000 rad showed lesions of the glomerular endothelium by 1 month [54]. This progresses to EC detachment and eventually to thrombosis of glomerular capillaries at 9–12 months [54]. These differences indicate that endothelia from different capillaries vary in their response to irradiation.

Several investigators [55–59] have shown an increase in vascular permeability following irradiation. They have used tracers such as radioiodinated serum albumin [55] or vital dyes such as pontamine sky blue [57] or ultrastructural observations, etc. [53]. In the lung of rats this increase in permeability appears to be biphasic: an initial moderate increase at 1 day after 1,100 or 1,800 rad SD to the thorax and a second larger increase peaking at 19 days [55]. The initial increase in vascular permeability may be diminished or even abolished (at least in rabbit skin) by intravenous administration of ε-amino-n-caproic acid [60].

While this increase in permeability seems to be well documented [55, 61], its significance is unclear. Is it just a transient local phenomenon without long-term significance, or does it lead to serious lesions (e.g. pulmonary hyaline membranes or fibrin accumulation in the stroma, with subsequent fibrosis)? Could the acute increase in vascular permeability explain the shock that occurs shortly after total-body high-dose accidental exposures [62]?

Relatively little is known about the effect of sublethal doses of radiation on the *functional integrity* of the endothelium. How does radiation affect the various roles of EC described in the previous pages (coagulation, inflammation-immunity, synthesis of stromal components, angiogenesis, specific metabolic activities, etc.)? Only some of these functions have been assessed in the irradiated EC, mostly in cultures.

The ACE activity decreased progressively as a function of time (over 72 h) in confluent bovine aortic EC following a single exposure of gamma radiation of 500 rad [63]. In the same experiments EC showed a marked increase in superoxide dismutase and lactic dehydrogenase with a shift from LDH_1 to LDH_4 and LDH_5. As expected, there was a consistent increased release of LDH into the culture medium [63]. A similar, but prolonged (up to 6 months) decrease in ACE has been demonstrated in the lungs of rats exposed to SD of 2,500 rad [64, 65]. *D*-Penicillamine initially ameliorates this deficiency [65].

As judged by the fibrinolytic activity of canine liver slices, fractionated doses of 4,600 rad/5 weeks produced an inhibition of the plasmin in EC, detectable as long as 18–30 months after exposure [66]. It is not clear from this experiment (or two others cited by the authors) whether this effect resulted from decreased PA synthesis (and/or release) or from increase in the inhibitor(s) of PA or from both mechanisms. This loss of activity was not caused by loss of EC: the histologic preparations showed no significant vascular lesions [66].

Reduced fibrinolytic activity was also observed in the lung of rats 1–6 months after SD of 2,500 rad [65, 67]. In these experiments PA inhibitors were measured, and it was felt that the decrease in fibrinolysis was mainly due to decreased PA activity rather than to increased inhibition of PA [67]. As in the case of ACE, *D*-penicillamine ameliorates initially the PA reduction and probably delays the fibrosis that occurs during the late phase of pulmonary radiation injury [65]. These studies on PA confirm observations made in irradiated canine lungs in 1962 [68] and offer a possible explanation for the hyaline membranes (made chiefly of fibrin) characteristic of radiation pneumonitis in humans [69].

Radiation produces a decrease in PGI_2 formation by EC in vitro [70] and in vivo [71]. There is a rapid drop of PGI_2 levels after irradiation of isolated segments of human umbilical arteries with SD of 200 rad [70]. Platelet thromboxane formation, however, is not affected by doses in the range of 200–2,000 rad [70]. In some vessels this depression of PGI_2 is long lasting: it is still significant up to 6 months after segmental exposure of rabbits' aortas to single doses of 1,000–5,000 rad [71]. In other vessels the long-term effect may be the opposite. An experiment has shown an acute (1 day) decrease in rat pulmonary PGI_2 (after 2,500 rad SD to the hemithorax) followed by a steady *increase*, reaching 2–3 times control values by 6 months [72]. Unlike in the intact EC, the decreased production of PGI_2 in some irradiated EC is not corrected by stimulation with platelet-derived growth factor [71].

An early consequence of therapeutic doses of gamma radiation is the inability of the EC plasma membrane to transport in vitro a sodium-dependent, nonmetabolizable amino acid, α-aminoisobutyric acid [73].

We were unable to demonstrate any qualitative modification in the density or in the pattern of distribution of v Will F in cultured bovine EC following SD radiation of 500–4,000 rad [Fajardo and Kelly, unpubl. observations]. The v Will F was stained using the peroxidase-antiperoxidase technique with an antibody specific for bovine v Will F [Fajardo and Kelly, unpubl. observations]. Release of v Will F into the medium was not measured in our experiments, but it was measured by other investigators using human umbilical vein EC exposed to SD of 1,000–4,000 rad [74]. They observed a significant increase in the amount of v Will F released, at 2,000 rad and above, which was not due to cell lysis [74]. Expecting to find variations in the plasma levels of v Will F after pulmonary irradiation, similar to those described in other forms of acquired, diffuse alveolar injury [75], we studied recently 14 patients undergoing thoracic irradiation (without chemotherapy): the plasma levels of v Will F showed no correlation with radiation dose (1,500–6,600 rad), irradiated lung volume, tumor burden, time interval after radiation, or, most importantly, with the presence or absence of clinical radiation pneumonitis [76]. The alkaline phosphatase activity, which is a non-specific marker of EC, has been studied in the myocardium of rats locally irradiated with SD of 1,000–2,500 rad [77]. Although rats do not develop the typical radiation-induced heart disease (pericardial fibrosis, pericardial effusion, and diffuse myocardial fibrosis) seen in humans and rabbits, heart failure does occur after large doses. In the above experiment there was a focal loss of alkaline phosphatase activity in myocardial capillaries starting 4 weeks after exposure and reaching a maximum by 200 days. This coincided with a decrease in capillary density. Recovery of both defects occurred at doses of 1,600 rad or below, but higher doses resulted in persistent loss of the enzyme and of the vessels [77], as would be expected from previous studies [36].

The damage to EC described above results, of course, in important physiologic alterations. One of these is the already mentioned increased vascular permeability. Other physiologic effects, demonstrated in the lungs of dogs, include a progressive (as long as 200 days) decrease in ventilation and compliance, after fractionated irradiation of one lung, and an initial (up to 40 days) increase in diffusion capacity, followed by a progressive decrease of the same [78].

The most important effect for most organs is probably obstruction or destruction (or both) of the microvasculature. This causes progressive ischemia and leads – depending on time and type of tissue – to necrosis, fibrosis, or replacement by adipocytes. Necrosis is seen in the central nervous system. Fibrosis is characteristic of tissues like skin, myocardium, and pulmonary parenchyma. Replacement by adipose tissue is typical of the hemopoietic marrow.

Again, endothelial (and thus, microvascular) injury appears to be the most consistent delayed effect and the most important mesenchymal lesion produced by radiation in mammalian tissues.

Acknowledgements

This work was supported in part by Veterans Administration Research Funds (MRIS 2735-01). Eric A. Jaffe, MD, Cornell University Medical College, reviewed the first portion of the manuscript and made useful suggestions. Donna L. Buckley assisted in the preparation of this review.

References

1 Palade, G. E.: Transport in quanta across the endothelium of blood capillaries. Anat. Rec. 1960;136:254–264.

2 Karnovsky, M. J.: The ultrastructural basis of capillary permeability studied with horseradish peroxidase. J. Cell Biol. 1967;35:213–236.

3 Booyse, F. M.; Bell, S.; Sedlak, B., et al.: Development of an in vitro vessel wall model for studying certain aspects of platelet-vessel (endothelial) interactions. Artery. 1975;1:518–539.

4 Moncada, S.; Gryglewski, R.; Bunting, S., et al.: An enzyme isolated from arteries transforms prostaglandin endoperoxides to an unstable substance that inhibits platelet aggregation. Nature. 1976;263:663–665.

5 Jaffe, E. A.; Nachman, R. L.; Becker, C. G.: Culture of human endothelial cells derived from umbilical veins: Identification by morphologic criteria. J. Clin. Invest. 1973;52:2745–2758.

6 Gospodarowicz, J.; Moran, J.; Braun, D., et al.: Clonal growth of bovine vascular endothelial cells: Fibroblast growth factor as a survival agent. Proc. Natl. Acad. Sci. USA. 1976;73:4120–4124.

7 Folkman, J.: Angiogenesis: Initiation and control. J. Cell Biol. 1982;104:212–227.

8 Gimbrone, M. H.; Cotran, R. S.; Folkman, J.: Tumor growth and neovascularization: An experimental model using the rabbit cornea. JNCI. 1974;52:413–419.

9 Folkman, J.; Klagsbrun, M.: A family of angiogenic peptides. Nature. 1987;329:671–672.
10 Auerbach, R.: Angiogenesis-inducing factors: A review; in Pick, E. (ed.): Lymphokines. New York, Academic Press, 1981, vol. IV, pp. 69–88.
11 Greenblatt, M.; Shubi, K. P.: Tumor angiogenesis: Transfilter diffusion studies in the hamster by the transparent chamber technique. JNCI. 1968;41:111–124.
12 Bevilaqua, M. P.; Pober, J. S.; Majeau, G. R., et al.: Interleukin (IL_1) induces biosynthesis and cell surface expression of procoagulant activity in human vascular endothelial cells. J. Exp. Med. 1984;160:618–623.
13 Naworth, P. P.; Stern, D. M.: Modulation of endothelial cell hemostatic properties by tumor necrosis factor. J. Exp. Med. 1986;163:740–745.
14 Cotran, R. S.: New roles for the endothelim in inflammation and immunity. Am. J. Pathol. 1987;129:407–413.
15 Jaffe, E. A.: Cell biology of endothelial cells. Hum. Pathol. 1987;18:234–239.
16 Cerveny, T. J.; Fass, D. N.; Mann, K. G.: Synthesis of coagulation factor V by cultured aortic endothelium. Blood 1984;63:1467–1474.
17 Emeis, J. J.; Koositra, T.: Interleukin 1 and lipopolysaccharide induce an inhibitor of tissue-type plasminogen activator in-vivo and in cultured endothelial cells. J. Exp. Med. 1986;163:1260–1265.
18 Palmer, R. M. J.; Ferrige, A. G.; Moncada, S.: Release of nitric oxide accounts for the biological activity of endothelium-derived relaxing factor. Nature 1987;327:524–526.
19 Jalkanen, S.; Steere, A. C.; Fox, R. I., et al.: A distinct endothelial recognition system controlling lymphocyte traffic into inflamed endothelium. Science 1986;233:556–558.
20 Streeter, P. R.; Berg, E. L.; Rouse, B. T. N., et al.: A tissue-specific endothelial cell molecule involved in lymphocyte homing. Nature 1988;331:41–46.
21 Pober, J. S.; Gimbrone, M. A.; Lapierre, L. A., et al.: Overlapping patterns of activation of human endothelial cells by interleukin 1, tumor necrosis factor, and immune interferon. J. Immunol. 1986;137:1893–1896.
22 Fajardo, L. F.; Kowalski, J.; Kwan, H. H., et al.: The disc angiogenesis system. Lab. Invest. 1988;58:718–724.
23 Furcht, L. T.: Critical factors controlling angiogenesis: Cell products, cell matrix and growth factors. Editorial Lab. Invest. 1986;55:505–509.
24 Sprugel, K. H.; McPherson, J. M.; Clowes, A. W., et al.: Effects of growth factors in vivo. I. Cell ingrowth into porous subcutaneous chambers. Am. J. Pathol. 1987;129:601–613.
25 Weiner, H. L.; Weiner, L. H.; Swain, J. L.: Tissue distribution and developmental expression of the messenger RNA encoding angiogenin. Science 1987;237:280–282.
26 Schor, A. M.; Schor, S. L.: Tumor angiogenesis. J. Pathol. 1983;141:385–413.
27 Schreiber, A. B.; Winkler, M. E.; Derinck, R.: Transforming growth factor alpha: A more potent angiogenic mediator than epidermal growth factor. Science 1986; 232:1250–1253.
28 Madri, J. A.; Williams, S. K.; Wyatt, T., et al.: Capillary endothelial cell cultures: Phenotypic modulation by matrix components. J. Cell Biol. 1983;97:153–165.
29 Doctrow, S. R.; Folkman, J.: Protein kinase C activators suppress stimulation of capillary endothelial cell growth by angiogenic endothelial mitogens. J. Cell Biol. 1987;104:679–687.
30 Laliberte, F., Laliberte, M. F.; Althen-Gelas, F., et al.: Cellular and subcellular localization of angiotensin-converting enzyme in rat adrenal gland. Lab. Invest. 1987;56:364–371.
31 Bar, R. S.; Peacock, M. L.; Spanheimer, R. C., et al.: Differential binding of insulin to

human arterial and venous endothelial cells in primary culture. Diabetes 1980;29:991–995.

32 King, G. L.; Buzney, S. M.; Kahn, C. R., et al.: Differential responsiveness to insulin of endothelial and support cells from micro and macrovessels. J. Clin. Invest. 1983;71:974–979.

33 Sage, H.: Collagen synthesis by endothelial cells in culture; in Jaffe, E. A. (ed.): Biology of Endothelial Cells. Boston, Martinus-Nijhoff, 1984, pp. 161–177.

34 Withers, H. R.; Peters, L. J.; Kogelnik, H. D.: The pathobiology of late effects of irradiation; in Meyn, E.; Withers, H. R. (eds.): Radiation Biology in Cancer Research. New York, Raven Press, 1980, pp. 439–448.

35 van den Brenk, H. A. S., Sharpington, C.; Orton, C., et al.: Effects of X-radiation on growth and function of the repair blastema. II. Measurement of angiogenesis in the Selye pouch in the rat. Int. J. Radiat. Biol. 1974;25:277–289.

36 Fajardo, L. F.; Stewart, J. R.: Pathogenesis of radiation-induced myocardial fibrosis. Lab. Invest. 1973;29:244–257.

37 Gillette, E. L.; Maurer, G. D.; Severin, G. A.: Endothelial repair of radiation damage following beta irradiation. Radiology 1975;116:175–177.

38 Hopewell, J. W.; Campling, D.; Calvo, W., et al.: Vascular irradiation damage: Its cellular basis and likely consequences. Br. J. Cancer 1986;53(suppl. VII):181–191.

39 Reinhold, H. S.: The influence of radiation on blood vessels and circulation. IV. Structural changes in blood vessels. Curr. Top. Radiat. Res. Q. 1974;10:58–74.

40 DeGowin, R. L.; Lewis, L. J.; Mason, R. E., et al.: Radiation-induced inhibition of human endothelial cells replicating in culture. Radiat. Res. 1976;68:244–250.

41 Johnson, L.; Longenecker, J. P.; Fajardo, L. F.: Differential radiation response of cultured endothelial cells and smooth myocytes. Anal. Quant. Cytol. 1982;4:188–198.

42 Kwock, L.; Davenport, W. C.; Clark, R. L., et al.: The effects of ionizing radiation on the pulmonary vasculature of intact rats and isolated pulmonary endothelium. Radiat Res. 1987;111:276–291.

43 Martin, D. F.; Fischer, J. J.: Radiation sensitivity of cultured rabbit aortic endothelial cells. Int. J. Radiat. Oncol. Biol. Phys. 1984;10:1903–1906.

44 Penhaligon, M.; Laverick, M.: Radiation response of endothelial cells in vitro. Br. J. Radiol. 1985;58:913–914.

45 Reinhold, H. S.; Buisman, G. H.: Radiosensitivity of capillary endothelium. Br. J. Radiol. 1973;46:54–57.

46 Rhee, J. G.; Lee, I.; Song, C. W.: The clonogenic response of bovine aortic endothelial cells in culture to radiation. Radiat. Res. 1986;106:182–189.

47 Fischer-Dzoga, K.; Dimitrievich, G. S.; Griem, M. L.: Radiosensitivity of vascular tissue. II. Differential radiosensitivity of aortic cells in vitro. Radiat. Res. 1984;99:536–546.

48 Moosavi, H.; McDonald, S.; Rubin, P., et al.: Early radiation dose-response in lung: An ultrastructural study. Int. J. Radiat. Oncol. Biol. Phys. 1977;2:921–931.

49 Narayan, K.; Cliff, W. J.: Morphology of irradiated microvasculature: A combined in vivo and electron microscopic study. Am. J. Pathol. 1982;106:47–62.

50 Stearner, S. P.; Sanderson, M. H.: Mechanisms of acute injury in the gamma-irradiated chicken: Effects of a protracted or a split-dose exposure on the fine structure of the microvasculature. Radiat. Res. 1972;49:328–350.

51 Adamson, I. Y. R.; Bowden, D. H.: Endothelial injury and repair in radiation-induced pulmonary fibrosis. Am. J. Pathol. 1983;112:224–230.

52 Phillips, T. L.: An ultrastructural study of the development of radiation injury in the lung. Radiology 1966;87:49–54.

53 Maisin, J. R.: The influence of radiation on blood vessels and circulation. III. Ultrastructure of the vessel wall. Curr. Top. Radiat. Res. 1974;10:29–57.
54 Fajardo, L. F.; Brown, J. M.; Glatstein, E.: Glomerular and juxtaglomerular lesions in radiation nephropathy. Radiat. Res. 1976;68:177–183.
55 Evans, M. L.; Graham, M. M.; Mahler, P. A., et al.: Changes in vascular permeability following thorax irradiation in the rat. Radiat. Res. 1986;107:262–271.
56 Gross, N. J.: Experimental radiation pneumonitis. IV. Leakage of circulatory proteins onto the alveolar surface. J. Lab. Clin. Med. 1980;95:19–31.
57 Jolles, B.; Harrison, R. G.: Enzymatic processes and vascular changes in the skin radiation reaction. Br. J. Radiol. 1966;39:12–18.
58 Law, M. P.; Thomlinson, R. H.: Vascular permeability in the ears of rats after X-irradiation. Br. J. Radiol. 1978;51:895–904.
59 Mount, D.; Bruce, W. R.: Local plasma volume and vascular permeability of rabbit skin after irradiation. Radiat. Res. 1964;23:430–445.
60 Eassa, E.-H. M.; Casarett, G. W.: Effect of epsilon-amino-n-caproic-acid (EACA) on radiation-induced increase in capillary permeability. Radiology 1973;106:679–688.
61 Reinhold, H. S.; Keyeux, A.; Dunjic, A., et al.: The influence of radiation on blood vessels and circulation. Chapter XII, Discussion and Conclusions. Curr. Top. Radiat. Res. Q. 1974;10:185–198.
62 Fanger, H.; Lushbaugh, C. C.: Radiation death from cardiovascular shock following a criticality accident. Arch. Pathol. 1967;83:446–460.
63 Rubin, D. B.; Drab, E. A.; Ward, W. F., et al.: Enzymatic responses to radiation in cultured vascular endothelial and smooth muscle cells. Radiat. Res. 1984;99:420–432.
64 Ward, W. F.; Solliday, N. H.; Molteni, A., et al.: Radiation injury in rat lung. II. Angiotensin converting enzyme activity. Radiat. Res. 1983;96:294–300.
65 Ward, W.; Molteni, A.; Ts'ao, C.-H., et al.: Radiation injury in rat lung. IV. Modification by *D*-penicillamine. Radiat. Res. 1984;98:397–406.
66 Henderson, B. W.; Bicher, H. I.; Johnson, R. J.: Loss of vascular fibrinolytic activity following irradiation of the liver. An aspect of late radiation damage. Radiat. Res. 1983;95:646–652.
67 Ts'ao, C.-H.; Ward, W. F.; Port, C. D.: Radiation injury in rat lung. III. Plasminogen activator and fibrinolytic inhibitor activities. Radiat. Res. 1983;96:301–308.
68 Fleming, W. H.; Szakacs, J. E.; King, E. R.: The effect of gamma irradiation on the fibrinolytic system of dog lung and its modification by certain drugs: Relationship to radiation pneumonitis and hyaline membrane formation in lung. J. Nucl. Med. 1962;3:341–351.
69 Fajardo, L. F.: Pathology of Radiation Injury. New York, Masson, 1982.
70 Allen, J. B.; Sagerman, R. H.; Stuart, M. J.: Irradiation decreases vascular prostacyclin formation with no concomitant effect on platelet thromboxane production. Lancet. 1981;ii:1193–1196.
71 Sinzinger, H.; Firbas, W.: Irradiation depresses prostacyclin generation upon stimulation with the platelet-derived growth factor. Br. J. Radiol. 1985;58:1023–1026.
72 Ts'ao, C.-H.; Ward, W. F.; Port, C. D.: Radiation injury in rat lung. I. Prostacyclin (PGI_2) production, arterial perfusion and ultrastructure. Radiat. Res. 1983;96:284–293.
73 Kwock, L.; Douglas, W. H. J.; Lin, P.-S., et al.: Endothelial cell damage after gamma-irradiation in vitro: Impaired uptake of alpha-amino isobutyric acid. Am. Rev. Respir. Dis. 1982;125:95–99.
74 Sporn, L. A.; Rubin, P.; Marder, V. J., et al.: Irradiation induces release of von Willebrand protein from endothelial cells in culture. Blood 1984;64:567–570.

75 Carvalho, A. C. A.; Bellman, S. M.; Saullo, V. J., et al.: Altered factor VIII in acute respiratory failure. N. Engl. J. Med. 1982;307:1113–1119.
76 Fajardo, L. F.; Donaldson, S. S.; Kelly, N. I.: von Willebrand Factor levels do not predict or diagnose radiation pneumonitis. Int. J. Radiat. Oncol. Biol. Phys. 1986; 12:107–110.
77 Lauk, S.: Endothelial alkaline phosphatase activity loss as an early stage in the development of radiation-induced heart disease in rats. Radiat. Res. 1987;110:118–128.
78 Teates, C. D.: Effects of unilateral thoracic irradiation on lung function. J. Appl. Physiol. 1965;20:628–636.
79 Spaet, T. H.; Lejnieks, I.: Mitotic activity of rabbit blood vessels. Proc. Soc. Exp. Biol. Med. 1967;125:1197–1201.
80 Tannock, I. F.; Hayashi, S.: The proliferation of capillary endothelial cells. Cancer Res. 1972;32:77–82.
81 Engerman, R. L.; Pfaffenbach, D.; Davis, M. D.: Cell turnover of capillaries. Lab. Invest. 1967;17:738–743.
82 Hobson, B.; Denekamp, J.: Endothelial proliferation in tumours and normal tissues: Continuous labelling studies. Br. J. Cancer 1984;49:405–413.
83 Bruns, R. R.; Palade, G. E.: Studies on blood capillaries. I. General organization of blood capillaries in muscle. J. Cell. Biol. 1968;37:244–276.
84 Weibel, E. R.; Palade, G. E.: New cytoplasmic components in arterial endothelia. J. Cell. Biol. 1964;2:101–112.
85 Turner, R. R.; Beckstead, J. H.; Warnke, R. A., et al.: Endothelial cell phenotypic diversity. Am. J. Clin. Pathol. 1987;87:569–575.
86 Charo, I. F.; Shak, S.; Karasek, M. A., et al.: Prostaglandin I_2 is not a major metabolite of arachidonic acid in cultured endothelial cells from human foreskin microvessels. J. Clin. Invest. 1984;74:914–919.
87 Johnson, C. M.; Fass, D. N.: Porcine cardiac valvular endothelial cells in culture. A relative deficiency of fibronectin synthesis *in vitro*. Lab. Invest. 1983;49:589–598.
88 Fajardo, L. F.; Brown, J. M.: Cardiac mural thrombi caused by radiation. Radiat. Res. 1973;55:387–389.
89 Stewart, J. R.; Fajardo, L. F.: Radiation induced heart disease. An update. Prog. Cardiovasc. Dis. 1984;27:173–194.
90 Fajardo, L. F.; Stewart, J. R.: Experimental radiation-induced heart disease. I. Light microscopic studies. Am. J. Pathol. 1970;59:299–315.
91 Trillo, A. A.; Pritchard, R. W.: Early endothelial changes in experimental primate atherosclerosis. Lab. Invest. 1979;41:294–302.

Luis F. Fajardo, MD, Professor of Pathology, Stanford University School of Medicine, and Chief of Laboratory Service, Veterans Administration Medical Center, 3801 Miranda Avenue, Palo Alto, CA 94304 (USA)

Vaeth JM, Meyer JL (eds): Radiation Tolerance of Normal Tissues.
Front Radiat Ther Oncol. Basel, Karger, 1989, vol 23, pp 113–130

Time-Dose Considerations for Normal-Tissue Tolerance

Howard D. Thames[a], *Lester J. Peters*[b], *Kian K. Ang*[b]

Divisions of [a]Biomathematics and [b]Radiotherapy, The University of Texas M.D. Anderson Cancer Center, Houston, Tex., USA

Introduction

Since the earliest days of radiotherapy, there has been lack of agreement as to optimum dose fractionation schedules for the treatment of various disease entities [24]. Regimens regarded as 'conventional' differ widely in different parts of the world. For example, in the Manchester School, radical (i.e., definitive) treatments are dispensed in 15 fractions over 3 weeks in increments of 3.3–3.6 Gy, while in the USA, most definitive treatments are administered in 35–40 fractions over 7–8 weeks in increments of 1.8–2.0 Gy. Many other variations exist in what is considered conventional therapy. To a large extent, the evolution of 'conventional' dose fractionation schedules reflects logistic and financial considerations, and the availability of equipment and staff, as much as any serious effort to determine by clinical trial which fractionation schedule maximizes the therapeutic radiation dose [21]. Notwithstanding this unfortunate fact, the range of dose fractionation schedules that has been used clinically over the years allows certain conclusions to be drawn concerning the effects of different fractionation parameters on the response of normal tissues to ionizing radiations. These clinical data, supported by a large body of experimental animal data, have established conclusively that changes in fractionation parameters differentially affect the response of tissues according to their organization and turnover rate, i.e., whether they manifest acute (early) or late reactions to radiations [26].

For any dose fractionation schedule, the maximum biologically effective dose that can be delivered is limited by normal-tissue tolerance of acute reactions or, more commonly within the USA, late reactions. Careful clinical observation has enabled radiotherapists familiar with a given fractionation regimen to establish the expected relationship between the severity of acute and late reactions. When a major change in fractionation is undertaken, this expected relationship is no longer valid, and it is therefore imperative that radiotherapists are aware of the changes in the proportionality between acute and late reactions that accompany changes in dose fractionation (fig. 1).

Time-Dose Parameters

The time-dose parameters that influence the tolerance of normal tissues are total dose, overall duration of treatment, size of dose per fraction, and spacing of dose fractions, the latter two determining the rate of dose accumulation, sometimes referred to as the weekly dose rate. The intensity of acute reactions in epithelia and other tissues organized into stem cell, maturation, and functional compartments (such as the bone marrow) reflects the balance between the rate of cell killing by irradiation and the rate of regeneration of surviving stem cells, and this will depend on the rate of dose accumulation. The fraction size is also a factor in determining the severity of acute reactions (large fractions being more damaging, cGy for cGy, than small ones), but to a lesser extent than is the case for late reactions. Healing of an acute reaction requires the survival of a certain minimum number of stem cells which may not occur if the rate of dose accumulation and/or total dose are too great. Under these circumstances, consequential late injury may result from what was primarily an acute radiation reaction.

Late reactions following radiation therapy occur in tissues characterized by little or no cellular turnover, such as mature connective tissues and the parenchymal cells of various organs. Since cellular depletion in such tissues is not manifested until after a typical course of radiation therapy is completed, there is no opportunity for regeneration to occur during treatment, and the rate of dose accumulation and overall duration of treatment are, therefore, of minor significance in determining the severity of late reactions. Conversely such reactions depend markedly on total dose and size of dose per fraction and, when dose fractions are closely spaced, on the interfraction interval. Intracellular repair in late-reacting tissues appears to proceed more slowly than in acutely reacting tissues [28], so that a greater interfraction interval (at least 6 h) is necessary to assure complete independence of effect of dose fractions.

Isoeffect Formulae

In an attempt to guide clinicians in the choice of fractionation parameters (other than those with which they are familiar) which will produce equivalent normal-tissue reactions, several formulae have been proposed, most notably the NSD (and its derivatives TDF and CRE), the modified CRE, and the alpha/beta formula [24, 29]. *None* of these for-

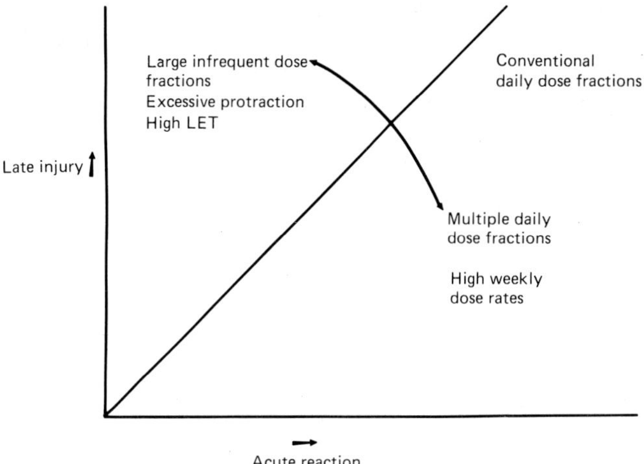

Fig. 1. Relative changes in acute and late reactions after altered dose fractionation and LET. The line denotes the balance between acute and late tolerance in conventional daily fractionation with low-LET irradiations: there are corresponding increases in acute and late reactions with increasing total dose if the overall time and dose per fraction are unchanged. Disproportionate increases in late effects can occur when the dose per fraction is increased, or the total dose *and* overall time are increased (protraction), or with high LET (upper curved arrow). By contrast, disproportionate increases in acute reactions can occur when the fraction size is reduced and the weekly rate of dose accumulation is increased (lower curved arrow).

mulae is sufficiently reliable to pre-empt clinical judgment. The NSD (and its derivatives), while breaking new ground by separating the effects of fraction number and overall time, has several major deficiencies [34] and has been shown clinically to result in significant overestimation of late normal-tissue tolerance with regimens using large doses per fraction [5]. The modified CRE and alpha/beta models are improvements in that they account for the different fractionation responses of different tissues and predict the differential effects of changes in dose fractionation for acute and late reactions. However, the accuracy of the coefficients in these models is inadequate to allow them to serve as more than guidelines for significant changes in clinical practice. Moreover, all the above isoeffect models assume complete repair between fractions which may not be applicable to multiple-fractions-per-day (MFD) regimens. A modification of the alpha/beta model to account for this factor has recently been proposed [24]. In the final analysis, each new fractionation schedule has to be tested clinically to establish its safety.

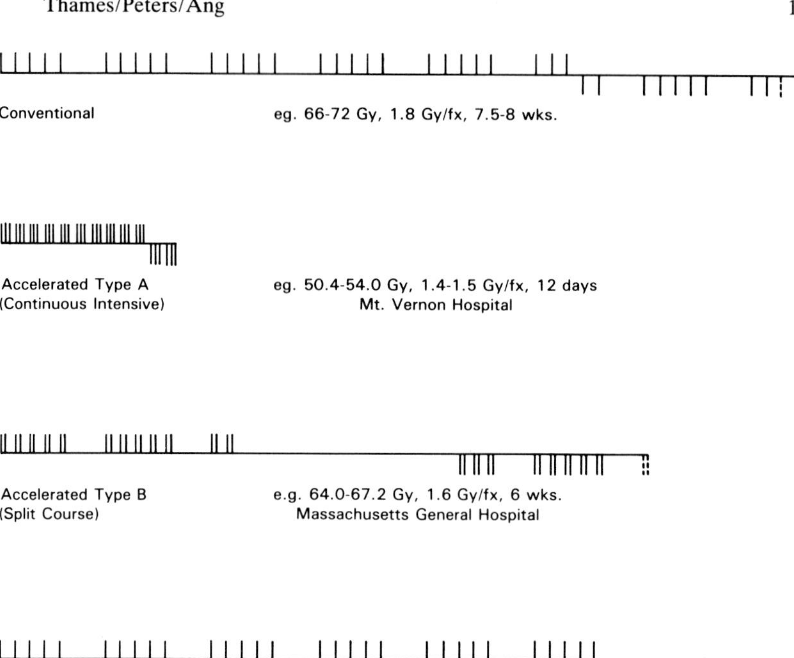

Fig. 2. Comparison of conventional and three prototypical accelerated fractionation schedules. For each schedule the bars above the line represent the large-field treatment, and the bars below the line represent the boost-field treatment. The dotted bars represent treatments omitted when total doses are lower. [From ref. 17, with permission.]

Time-Dose Considerations for MFD Regimens

In recent years, a variety of fractionation schedules using two or more dose fractions per day has been proposed and tested in an effort to improve the therapeutic ratio. Generically, these regimens may be categorized as hyperfractionation or accelerated fractionation according to whether their primary rationale is a reduction in size of dose per fraction or a reduction in overall treatment time [18, 25]. Some of the regimens tested clinically were based on radiobiological predictions, while others were empirically derived.

In this paper we review normal-tissue reactions encountered with MFD regimens to illustrate the fractionation parameters determining acute and late reactions and to highlight the caution required in implementing radically new fractionation regimens.

Table I. Predominantly accelerated fractionation regimens

Site	References
Head and neck	Ang and Peters [unpubl observations], 1, 3, 8, 9, 16, 20, 23, 31
Prostate	30
Lung	19, 20, 23
Breast	2, 23
Brain	8
Melanoma (brain metastases)	4

Table II. Predominantly hyperfractionated regimens

Site	References
Head and neck	8, 10–13, 15, Wendt and Peters [unpubl. observations]
Bladder	5, 7
Lung	5, 22
Brain	6, 14, 33

Materials and Methods

Under the category of accelerated fractionation we include regimens designed primarily to reduce the duration of conventional treatment with daily fractions of 1.8–2 Gy, 5 days/week by the delivery of two or more treatments usually in the range of 1.5–2.0 Gy on some or all of the treatment days. Examples of three prototypical schedules of accelerated fractionation currently in use in the treatment of advanced squamous cell carcinomas of the head and neck region are illustrated in figure 2. Schedules of type A consist of an intensive course of treatment in which the overall duration of treatment is markedly reduced with a corresponding substantial decrease in the total dose. Schedules of types B and C represent techniques where the duration of treatment is more modestly reduced, but the total dose is kept in the same range as for a conventional treatment. This is accomplished by using either an MFD split course or concomitant boost technique, i.e., giving the boost as a second daily dose during the basic treatment course. These techniques are conveniently distinguished on the basis of the strategy adopted to circumvent intolerable acute reactions: A reduction in total dose, B break in treatment, and C reduction in volume exposed to accelerated treatment. Recent use of accelerated fractionation of these types is illustrated in table I. It is clear that the preponderance of these studies involves head and neck tumors.

We classify as hyperfractionation, schedules designed primarily to exploit small doses per fraction (usually less than 1.3 Gy) given two or more times on each treatment day with overall times similar to or somewhat less than with conventional treatment. With one exception, the total dose is larger than conventional. Recent applications of hyperfractionation are listed in table II, head and neck tumors again being the most frequently treated.

Not all the studies listed in tables I and II lend themselves to analysis of the effects of time-dose parameters on normal tissue reactions. We have, therefore, focused our attention on reports meeting two criteria: (1) the patient population was sufficiently homogeneous in regard to site and stage of disease, and (2) quantitative data on patients treated according to specified protocols were provided. For the remaining reports, qualitative observations concerning normal–tissue reactions are cited as quoted by the authors. Since this analysis was directed towards normal-tissue reactions, no attempt has been made to compare the therapeutic efficacy of the various schedules.

Results

Accelerated Fractionation

Type A Schedules Examples of treatment using type A schedules are set out in table III. In a study of intensive treatment acceleration, Saunders et al. [20] reported the results of 3 × 1.4–1.5 Gy/day over a continuous period of 12 days (weekend included) to total doses of 50.4–54.0 Gy. The field size was reduced after about 38 Gy. Acute reactions were dose limiting: almost all patients were obliged after completion of treatment to be hospitalized 2 weeks, while mucosal reactions resolved. With the qualification that follow-up times have been short, however, late complications have been mild.

Svoboda [23] reported on results of 59 head and neck tumors. Initially treatment volumes were small, and the acute tolerance was satisfactory; when larger volumes (including elective nodal irradiation) were treated, it became necessary to limit the size of dose per fraction to 1.7 Gy. The response rate was high (86%), but nine moderate-to-severe late complications were reported. By contrast, Peracchia and Salti [16] reported very severe acute and consequential late reactions in 12 of 22 patients receiving 3 × 2 Gy/day to doses as high as 54 Gy in 9–11 days. It is noteworthy that the interfraction interval was significantly higher in the treatments described by Saunders et al. [20]. Svoboda [23] treated 39 inoperable carcinomas of the breast by type A acceleration. The size of dose per fraction was most important for the late effects; acute effects were not dose limiting because of megavoltage skin sparing.

Barker et al. [2] reported their experience with radiotherapy of inflammatory carcinoma of the breast using twice daily fractionation. With 2 × 1.25–1.35 Gy/day to total doses of 51–54 Gy within 4 weeks, there was a 7% incidence of severe fibrosis and a 10% incidence of short-term pneumonitis. Choi et al. [4] used accelerated treatment for metastatic melanoma in the brain: 30–37 Gy within 1 week or 37–38 Gy within 2 weeks. Acute reactions were not reported. The major causes of death included one radiation edema. Von Rottkay [19] used accelerated fractionation for non-small-cell lung tumors. A treatment period of less than

4 weeks caused considerable acute and persistent esophageal reactions. With treatment times longer than 5 weeks, there was less toxicity. Arcangeli et al. [1] used three times daily treatment of 111 multiple neck node metastases. The schedule was 2 + 1.5 + 1.5 Gy/day at 4-hour intervals to a total dose of 60 Gy. No data on complications were reported.

Type B Schedules Some results of using type B schedules are illustrated in table III. These schedules have evolved in Europe [3] and in the USA [31, 32] and were motivated by the necessity to allow acute mucosal responses to subside before continuation of treatment. A randomized trial was carried out by the EORTC Radiotherapy Group [3] to compare the results of conventional 70 Gy/7 weeks to MFD 3 × 1.6 Gy/day for 10 days, 3 weeks rest, followed by a boost to 67.2–72 Gy with or without misonidazole. The early mucosal reactions were more severe in the MFD arms, and 5 patients died of pharyngeal hemorrhages that resulted from rapid regression of the tumor. However, the incidence of fibrosis and edema was the same in all three arms.

After having begun with a b.i.d./q.d. schedule, Wang et al. [31] and Wang [32] changed to a 'twice daily/twice daily' treatment where patients with head and neck tumors were treated before and after the 2-week rest with 2 × 1.6 Gy/day to 64 Gy within 6 weeks. Acute effects consisted of patchy to confluent mucositis that decreased rapidly during the 2 weeks of rest; reactions were generally less severe after the second course. Late effects were deemed insignificant though no specific data were cited.

Late complications associated with two different MFD irradiation schedules used for the treatment of prostate cancer were analyzed in 91 patients [30]. The initial treatment of two 30-Gy courses was modified on account of severe acute complications to three courses of 20 Gy. Complications were generally localized in the urinary system and consisted mainly of chronic cystitis and incontinence. There were few exclusive gastrointestinal problems.

Horiot et al. [8] reported a randomized trial of the treatment of high-grade malignant gliomas by single or three daily fractions (with and without misonidazole).

Type C Schedules Examples of type C schedules are set out in table III. The concomitant boost technique (type C) is a variant of accelerated fractionation in which the boost is delivered as a second daily fraction during the basic treatment course. By this means the duration of treatment can be reduced by the time usually taken for the boost (1.5–2 weeks). Favorable results in a pilot study [9] prompted initiation of a randomized phase II study in 1984 to evaluate three different schedules for the boost. All three arms required the delivery of a basic treatment

Table III. Complications after accelerated fractionation

Site	Patients evaluable	Factionation	Δt h	Complications
Type A regimens				
Head and neck	17	3 × 1.4–1.5 Gy/day 50.4–54 Gy/12 days	6	minor xerostomia, maximum mucosal irradiations after treatment, most patients hospitalized for 2 weeks, no late toxicity data [20]
Head and neck	59	3 × 1.7–2.3 Gy/day 50–55 Gy/10–14 days	≥3	peak mucositis 5–10 days after treatment, sometimes requiring hospitalization; symptoms subsided after 2–3 weeks; 15% severe late damage with small tumors, 22% with large tumors (cartilage necrosis, stenosis) [23]
Head and neck	22	3 × 2 Gy/day 48–54 Gy/9–11 days	4	55% mucosal necrosis, 100% confluent mucositis requiring 4–5 months of healing, 13 treatment-related deaths [16]
Breast	39	3 × 1.4–3 Gy/day 40–47.5 Gy/5–14 days	>3	minimal changes for dose <45 Gy or if dose/fraction <1.6 Gy; thickening, shrinkage for dose >45 Gy and dose/fraction >1.6 Gy; leathering, necrosis if dose >45 Gy and dose/fraction >3 Gy [23]
Breast (inflammatory)	42	2 × 1.27–1.35 Gy/day 51–54 Gy/4 weeks	≥3	3/42 severe fibrosis; 10% short-term pneumonitis [2]
Brain metastases	59	30–37.5 Gy/10 fractions/1 week 37.5–48 Gy/10 fractions/2 weeks	≥4	1 fatal radiation edema [4]
Lung	55	17 patients: 2 × 1.8–2 Gy/day 66 Gy/<4 weeks; 15 patients; 1–2 × 1.8–2 Gy/day 66 Gy/29–35 days; 23 patients: 1–2 × 1.8–2 Gy/day 66 Gy/>35 days	~3	treatment <4 weeks led to marked (100%) acute and long-term esophagitis; other complications with treatment <4 weeks: 2/17 stenosis, 1/17 fistula (esophagus), 1/17/ lethal pneumonitis, [15]

Type B regimens				
Head and Neck	179	3 × 1.6 Gy/day 67.2–72 Gy/6–7 weeks (48 Gy + 3–4 weeks rest + remainder)	4	heavy mucosal irradiations after 1st session; late reactions similar to conventional; 9% complication-related deaths (5 pharyngeal hemorrhage due to rapid regression) [3]
Head and neck	106	2 × 1.6 Gy/day 64 Gy/6 weeks (2 weeks rest after 38 Gy)	≥4	acute mucosal irradiations more severe in patients treated twice daily; late effects comparable to fractions
Prostate	91	3 × 2 Gy/day 30 Gy/1 week + (83>1 year 47>2 years) 3–4 weeks rest + repeat (17 patients) 3 × 2 Gy/day 20 Gy/1 week + 17 days + repeat + 17 days + repeat (74 patients)	≥4	19% severe complications (incontinence and/or hematuria 9/91, ureteral obstruction 3/91, intractable pain 1/91, fistual (fatal) 2/91, rectal ulcer or stenosis 2/91); acute reactions more severe in the 2 × 30-Gy regimen [30]
Brain	295	3 × 2 Gy/day, 30 Gy/week + 2 weeks rest and repeat ± misonidazole versus 1 × 2 Gy/day 60 Gy/6 weeks (randomized phase III)	≥4	no difference in brain necrosis in the three arms [8]
Type C regimens				
Head and neck	53	1 × 1.8–2 Gy/day + 1.2–1.5 Gy boost 2–3 times weekly (17Gy in 12 fraction boost) 70–74 Gy/6 weeks	3–6	severe mucosal reactions (35%) when boost included mucosa; 14/53 moderate-severe late radiations; 6/53 XRT only [9]
Head and neck	63	30 × 1.8 Gy, 54 Gy/6 weeks (basic course) + 10–20 × 1.5 Gy (boost dose) during 1st 2 weeks (I), last 2 weeks (II), or 2/weakly throughout basic course (III), 69–72 Gy/6 weeks	4–6	acute radiations: NG tube: 5/21 (I) 3/28 (II), 1/14 (III); persistent mucositis >4 weeks after treatment: 2/21 (I), 2/28 (II), 0/14 (III); late effects: 1 carotid rupture after salvage surgery (I); 1 patient in each arm with transient bone exposure secondary to severe acute reactions [Ang and Peters, unpubl. data]

dose of 54 Gy in 30 fractions of 1.8 Gy over 6 weeks. The boost was given either during the first 2 weeks, the last 2 weeks, or uniformly throughout the basic treatment. All patients have completed the treatment without interruption, even though acute reactions have been more severe than with conventional treatment [Ang and Peters unpubl. data], as detailed in table III. Late effects have been limited to one carotid rupture that occurred after salvage surgery.

Hyperfractionation

A summary of the complications attending hyperfractionated radiotherapy in three randomized phase-III trials is set out in table IV. From 1979 to 1983 the RTOG [10] conducted a prospective phase III study for advanced head and neck tumors that compared a standard schedule with a twice-a-day schedule in which the total dose, instead of being higher as required for a therapeutic gain, was lower than in the conventional arm. In spite of the lower total dose, acute reactions were more severe with the hyperfractionation schedule. The incidence of late effects was similar in the two groups. There was a tendency toward more severe acute and late reactions when the interfraction interval was less than 4.5 vs. greater than 4.5 h.

A prospective randomized study by the EORTC [8] in patients with T2–3 NO–1 squamous carcinoma of the oropharynx was closed in 1987. Mucosal reactions were somewhat worse in the hyperfractionated arm, while late reactions were similar.

At the Radiumhemmet in Stockholm [7] 168 patients with bladder cancer were treated in a randomized trial with either 64 Gy in 2-Gy fractions within $6\frac{1}{2}$ weeks or with 84 Gy in fractions of 3 × 1 Gy/day in a split course lasting $8–8\frac{1}{2}$ weeks. The split was necessary in the hyperfractionated arm to avoid excessive acute reactions. There was a higher incidence of severe late reactions in the hyperfractionation arm, but this was insignificant after allowance was made for the 50% higher survival of patients in this arm (table IV).

A nonrandomized study at the University of Florida showing encouraging results with hyperfractionation for head and neck cancer has recently been updated by Parsons et al. [15]. As shown in table IV, acute mucosal reactions were more severe than with conventional treatment, but late sequelae were overall similar to or less than expected with conventional treatment.

Meoz et al. [12] reported the treatment of 65 patients with advanced squamous cell tumors of the head and neck region with hyperfractionation. The incidence of late complications was 17%, of which 3 cases were fatal. A high incidence of severe mucositis was observed. A subsequent prospective study at The University of Texas M.D. Anderson Cancer Center using twice daily treatments for laryngeal and hypopharyngeal cancer was begun in 1982 [Wendt and Peters, unpubl. data]. Mucosal reactions were severe, but late complications have not exceeded those experienced with conventional treatment.

Medini et al. [11] treated 21 patients with head and neck cancer using hyperfractionation (2 × 1.1 Gy/day to 74.8 Gy/6.5 weeks). No difference was observed between the mucosal or skin reactions as compared with conventional treatment, and there was no evidence of cartilage necrosis.

Late effects were analyzed by Nguyen et al. [13] in a series of 39 patients with 2-year minimum follow-up who had been treated by rapid hyperfractionation using 6–8 fractions/day with a 2-hour interfraction interval (table IV). Seventy percent of the patients experienced late complications (cervical fibrosis, necrosis, and edema), and in 54% these were severe. Comparing these results to what would be expected from conventional treatment to similar total doses, the authors concluded that the interfraction interval was too short for complete repair in the late-responding normal tissues. Douglas and Worth [6] used hyperfractionation (3 × 1 Gy/day whole brain with a 3- to 3.5-hour interfraction interval to 45–60 Gy plus a 10-Gy/5 fractions boost to the tumor volume) in the treatment of 30 glioblastomas. There was no evidence of pathologic brain injury in the patients who were autopsied.

There has been a number of phase I–II trials of hyperfractionation using dose escalation to determine maximum tolerated doses. Two of these [14, 33] involved treatment of brain stem gliomas in children. No acute or subacute neurologic toxicity was seen in the study of Packer et al. [14]; there were 2 patients with signs of neurologic deterioration in the study of Wara et al. [33]. However, long-term effects on the brain could not be assessed.

In the study of Seydel et al. [22] patients with localized unresectable non-oat cell carcinoma of the lung were entered into a dose escalation trial (table IV). Ten patients received 50.4 Gy, 20 received 60, 79 received 69.6, and 11 received 74.4 Gy. The treatment was discontinued or stopped in 14 patients because of early death or deterioration in condition. The median survival was 7.2 months. There were 6 cases of severe and 2 of life-threatening toxicity, but this was considered less than in previous experience with this tumor.

The RTOG has recently undertaken dose escalation studies for determining the maximum tolerable doses using hyperfractionation at 1.2 Gy twice daily in the treatment of cancer of the brain, lung, head and neck, and bladder (table V). Five total dose levels were chosen, and patients were accrued at levels A–C until it was determined that dose C was toler-

Table IV. Complications after Hyperfractionation

Site	Patients evaluable	Factionation	Δt h	Complications
Randomized trials				
Head and neck	187	2 × 1.2 Gy/day 60 Gy/5 weeks versus 1.8–2 Gy/day 66–73.8 Gy/7–8 weeks	3–6	more severe mucositis with hyperfractionation; similar late reactions; acute and late radiations worse for $\Delta t<4.5$ h verus $\Delta t>4.5$ h ($p<.05$) [10]
Head and neck (oropharynx)	254	2 × 1.15 Gy/day 80.5 Gy/7 weeks versus 2 Gy/day 70 Gy/7 weeks	4–6	severe mucosal irradiations required increased T in 8% (conventional) versus 12% (hyperfractionation); late edema 36% (conventional) versus 52% (hyperfractionation), not significant; other late reactions similar [8]
Bladder	168	3 × 1 Gy/day 84 Gy/8 weeks (2-week split) versus 2 Gy/day 64 Gy/6.5 weeks	4	severe late reactions (intestinal obstruction, fistulae, bleeding) in 10/83 (hyperfractionation) versus 4/85 (conventional); estimated complication rate biased by 50% higher survival at 3 years in hyperfractionation arm [7]
Nonrandomized trials				
Head and neck	132	2 × 1.2 Gy/day 74.4–79.2 Gy/6 weeks	4–6	20% severe mucosal irradiations: 15/132 NG tube, 2 treatment interruptions, 1 tracheostomy; late reactions: 15/132 mild, 5 moderate, 7 severe (necrosis, stricture, permanent NG tube); overall ≤ conventional treatment [15]
Head and neck	65	2 × 1.1–1.2 Gy/day 60–75 Gy/5–6.5 weeks	3–6	22% severe mucositis; late reactions 17% (11/65), 3 fatal (1 surgical) [12]

Head and neck	89	2 × 1.2 Gy/day 72–80.6 Gy/6–7 weeks	≥4	18% severe acute effect (>10% weight loss), NG tube, persistent (>2 months) mucositis); 7% severe late effects (necrosis, stricture, edema) [Wendt and Peters, unpubl.]
Head and neck	21	2 × 1.1 Gy/day 74.8 Gy/6.5 weeks	≥4	complications similar to conventional treatment [11]
Head and neck	178 (39 with 2-year follow-up)	6–8 × 1.1–0.9 Gy/day 66–72 Gy/4–6 weeks (2 series of 33–36 Gy with 2–4 weeks rest)	2	54% severe late reactions (cervical fibrosis, mucosal and bone necrosis, trismus, edema); 13% treatment-related deaths [13]
Brain stem	16	2 × 1.2 Gy/day 64.8 Gy/5.5 weeks	4–8	no evidence of radionecrosis [14]
Brain stem	45	2 × 1 Gy/day 72 Gy/7 weeks	4	2/45 local tumor necrosis and neurologic deterioration [33]
Brain	30	3 × 1 Gy/day 45–60 Gy/4–5 weeks + boost (2 Gy/day, 10 Gy/1 week)	3–3.5	moist desquamation behind ears; no evidence of high-dose effects from autopsies [6]
Lung	96	2 × 1.2 Gy/day 50.4–74.4/4.5–6.5 weeks (dose escalation)	4–6	10% (7/71) severe to life-threatening late complication in patients receiving >60 Gy; compares with 16% for 60 Gy in 2-Gy fractions in protocol RTOG 73–01 [22]

Table V. Total doses in phase I/II hyperfractionation trials of the RTOG [from ref. 5]

Arm	Glioma[a]	Total doses Gy		
		upper respiratory/ digestive tract	lung	bladder
A	67.2	67.2	60	60
B	72.0	72.0	64.8	64.8
C	76.8	76.8	69.6	69.6
D	81.6	81.6	74.4	74.4
E	no plan	86.4	79.2	79.2

[a] Study closed due to slow accrual with total doses limited to A, B, and C.

able. The results so far suggest that current modeling of differences in acute and late effects is correct [5].

Discussion

This survey has shown that MFD treatment, whether with accelerated fractionation or hyperfractionation, is in general associated with an increased severity of acute effects; late effects were increased in some of the accelerated treatment studies, but not in others, and were generally equivalent or reduced in the hyperfractionated regimens. Specific predictions made on biological grounds can be partly substantiated by the clinical data:

(1) Acute reactions are limited by the rate of dose accumulation, i.e., the weekly dose rate. This statement is borne out by most of the accelerated fractionation studies. It is unlikely that the mucous membranes of the head and neck can tolerate in excess of 55 Gy in 2 weeks, regardless of fractionation schedule. In particular, doses per fraction of 2 Gy or more given three times daily cannot be tolerated, unless very small field sizes are used. The limitation imposed by the weekly dose rate is a reflection of the biological fact that acute reactions represent a deficit in the balance between the rate of cell killing by irradiation and cell regeneration from surviving stem cells. Once the stem cell population is depleted to the point where it is unable to renew the functional layers of the epithelium, the acute reaction peaks, and further depopulation produces no increase in severity of the reaction. As a corollary it might be expected that the intensity of acute reactions would be more influenced by the rate of dose accumulation than by the total dose, once a certain threshold of total dose

has been reached. This is corroborated at least partly by a comparison of the type A schedules and the type B schedule [3]; although the issue is clouded somewhat by the split, it is clear that a significant boost in total dose in the latter study did not result in noticeably worse acute responses, even though the same dose (48–50 Gy) had been given in the first 2 weeks, and no further dose was given in the type A schedules. This point is also borne out by the study of Marcial et al. [10] where acute reactions were more severe with the hyperfractionated regimen than with standard fractionation in spite of a lower total dose being given in the hyperfractionated arm.

Conversely, the time taken to heal, as opposed to the severity of, the acute reaction, is dependent on the total dose, provided the weekly dose rate exceeds the regenerative ability of the surviving mucosal stem cells. This is because healing is a function of the absolute number of stem cells surviving the course of treatment, and the higher the total dose, the fewer stem cells will survive. Clinical data illustrating this point are found in the reports of Parsons et al. [15] and Wendt and Peters [unpubl. data] where prolonged healing times were associated with hyperfractionated doses in excess of 76.8 Gy.

(2) The weekly dose rate may be of significance for late effects: The studies of Svoboda [23], Peracchia and Salti [16], and van den Bogaert et al. [3], where total doses were less than or similar to conventional regimens, showed a higher incidence of late reactions. Here, however, a distinction needs to be drawn between 'true' late effects and consequential late reactions [17]. Many of the late effects seen in these studies can be attributed to severe and prolonged epithelial denudation rather than to injury of the mesenchymal tissues normally associated with late reactions. The study of Nguyen et al. [13] could be taken as another example, but the interfraction interval was very short, and this confounds the influence of overall time.

(3) Late effects are limited by fraction size and interfraction interval: The analysis of Marcial et al. [10] establishes rigorously the important role of interfraction interval, late complications being worse after intervals less than 4.5 h versus greater than 4.5 h. This was also true of acute effects. However, the fraction size affects late effects more strongly than acute effects, as has been amply documented [26], and recently attention has been focused on the importance of interfraction interval and tissue repair kinetics [24]. The experience of Nguyen et al. [13] clearly demonstrates that short intervals can greatly intensify the biological effect of total doses (66–72 Gy) that, given in such small fractional doses (0.9–1.1 Gy), would have been expected to yield milder than conventional late reactions if repair had been near completion. This is corroborated by

the results of Marcial et al. [10], showing that 4.5 h may not be sufficient to approach complete repair, in either acutely or late-reacting normal tissues in humans.

Acknowledgements

The authors are grateful to Ms. C. Seifert and Ms. B. Foremsky for expert assistance in preparing the manuscript. This work was supported in part by grants CA-29026, CA-06294, and CA-16672 from the National Cancer Institute, Department of Health and Human Services.

References

1 Arcangeli, G.; Nervi, C.; Cividalli, A.; Mauro, F.; Pardini, M.: Clinical implications of the radiobiological data in multiple fractions per day (MFD) radiotherapy. Proc. Varian's 4th Eur. Clinac Users Meet., Malta 1984, pp. 36–43 (Varian, Zug, 1984).

2 Barker, J.; Montague, E.; Peters, L.: Clinical experience with irradiation of inflammatory carcinoma of the breast with and without elective chemotherapy. Cancer *45:* 625–629 (1980).

3 Bogaert, W. van den; Schueren, E. van der; Horiot, J.; Chaplain, G.; Devilhena, M.; Raposo, S.; Leonor, J.; Schraub, S.; Chenal, C.; Barthelme, E.; Daban, A.; Eschwege, F.; Gonzalez, D.; Leer, J.; Hamers, H.; Svoboda, V.; Rigon, A.; Arcangeli, G.; Sack, H.; De Pauw, M.; Glabbeke, M. van: Early results of the EORTC randomized clinical trial on multiple fractions per day (MFD) and misonidazole in advanced head and neck cancer. Int. J. Radiat. Oncol. Biol. Phys. *12:* 587–591 (1986).

4 Choi, K.; Withers, H.; Rotman, M.: Metastatic melanoma in brain: rapid treatment or large dose fractions. Cancer *56:* 10–15 (1985).

5 Cox, J.: Presidential address: fractionation: a paradigm for clinical research in radiation oncology. Int. J. Radiat. Oncol. Biol. Phys. *13:* 1271–1281 (1987).

6 Douglas, B.; Worth, A.: Superfractionation in glioblastoma multiforme: results of a phase II study. Int. J. Radiat. Oncol. Biol. Phys. *8:* 1787–1794 (1982).

7 Edsmyr, F.; Andersson, L.; Esposti, P.; Littbrand, B.; Nilsson, B.: Irradiation therapy with multiple small fractions per day in urinary bladder cancer. Radiother. Oncol. *4:* 197–203 (1985).

8 Horiot, J.; Bogaert, W. van den; Ang, K. K.; Schueren, E. van der; Bartelink, H.; Gonzalez, D.; Pauw, M. de; Glabbeke, M. van: European Organization for Research on Treatment of Cancer Trials Using Radiotherapy with Multiple Fractions Per Day. A 1978–1987 survey; in Vaeth, Meyer, Time, dose and fractionation in the radiation therapy of Cancer. Front. Radiat. Ther. Onc., vol. 22, pp. 149–161 (Karger, Basel 1988).

9 Knee, R.; Fields, R.; Peters, L.: Concomitant boost radiotherapy for advanced squamous cell carcinoma of the head and neck. Radiother. Oncol. *4:* 1–7 (1985).

10 Marcial, V.; Pajak, T.; Chang, C.; Tupchong, L.; Stetz, J.: Hyperfractionated photon radiation therapy in the treatment of advanced squamous cell carcinoma of the oral cavity, pharynx, larynx, and sinuses, using radiation therapy as the only planned mod-

ality. Preliminary report by the Radiation Therapy Oncology Group (RTOG). Int. J. Radiat. Oncol. Biol. Phys. *13:* 41–47 (1987).

11 Medini, E.; Rao, Y.; Kim, T.; Levitt, S.: Radiation therapy for advanced head and neck squamous cell carcinoma using twice-a-day fractionation. Am. J. Oncol. *8:* 65–68 (1985).

12 Meoz, R.; Fletcher, G.; Peters, L.: Barkley, H.; Thames, H.: Twice-daily fractionation schemes for advanced head and neck cancer. Int. J. Radiat. Oncol. Biol. Phys. *10:* 831–836 (1984).

13 Nguyen, T.; Panis, X.; Proissart, D.; Legros, M.; Coninx, P.; Loirette, M.: Analysis of late complications after rapid hyperfractionated radiotherapy in advanced head and neck cancers. Int. J. Radiat. Oncol. Biol. Phys. *14:* 23–25 (1988).

14 Packer, R.; Littman, P.; Sposto, R.; D'Angio, G.; Priest, J.; Heideman, R.; Bruce, D.; Nelson, D.: Results of a pilot study of hyperfractionated radiation therapy for children with brain stem gliomas. Int. J. Radiat. Oncol. Biol. Phys. *13:* 1647–1651 (1987).

15 Parsons, J.; Mendenhall, W.; Cassisi, N.; Isaacs, J., Jr.; Million, R.: Accelerated hyperfractionation for head and neck cancer. Int. J. Radiat. Oncol. Biol. Phys. *14:* 649–658 (1988).

16 Peracchia, G.; Salti, C.: Radiotherapy with thrice-a-day fractionation in a short overall time: clinical experiences. Int. J. Radiat. Oncol. Biol. Phys. *7:* 99–104 (1981).

17 Peters, L.; Ang, K.; Thames, H.: Accelerated fractionation in the treatment of head and neck cancer: a critical comparison of different strategies. Acta oncologica *27:* 185–194 (1988).

18 Peters, L.; Withers, H.; Thames, H.: Radiobiological bases for multiple daily fractionation; in Karcher, Kogelnik, Reinartz, Progress in radio-oncology, vol. II, pp. 317–323 (Raven, New York, 1982).

19 Rottkay, P. von: Remissionen und akute Toxizität bei beschleunigt fraktionierter Bestrahlung nichtkleinzelliger Bronchialkarzinome. Strahlenther. Onkol. *162:* 300–307 (1986).

20 Saunders, M.; Dische, S.; Fowler, J.; Denekamp, J.; Dunphy, E.; Grosch, E.; Fermont, D.; Ashford, R.; Maher, J.; Des Rocher, C.: Radiotherapy with three fractions per day for twelve consecutive days for tumors of the thorax, head and neck; in Vaeth, Meyer, Time, dose and Fractionation in the radiation therapy of cancer. Front. Radiat. Ther. Onc., vol. 22, pp. 99–104 (Karger, Basel 1988).

21 Scott, O.: Divergence of opinion over the linear-quadratic model. Br. J. Radiol. *60:* 1042–1043 (1987).

22 Seydel, H.; Diener-West, M.; Urtasun, R.; Podolsky, W.; Cox, J.; Zinninger, M.; Francis, M.; Radiation Therapy Oncology Group (RTOG): Hyperfractionation in the radiation therapy of unresectable non-oat cell carcinoma of the lung: preliminary report of a RTOG pilot study. Int. J. Radiat. Oncol. Biol. Phys. *11:* 1841–1847 (1985).

23 Svoboda, V.: Accelerated fractionation: the Portsmouth experience 1972–1984. Proc. Varian's 4th Eur. Clinac Users Meet., Malta 1984, pp. 70–75 (Varian, Zug 1984).

24 Thames, H.; Hendry, J.: Fractionation in radiotherapy. (Taylor and Francis, London 1987).

25 Thames, H.; Peters, L.; Withers, H.; Fletcher, G.: Accelerated fractionation vs. hyperfractionation: rationales for several treatments per day. Int. J. Radit. Oncol. Biol. Phys. *9:* 127–138 (1983).

26 Thames, H.; Withers, H.; Peters, L.; Fletcher, G.: Changes in early and late radiation responses with altered dose fractionation: implications for dose-survival relationships. Int. J. Radiat. Oncol. Biol. Phys. *8:* 219–226 (1982).

27 Thames, H.: An 'incomplete-repair' model for survival after fractionated and continuous irradiations. Int. J. Radiat. Biol. *47:* 319–339 (1985).

28 Turesson, I.; Thames, H.: Repair capacity and kinetics of human skin during fractionated radiotherapy: erythema, desquamation, and telangiectasia after 3 and 5 year's follow-up. Radiother. Oncol. (submitted 1988).

29 Turesson, I.; Notter, G.: Control of dose administered once-a-week and three times a day according to schedules calculated by the CRE-formula, using skin reaction as a biological parameter. Radiology *120:* 399–404 (1976).

30 Van Uytsel, L.; Ang, K.; Vandenbussche, L.; Vereecken, R.; Schueren, E. van der: Radiotherapy in multiple fractions per day for prostatic carcinoma: late complications. Int. J. Radiat. Oncol. Biol. Phys. *12:* 1589–1595 (1986).

31 Wang, C.; Suit, H.; Blitzer, P.: Twice-a-day radiation therapy for supraglottic carcinoma. Int. J. Radiat. Oncol. Biol. Phys. *12:* 307 (1986).

32 Wang, C.: Improved local control for advanced oropharyngeal carcinoma following twice daily radiation therapy. Am. J. clin. Oncol. *8:* 512–516 (1985).

33 Wara, W.; Edwards, M.; Levin, V.; Heideman, R.; Urtasun, R.; Diaz, R.; Silver, P.; Sposto, R.: A new treatment regimen for brain stem glioma: a pilot study of the Brain Tumor Research Center and Children's Cancer Study Group (Abstract). Int. J. Radiat. Oncol. Biol. Phys. *12:* suppl. 1, p. 143 (1986).

34 Withers, H.; Peters, L.: Biologic aspects of radiotherapy; in Fletcher, Textbook of radiotherapy, (Lea & Febiger, Philadelphia 1980).

Howard D. Thames, PhD, Division of Biomathematics, The University of Texas M.D. Anderson Cancer Center, Houston, TX 77030 (USA)

Vaeth JM, Meyer JL (eds): Radiation Tolerance of Normal Tissues.
Front Radiat Ther Oncol. Basel, Karger, 1989, vol 23, pp 131–139

Modulation of the Oncogenic Potential of Various Anticancer Modalities[1]

Eric J. Hall, Tom K. Hei, Richard C. Miller

Radiological Research Laboratory, Department of Radiation Oncology,
College of Physicians and Surgeons, Columbia University, New York, N.Y., USA

Introduction

While the treatment of human tumors by chemotherapy has become increasingly effective through the years, many agents used to treat cancer are known also to be carcinogenic and, therefore, pose the risk that they may induce secondary malignancies. This is particularly true for patients with lymphoma and pediatric cancer who are treated aggressively with radiotherapy and chemotherapy [1–3]. This is of mounting concern as combined modality therapy leads to an increased number of long-term survivors among oncology patients.

There is considerable variability in the efficiency with which agents, used primarily in the therapy of cancer, can induce secondary malignancies. In addition, compounds have been identified that can block the phenotypic expression of tumor cells *in vitro* [4, 5] and inhibit growth or induce cellular differentiation in many animal and human cell types [6–8]. This has led to the suggestion of chemoprevention in populations at high risk for cancer development [9].

Due to the length of the latent period for cancer induction in humans, by either radiation or chemotherapy agents, and the large population base required to compare the effectiveness of different agents to induce secondary malignancies, model systems that give quick answers are clearly needed. *In vitro* assays of oncogenic transformation, based on established cell lines of rodent origin, make possible a quantitative assessment at the cellular level of the oncogenic potential of a variety of physical, chemical, and viral agents [see ref. 10 for a review]. These systems, free of host-mediated homeostatic influence, afford the opportunity to study

[1] This investigaton was supported by grants No. CA 12536 and CA 43194 awarded by National Cancer Institute.

dose-related and time-dependent interactions of radiation with chemotherapeutic agents and to identify factors and conditions that may prevent or enhance such interactions.

Oncogenic Transformation by Chemotherapeutic Agents

Many different chemotherapeutic agents have been tested for their ability to induce transformed foci [10–13]. Figure 1 summarizes some of the data currently available. The plot of transformation frequency versus cell-surviving fraction allows one to examine the ability of each agent to produce transformed foci at doses that result in similar levels of cell killing. The known chemical carcinogen Benzo (a) pyrene (BaP) is included as a reference point to the other agents used. It is evident from figure 1 that there is a range of oncogenic transforming abilities among the various chemotherapeutic agents. Some agents, such as BCNU and actinomycin D, produce higher incidences of transformation for any given level of cell killing. α-particles, also, produce substantially more transformation than γ-rays at comparable levels of cell killing.

Modulation of Survivial versus Transformation

With cell lethality as an end point, the biological effectiveness of a given dose of radiation can be modulated (increased or decreased) by a variety of factors, including radiation quality, dose rate, oxygen tension, the presence of free radical scavengers, or sensitizers. In general, cells must be exposed to modulators at the time of irradiation in order for cell lethality to be affected. An exception to the generalization occurs with manipulation of the postirradiation environment that inhibits cell division and allows repair of potentially lethal damage, leading to an increase in cell survival [14]. In general, this is a relatively small effect. In contrast, many agents have been identified that can dramatically influence the oncogenic transformation potential of a given dose of radiation when added after the radiation exposure. Results of a series of experiments along these lines are summarized in figures 2 and 3.

Modulation by Hormones and Vitamins

It is interesting to note that manipulation of hormonal levels can dramatically alter the transformation incidence (fig. 2), demonstrating

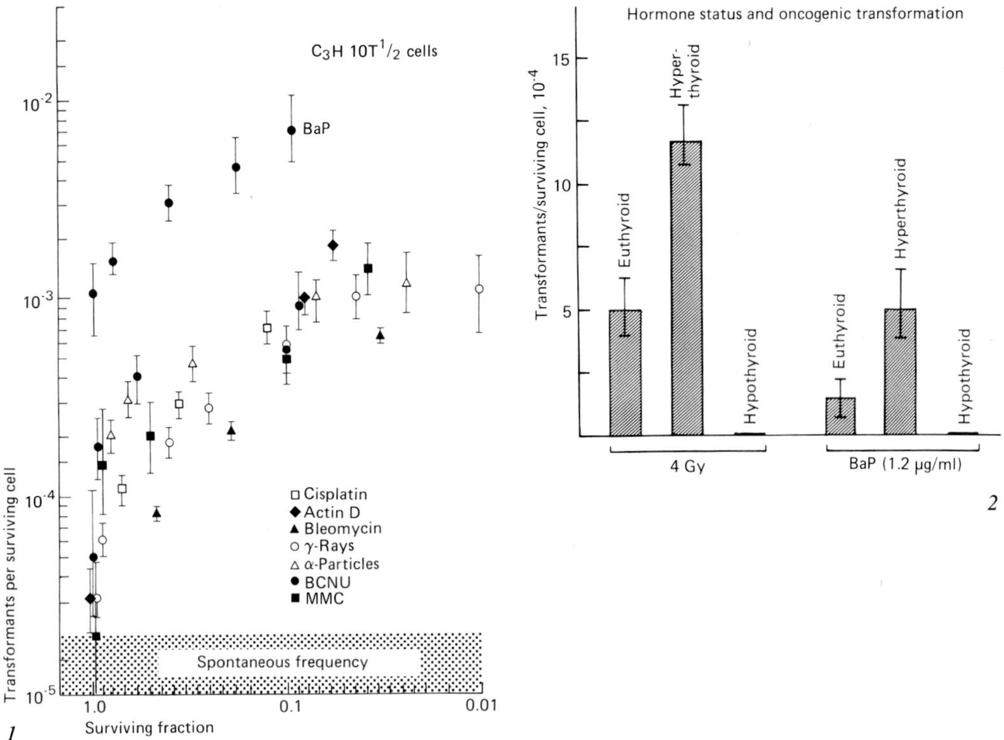

Fig. 1. Transformation per surviving cell versus surviving fraction for BaP, X-rays, α-particles, and a series of chemotherapeutic agents. MMC = mitomycin-C.

Fig. 2. Effects of thyroid hormone status on radiation and chemically induced transformation frequencies in C_3H $10T^1/_2$ cells.

in the Petri dish what is evident from experiments with both humans and animals [15, 16]. Under hypothyroid conditions neither X-rays- nor BaP-induced transformations are expressed [17, 18]. When thyroid hormone (triiodothyronine) is added to the medium, oncogenic transformation is expressed in a dose-dependent fashion. The induction of cellular transformation protein by thyroid hormone, and its effect on the oxidative state of cells, is thought to influence the transformation induction in cells [18].

In the context of chemoprevention, i.e., adding a compound to a group of people at high risk of developing cancer, such as patients 'cured' of their first malignancies by a combination of radiation and chemother-

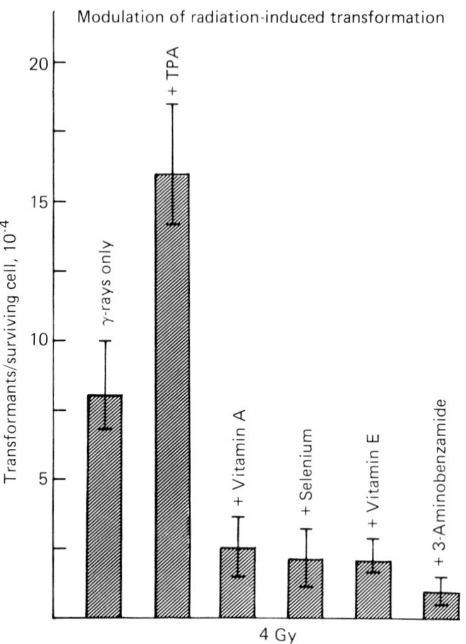

Fig. 3. Transformation incidence in C_3H $10T^{1}/_{2}$ cells by 4 Gy of γ-rays and its modulation by various chemical and dietary factors. TPA = 12-O-tetradecanoyl-phorbol-13 acetate.

apy, retinoids would appear to be particularly promising and appropriate. The term retinoid has been used for a group of compounds that include vitamin A and its natural and synthetic analogues. Retinoids have been found to frequently block the phenotypic expression of tumor cells *in vitro* [4]; they also inhibit growth and induce differentiation in many animal and human malignant cell types [4]. The mechanism of retinoid action that has been proposed involves the protein kinase-C cascade system. This system may mediate the many diverse actions of retinoids, including their effects on enzyme synthesis, membrane properties, growth factors, binding proteins, genomic and postgenomic expression, the extracellular matrix, and immunologic response [for reviews see refs. 19, 20]. Figure 3 illustrates the suppression of radiation-induced transformation by vitamin A analogues, shown more than 10 years ago [21]. A large body of data has accumulated with regard to the importance of retinoids for chemoprevention of cancer, whether it be caused by irradiation, chemical carcinogens, or viral transforming factors [4, 19]. Experimental studies have shown that chemoprevention with retinoids inhibits the development of neoplastic or transformed cell populations *in vitro* as well as in tumor models such as skin, bladder, and mammary glands in mice and rats [20]. Some of the retinoids have been found to be effective in inhibiting the recurrence of these tumors. More work is needed to determine whether retinoids inhibit the transformation process *per se* or whether they simply inhibit the clonal expansion of initiated or transformed cells.

The modulation of transformation by other compounds is also illustrated in figure 3. Selenium is a microcomponent of the diet and a cofactor for glutathione peroxidase, illustrating again the substantial impact that dietary factors may have in the cancer incidence resulting from physical or chemical insults. Vitamin E is principally an antioxidant, while 3-amino-benzamide is an inhibitor of the enzyme poly-ADP-ribose polymerase and prevents DNA repair by interferring with the ligation process.

Modulation by Hyperthermia

Hyperthermia is about the only cancer therapy, apart from the surgeon's knife, that has not been implicated in the induction of cancer as well as its cure. Using the transformation assay, hyperthermia has been shown to reduce the incidence of radiation-induced transformed foci [22]. Figure 4 shows that concurrent exposure of cells to chemotherapeutic drugs and hyperthermia also *reduces* the transformation incidence produced by some chemotherapy agents, while it has no apparent effect on others [12, 13]. The mechanism by which concurrently administered heat modulates the cytotoxicity and oncogenic transforming potential of chemotherapeutic agents is not clear. It has been suggested that changes in cellular metabolism of the drugs, abnormalities in membrane permeability, and cellular transport induced by hyperthermia may partially explain the differences [12, 23]. Furthermore, heat has been postulated to alter intracellular drug concentrations by either increasing the influx or blocking the effluence of drugs, thus affecting toxicity and, perhaps, oncogenicity of the drugs, depending on the heat-drug sequence.

Modulation by Radiation

The interaction between chemotherapeutic agents and radiations on the induction of oncogenic transformation has not been well defined.

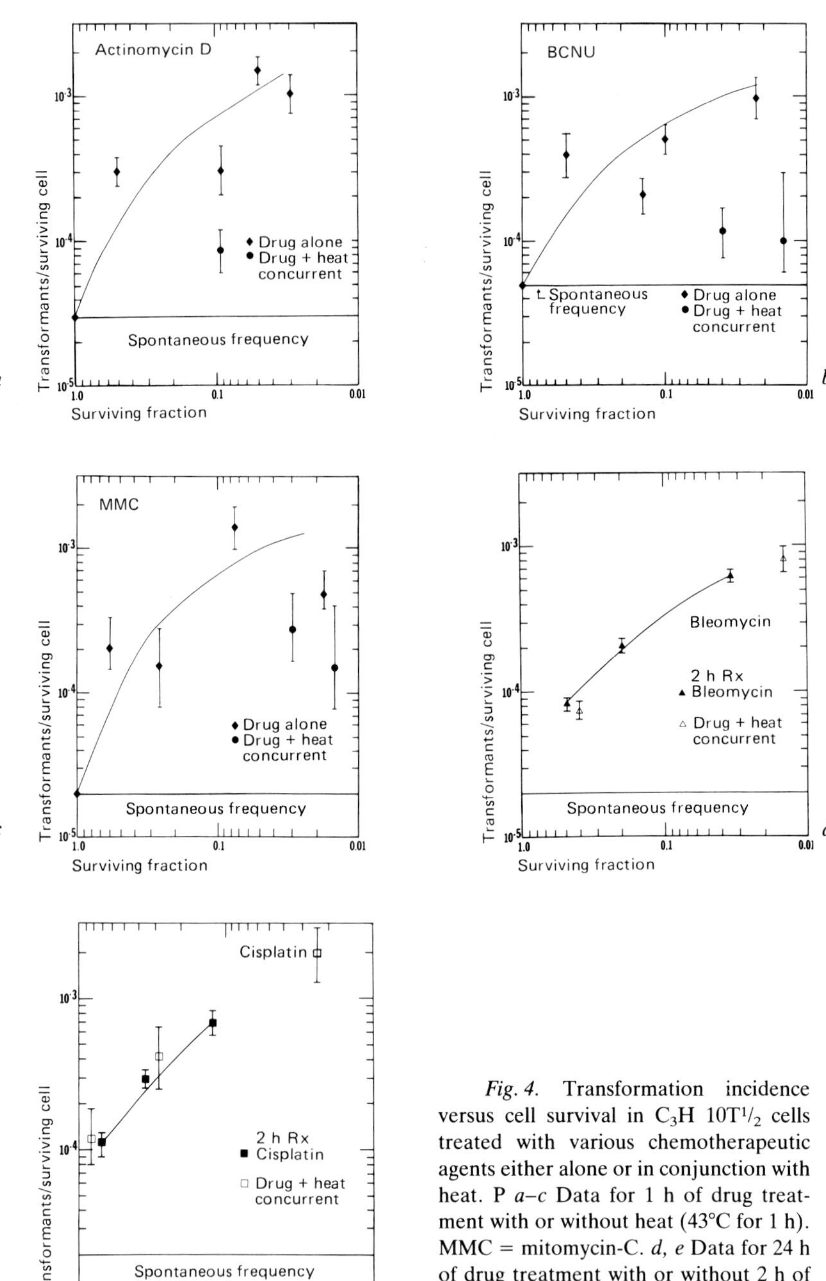

Fig. 4. Transformation incidence versus cell survival in C_3H 10T$^1/_2$ cells treated with various chemotherapeutic agents either alone or in conjunction with heat. P *a–c* Data for 1 h of drug treatment with or without heat (43°C for 1 h). MMC = mitomycin-C. *d, e* Data for 24 h of drug treatment with or without 2 h of hyperthermia (Rx) treatment at 42°C. [See refs. 12 and 13 for details.]

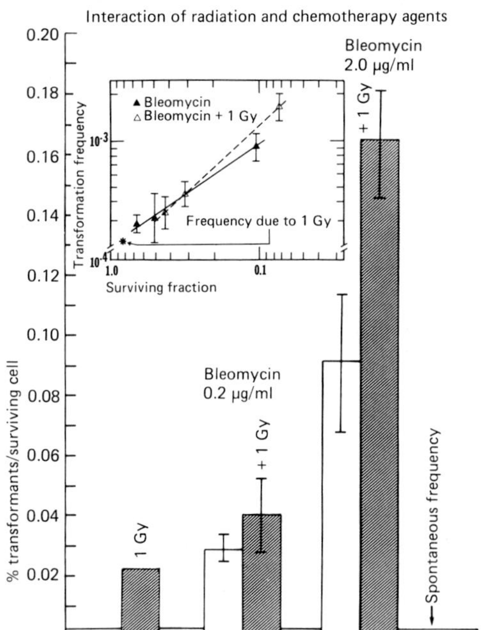

Fig. 5. Oncogenic transformation incidence in C_3H $10T^1/_2$ cells treated with bleomycin sulfate either alone or in combination with 1-Gy γ-rays. Open columns represent frequencies obtained from drug treatment alone. Hatched columns represent frequencies obtained from combined radiation and drug treatment. There is a substantial enhancement in transformation incidence by radiation at higher drug concentration. Inset: replot of the transformation data versus surviving fraction, indicating a real difference in transformation incidence at higher cytotoxic dose of the drug.

While radiations and drugs have shown enhanced toxicities *in vitro*, data on transformation incidence are scarce [24]. Figure 5 shows the oncogenic transforming effects of 1 Gy of γ-rays delivered concurrently with bleomycin. While radiation and low doses of bleomycin result in transformation yields that are simply additive, at higher drug concentrations a supra-additive effect is apparent. Qualitatively, similar findings have been reported for mutation frequencies at the thymidine kinase locus in human lymphoblastoid cells [25]. The kinetics of interaction depend not only on the doses used, but also on the type of drug used and the treatment protocol.

Conclusion

In vitro assays for oncogenic transformation allow a rapid and relatively inexpensive comparison to be made of the relative oncogenic potential of a variety of anticancer modalities. They also illustrate the effectiveness of agents such as the retinoids in inhibiting the expression of transformation induced by radiation and chemicals, emphasizing the possible role of chemoprevention in reducing the induction of secondary malignancies in patients cured of their first cancer. Lastly, they show that the combination of heat and some chemotherapy agents results in a lower transformation incidence for a given level of cell kill than the use of the chemotherapy agent alone.

References

1 Rubin P., Zagars G., Chuang C., et. al.: Hodgkin's disease: Is there a price for successful treatment? A 25 year experience. Int. J. Radiat. Oncol. Biol. Phy. 1986; *12:* 153–166.

2 Norman Coleman C.: Secondary neoplasms in patients treated for cancer: Etiology and perspective. Radiat. Res. 1982; *92:* 188–200.

3 Kyel R. A.: Second malignancies associated with chemotherapeutic agents. Semin. Oncol. 1982; *9:* 131–142.

4 Lotan R.: Effects of vitamin A and its analogs on normal and neoplastic cells. Biochim. Biophys. Acta. 1980: 33–91.

5 Borek C.: Vitamin and micronutrients modify carcinogenesis and tumor promotion in vitro; in Arnott M. S., Van Eys J., Wang Y.M. (eds): Molecular Interactions of Nutrition and Cancer. Raven Press, New York, pp. 337–350, 1982.

6 Sachs L.: Control of normal cell differentiation and the phenotypic reversion of malignancy in myeloid leukemia. Nature 1978; *274:* 535–539.

7 Reuben R. C., Wife R. L., Breslow R., et. al.: A new group of potent inducers of differentiation in murine erythroleukemia cells.

8 Marks P. A., Sheffery M., Rifkind R. A.: Induction of transformed cells to terminal differentiation and the modulation of gene expression. Cancer Res. 1987; *47:* 659–666.

9 Griffin A. C.: Role of selenium in chemoprevention of cancer. Adv. Cancer Res. 1970; *34:* 419–442.

10 Hall E. J., Hei T. K.: Oncogenic transformation of cells in culture: Pragmatic comparisons of oncogenicity, cellular and molecular mechanisms. Int. J. Radiat. Oncol. Biol. Phys. 1986; *12:* 1909–1921.

11 Hall E. J., Miller R. C., Osmak R., et. al.: Comparison of the incidence of oncogenic transformation produced by X-rays, midonidazole and chemotherapeutic agents. Radiology 1982; *145:* 521–526.

12 Hei T. K., Hall E. J., Kushner S., et. al.: Hyperthermia, chemotherapeutic agents and oncogenic transformation. Int. J. Hyperthermia 1986; *2:* 311–320.

13 Komatsu K., Miller R. C., Hall E. J.: The oncogenic potential pof a combination of hyperthermia and chemotherapeutic agents. Br. J. Cancer, in press.

14 Little J. B., Han G. M., Frindel E., et. al.: Repair of potentially lethal damage in vitro and in vivo. Radiology 1973; *106:* 689–694.
15 Henderson B. E., Ross R. K., Pike M. C., et. al.: Endogenous hormones as a major factor in human cancer. Cancer Res 1982; *43:* 3232–3239.
16 Erdstein J., Guyda H. J., Mishkin S.: Effects of hypophysectomy and hormone replacement on the local and metastatic growth of Morris hepatoma 44. Cancer Res. 1984; *44:* 2936–2941.
17 Guernsey D. L., Ong A., Borek C.: Modulation of X-ray-induced neoplastic transformation in vitro by thyroid hormone. Nature 1980; *228:* 591–592.
18 Borek C.: The induction and control of radiogenic transformation in vitro: Cellular and molecular mechanisms. Pharmacol. Ther. 1985; *27:* 99–142.
19 Bertram J. S., Kolonel L. N., Meysken F. L.: Rationale and strategies for chemoprevention of cancer in humans. Cancer Res. 1987; *47:* 3012–3031.
20 Moon R. C., Itri L. M.: Retinoids and cancer; in Sporn M. B., Roberts A. B., Goodman D. S. (eds.): The Retinoids. New York, Academic Press, 1984, vol. 2, pp. 327–371.
21 Harisiadis L., Miller R. C., Hall E. J., et. al.: Vitamin A analog inhibits radiation induced oncogenic transformation. Nature 1978; *274:* 486–487.
22 Hall E. J.: Oncogenic transformation studies with hyperthermia and X-rays; in Overgaard J. (ed.): Hyperthermia Oncology 1984. London, Taylor & Francis, 1984, vol. 1, pp. 479–483.
23 Dewey W. C.: Interaction of heat with radiation and chemotherapy. Cancer Res. 1984; *44(suppl):* 4714–4720.
24 Hei T. K., Hall E. J.: Radiation, chemotherapeutic agents and oncogenic transformation. Proc. Am. Assoc. Cancer Res. 1987; *28:* 470.
25 Loeffler J. S.: personal communication.

Eric J. Hall, DSc, Radiological Research Laboratory,
Department of Radiation Oncology, College of Physicians and Surgeons,
Columbia University, New York, NY 10032 (USA)

Vaeth JM, Meyer JL (eds): Radiation Tolerance of Normal Tissues.
Front Radiat Ther Oncol. Basel, Karger, 1989, vol 23, pp 140–149

Effects of Irradiation on the Human Immune System

Richard T. Hoppe
Department of Radiation Oncology, Stanford University, Stanford, Calif., USA

The human immune system consists of an intricate network of lymphoid tissues, organs, and circulating cells. The cells of the immune system, including the lymphocytes, monocytes-macrophages, and granulocytes, circulate in the peripheral blood and lymphatic systems and in addition have a ubiquitous presence in extravascular sites. Extranodal lymphoid aggregates are present in many regions, most notably the Peyer's patches of the small intestine and the Waldeyer lymphoid tissue. The organ components of the immune system include lymph nodes, spleen, thymus, and bone marrow.

Although the effects of irradiation on the human immune system may be profound, the multiplicity of organ and cellular components of the immune system, their complex interactions, and patterns of cellular migration have made the precise characterization of these abnormalities difficult.

Studies performed *in vitro* ignore the effects of cell interactions, the influence of lymphokines, and the impact of cell repopulation. *In vivo* studies are complicated by numerous and often uncontrollable variables. Irradiation may be directed at the entire body (with treatment of the entire immune system), it may be concentrated on the organ components of the immune system (total lymphoid irradiation), or it may be limited to regional sites which fortuitously include parts of the immune system such as lymph nodes or the circulating lymphocyte pool. Dose and fractionation are important variables, for which it is difficult to control in *in vivo* studies. For example, fractionated doses of whole-body irradiation (WBI) totaling as little as 1.5 Gy may be used in the management of low-grade lymphomas, while single doses as high as 8–10 Gy or fractionated doses in excess of 13.20 Gy may be used prior to bone marrow transplantation. For total lymphoid irradiation (TLI), fractionated doses of 18–44 Gy have been used in different situations. In the treatment of regional fields, even higher therapeutic doses may be utilized (60.00–65.00 Gy).

The characterization of *in vivo* effects is further complicated because many patients undergoing these treatment programs (such as in Hodgkin's disease) may have preexisting abnormalities of the immune system or may suffer from alterations of the immune system secondary to cytotoxic chemotherapy.

Despite the complexity of these problems, both empirical observations and careful laboratory studies have documented a variety of immune dysfunctions following therapeutic irradiation. Furthermore, the selected use of irradiation directed at the immune system (TLI) has proved to be a means of immunomanipulation to enhance transplantation tolerance and to manage patients with certain autoimmune diseases.

In vitro *Effects of Irradiation on Lymphocytes*

The survival curve for irradiated lymphocytes demonstrates a linear decrease in survival with increasing dose, expressed on a semi-log plot. There is little, if any, shoulder on the cell survival curve, indicating that lymphocytes are deficient in their ability to repair sublethal damage. The D_0 is 1.0–1.4 Gy, suggesting exquisite radiosensitivity [1]. Irradiated lymphocytes may undergo an interphase death, i.e., death during the G_0 phase of the cell cycle. The exact mechanism of interphase death is not known. It may not be related to an event at the DNA level, but perhaps to an effect on the cell surface membrane [2].

Lymphocytes undergo visible microscopic changes within 30 min after irradiation exposure [3]. Initially cytoplasmic swelling is noted. This is followed by dispersion of the chromatin to the periphery of the nucleus with development of a nuclear vacuole. Subsequently, there is nuclear phknosis and fragmentation and, finally, cytoplasmic disintegration. These changes may be detected with doses as low as 3.5 Gy [3].

Among different lymphocyte subpopulations, there is variation in *in vitro* radiosensitivity. B cells are more radiosensitive than T cells. The radiation sensitivity decreases following exposure to antigens, and committed B cells (i.e., plasma cells) are quite radioresistant, with no apparent effect of single doses as great as 8.0 Gy *in vitro* [3]. The decreased radiosensitivity of lymphocytes which have been exposed to antigen explains the relative radioresistance of the secondary antibody response compared to the primary antibody response. The nonlymphoid cells of the immune system, such as granulocytes and macrophages, also are relatively radioresistant, although their precursors may not be [3].

The relative radiosensitivity of different lymphocyte populations when measured *in vitro* does not necessarily correspond to *in vivo* observations. This is probably a result of repopulation kinetics which can have important effects *in vivo*, but are absent *in vitro*.

In vivo *Effects of Irradiation on Human Lymphoid Tissues*

Fractionated doses of irradiation in the range of 40–50 Gy may produce long-lasting changes in the histologic appearance of lymph nodes [3]. There may be cortical and follicular depletion of lymphocytes. When the depletion is extensive, the sinusoidal pattern within the lymph node may become more apparent. Occasionally, adipose cells may infiltrate the cortex of the node [3].

Long-term changes in the microscopic appearance of the spleen are apparent after fractionated doses in the therapeutic range (40 Gy) [4]. There may be capsular thickening, loss of parenchyma, fibrosis of the red pulp, loss of the white pulp, and myointimal proliferation of the arteries. These changes may be manifest grossly as splenic atrophy, with decreased splenic size and weight [4].

The changes induced by irradiation of the human thymus gland have not been described well. In adults the thymus is present as only a remnant, and the opportunity to observe histologic change is rare. However, in infants who received mediastinal irradiation, a rapid decrease in size of the thymus can be observed radiographically.

In vivo *Effects of Irradiation on Lymphocyte Subpopulations*

Whole-Body Irradiation

WBI leads to rapid depletion of peripheral blood lymphocytes. The severity of the depletion is dose related and is evident within 4 h after a dose of only 0.50 Gy [5]. Several investigators have looked at the kinetics of peripheral blood lymphocyte depletion among patients undergoing either fractionated or single-dose WBI in preparation for bone marrow transplantation [6, 7].

Dutreix et al. [6] examined peripheral blood lymphocyte counts before, during, and after single-dose and fractionated WBI and compared their observation with lymphocyte survival *in vitro* for the same patients. These were all patients with leukemia in remission, and the period of observation was limited to the time before which they received cytotoxic chemotherapy for their bone marrow transplantation. Seven patients were evaluated who received a single fraction of 10 Gy over a period of 4 h. Changes in total lymphocyte numbers were detectable at 2 h, after 5 Gy had been applied. At that time lymphocyte counts were 75% of pretreatment values. By 4 h (10 Gy total dose), the lymphocyte count had decreased to 60% of its baseline, at 8 h to 39, at 24 h to 26, at 48 h to 16, and at 72 h to 11%. In contrast, the *in vitro* decrement in lymphocyte counts was less marked. At 24 h, 76% of the lymphocytes were still viable, at 48 h 74, and at 72 h 53%. The authors speculated that the lymphocytes which die an interphase death are probably removed quite promptly *in vivo* by some unknown mechanism, and this accounts for the more rapid depletion of lymphocytes *in vivo* than in *in vitro*.

The same investigators studied peripheral blood lymphocyte counts in 18 patients who were undergoing fractionated WBI [6]. These patients received three 1.20-Gy fractions per day, each separated by approximately 5 h, for a total dose of 13.20 Gy. The total lymphocyte counts decreased to 58% of baseline values within 13 h after a single fraction of 1.20 Gy. As subsequent 1.20-Gy fractions were administered, the lymphocyte count continued to decrease exponentially, such that it was 45% at 24 h (after 3.60 Gy total dose), 25 at 48 h (after 7.20 Gy), and 8% at the time of completion of 13.20 Gy.

Based on their *in vivo* observations, these authors concluded that lymphocytes had a D_0 of approximately 1.20 Gy [6]. This observation is consistent with many *in vitro* observations.

Lymphocyte subsets were evaluated in a small group of patients tested 13–37 h after a single 1.20-Gy WBI [6]. No significant difference was detected between decreases in the T and B lymphocyte populations, nor was any difference detectable within the T cell population, when monoclonal antibody stains were employed to look at helper/inducer versus cytotoxic/suppressor cell populations.

Regional Irradiation

Regional irradiation, as commonly used in the treatment of cancer, has long been known to have lymphopenic effects [8, 9]. Although these lymphopenic effects are not generally as profound as those observed with WBI, it has been possible to follow these effects for a much longer period of time than after WBI. Several recent studies have looked at the effects of regional irradiation on lymphocyte subpopulations utilizing monoclonal antibody techniques [10, 11].

Rotstein et al. [11] examined the lymphocyte counts and lymphocyte subsets in a group of women who participated in a randomized trial comparing the management of breast cancer with surgery alone versus preoperative irradiation plus surgery versus surgery plus postoperative irradiation. The patients who were treated with surgery alone served as a control population. These investigators noted that the total lymphocyte counts were still depressed in the irradiated patients as long as 10–11 years after treatment. This decrease primarily was due to a decrease in the helper T cell population, while the B cells showed no significant decrease compared to the controls. Within the T cell population, the suppressor/cytotoxic population recovered to normal values within 5–6 years after completion of treatment, while those cells with the helper/inducer phenotype were still significantly decreased compared to the control population after 10–11 years. This observation is different from that of the WBI experience reported above [6], perhaps because of the duration of time after treatment when the lymphocytes were quantitated and repopulation effects.

Total Lymphoid Irradiation

Perhaps the best-studied effects of irradiation on the immune system relate to the alterations of lymphocyte subpopulations after fractionated TLI. These changes have been studied in patients undergoing TLI for the treatment of neoplastic diseases such as Hodgkin's disease and also in those who have undergone TLI for the management of autoimmune diseases.

Patients treated with fractionated TLI for Hodgkin's disease develop a marked lymphopenia during the course of TLI [12]. While the lymphocyte counts of some patients will eventually return to normal, many remain depressed for 10 or more years. However, even among patients who have recovery of the total lymphocyte count, there are long-term alterations of lymphocyte subsets. The B cells return to normal or even occasionally supranormal levels, while T cells remained depressed [12]. Examination of T lymphocyte subsets in these patients reveals a decrease in the percentage and/or absolute number of helper/inducer T cells and an increased percentage of suppressor/cytotoxic T cells [13, 14]. Patients treated with TLI for Hodgkin's disease also demonstrate an impaired ability to develop delayed hypersensitivity reactions, e.g., an inability to become sensitized to and respond to a challenge with dinitrochlorobenzene. In addition, the lymphocytes of these patients respond subnormally *in vitro* in the mixed lymphocyte reaction and in response to mitogens such as phytohemagglutinin and concanavalin A [12].

The alterations of lymphocyte subsets seen after high-dose fractionated TLI for Hodgkin's disease are mimicked in patients who have received low-dose fractionated TLI for the treatment of autoimmune diseases. Tanay et al. [15] studied the alterations of lymphocyte subsets and lymphocyte function in 32 patients who were treated with 20.00 Gy fractionated TLI for rheumatoid arthritis. The allogeneic mixed lymphocyte reaction and *in vitro* responses to phytohemagglutinin and pokeweed mitogen stimulated IGg secretion were markedly suppressed after the completion of TLI. Although gradual recovery of the mixed lymphocyte reaction was suggested after 3 years of observation, this function was still subnormal. There was no indication of recovery of the other functional assays. The absolute lymphocyte count in these patients was markedly depressed within the 1st month after TLI. Although the absolute lymphocyte count began to recover thereafter, it was still at only 50% of pretreatment value 1–4 years after TLI. The reduction in the helper/inducer population of T lymphocytes was more marked (75% reduction) than that of the suppressor/cytotoxic population (25% reduction). These abnormalities persisted for up to 3 years, after which the population of suppressor/cytotoxic cells was observed to recover to the pretreatment level, while that of the helper/inducer population remained reduced.

Clinical Implications of Radiation Immunosuppression

Radiation Complications

There are potential complications from radiation-induced immunosuppression. The primary effect is increased susceptibility to infection. In patients who are undergoing preparation for bone marrow transplantation, the intent of the WBI combined with high doses of chemotherapy is to paralyze the immune system. It is difficult to measure the relative impact of the irradiation and chemotherapy in achieving this end, but each modality certainly contributes. In the immediate posttransplant state, patients are at very high risk for developing viral infections with herpes-type viruses, especially herpes simplex, and later with cytomegalovirus. Herpes zoster may develop up to even several years after bone marrow transplantation. Bacterial infections are also common in the immediate posttransplant period, largely secondary to granulocytopenia.

After total lymphoid irradiation for the treatment of Hodgkin's disease, there appears to be an increased risk for the development of herpes zoster infections, but not other viral diseases. After treatment with irradiation alone, the risk for development of herpes zoster is approximately 10% during the first 2 years of observation [16]. Although herpes zoster has been reported to be common even in untreated patients with Hodgkin's disease due to abnormalities of cell-mediated immunity, the rate after treatment is probably higher than the background rate of infection. In addition, the frequency of development of herpes zoster has been reported to be higher than 25% for patients treated with low-dose TLI for autoimmune diseases [17].

Table I. Immunomanipulation with TLI for renal transplantation

Institution	Number of patients	Dose Gy	Drugs
University of Minnesota, Minneapolis, Minn., USA [19]	22	10.50–40.50	azathioprine, prednisolone
University of Leuven, Belgium [20]	24	20.00–30.00	prednisolone
Pacific Medical Center, Stanford University, Calif., USA [21]	50	20.00	antithymocyte globulin, prednisolone
	6	20.00	Anti-OKT3, prednisolone
University of Rome, Italy [22]	6	25.00–35.00	antilymphocyte globulin, azathioprine, prednisolone.
	14	15.00–20.00	cyclosporin A
University of Witwatersrand, South Africa [23]	8	21.00–32.00	prednisolone
	12	8.00–12.20	cyclosporin A, prednisolone

Table II. Immunomanipulation with TLI for autoimmune diseases

	Number of patients	Dose Gy	Institution
Rheumatoid arthritis	32	20.00	Stanford University, Stanford, Calif., USA [15]
	11	20.00	University of Erlangen, FRG [24]
	20	20.00, 7.50	St. Vincent's, Dublin, Ireland [25]
	12	30.00	Joint Center, Boston, Mass., USA [26]
Lupus nephritis	15	20.00	Stanford University [17]
Systemic lupus erythematosus	2	20.00	Hadassah University, Jerusalem, Israel [27]
Multiple sclerosis	20	19.80	Univ. Med. Dent. N.J. 7, USA [28]
Chronic demyelinating polyneuropathy	3	20.00	University of Colorado, Denver, Colo., USA [29]

Irradiation of the spleen, which is usually included in TLI fields, may also have effects on immune function. High-dose fractionated irradiation (40.0 Gy) may induce splenic atrophy, resulting in splenic hypofunction. Thery may be an increased risk for fatal sepsis, especially with gram-positive encapsulated organisms [4].

Immunomanipulation with TLI

The detailed characterization of the nature of the immune impairment induced by fractionated TLI in man led to a large number of laboratory investigations in animals, studying the potential effects of fractionated TLI on the course of autoimmune diseases and for the induction of transplantation tolerance [18]. These animal studies have now been extended into human clinical trials. In the realm of human renal transplantation TLI has been used by several investigators as an adjunct to standard immunosuppressive therapy or for patients at high risk for rejection [19–23]. These studies are summarized in table I. The most commonly treated autoimmune diseases have included rheumatoid arthritis, lupus nephritis, and multiple sclerosis (table II) [15, 17, 24–29].

Acknowledgements

The author is grateful to Marge Keskin who assisted in the preparation of the manuscript. This work was supported in part by grants CA 34233 and AI 11313 from the National Institutes of Health.

References

1 James S.E., Arlett C.F., Green M.H.L., et al.: Radiosensitivity of human T-lymphocytes proliferating in long-term culture. Int. J. Radiat. Oncol. Biol. Phys. 1983; *44:* 417–422.

2 Strober S., Weissman I.L.: Immunosuppressive and tolerogenic effects of whole-body, total lymphoid, and regional irradiation; in Salaman J.R. (ed): Immunosuppressive Therapy. J.B. Philadelphia, Lippincott, 1981, pp. 19–53.

3 Fajardo L.F.: Pathology of Radiation Injury. New York, Masson, 1982, pp. 147–165.

4 Dailey M.O., Coleman C.N., Kaplan H.S.: Radiation-induced splenic atrophy in patients with Hodgkin's disease and non-Hodgkin's lymphomas. N. Engl. J. Med. 1980; *302:* 215–217.

5 Anderson R.E., Standefer J.C., Tokuda S.: The structural and functional assessment of cytotoxic injury of the immune system with particular reference to the effects of ionizing radiation and cyclophosphamide. Br. J. Cancer. 1986; *53:* (suppl VII): 140–160.

6 Dutreix J., Girinski T., Cosset J.M., et al.: Blood cell kinetics and total body irradiation. Radiother Oncol 1987; *9:* 119–129.

7 Shank B., Andreeff M., Li D.: Cell survival kinetics in peripheral blood and bone marrow transplantation. Int. J. Radiat. Oncol. Biol. Phys. 1983; *9:* 1613–1623.

8 Stjernswärd J., Jondal M., Vanky F., et al.: Lymphopenia and change in distribution of human B- and T-lymphocytes in peripheral blood induced by irradiation for mammary carcinoma. Lancet 1972; *i:* 1352–1356.

9 Hoppe R.T., Fuks Z., Strober S., et al.: Long-term effects of radiation on T and B

lymphocytes in the peripheral blood after regional irradiation. Cancer 1977; *40:* 2071–2078.

10 Job G., Pfreundschuh M., Bauer M., et al.: The influence of radiation therapy on T-lymphocyte subpopulations defined by monoclonal antibodies. Int. J. Radiat. Oncol. Biol. Phys. 1984; *10:* 2077–2081.

11 Rotstein S., Blomgren H., Petrini B., et al.: Long-term effects on the immune system following local radiation therapy for breast cancer. I. cellular composition of the peripheral blood lymphocyte population. Int. J. Radiat. Oncol. Biol. Phys. 1985; *11:* 921–925.

12 Fuks Z., Strober S., Bobrove A. M., et al.: Long-term effects of radiation on T and B lymphocytes in peripheral blood of patients with Hodgkin's disease. J. Clin. Invest. 1976; *58:* 803–814.

13 Posner M. R., Reinherz E., Lane H., et al.: Circulating lymphocyte populations in Hodgkin's disease after mantle and para-aortic irradiation. Blood 1983; *61:* 705–708.

14 Schoeppel S., Hoppe R. T., Engleman E., et al.: Lymphocyte subsets in Hodgkin's disease patients treated with irradiation (abstract). Proc. AACR 1986; *27:* 329.

15 Tanay A., Field E. H., Hoppe R. T., et al.: Long-term follow-up of rheumatoid arthritis patients treated with total lymphoid irradiation. Arthritis Rheum 1987; *30:* 1–10.

16 Guinee V. F., Guido J. J., Pfalzgraf K. A., et al.: The incidence of herpes zoster in patients with Hodgkin's disease. An analysis of prognostic factors. Cancer 1985; *56:* 642–648.

17 Strober S., Farinas M. C., Field E. H., et al.: Lupus nephritis after total lymphoid irradiation: Persistent improvement and reduction of steroid therapy. Ann. Intern. Med. 1987; *107:* 689–690.

18 Hoppe R. T., Strober S.: Total lymphoid irradiation for immunosuppression; in Withers H. R., Peters L. (eds): Innovations in Radiation Oncology. Heidelberg, Springer, 1987, pp. 113–119.

19 Najarian J. S., Ferguson R. M., Sutherland D. E. R., et al.: Fractionated total lymphoid irradiation as preparative immunosuppression in high-risk renal transplantation. Clinical and immunological studies. Ann. Surg. 1982; *196:* 442–452.

20 Ang K. K., Vanrenterghem Y., Waer M., et al.: Kidney allograft tolerance in diabetic patients after total lymphoid irradiation (TLI). Radiother. Oncol. 1985; *3:* 193–199.

21 Levin B., Hoppe R. T., Collins G., et al.: Treatment of cadaveric renal transplant recipients with total lymphoid irradiation, antithymocyte globulin, and low-dose prednisone. Lancet 1985; *ii:* 1321–1325.

22 Cortesini R., Molajoni E. R., Monari C., et al.: Total lymphoid irradiation in clinical transplantation: Experience in 30 high-risk patients. Transplant. Proc. 1985; *17:* 1291–1293.

23 Myburgh J. A., Smit J. A., Meyers A. M., et al.: Total lymphoid irradiation in renal transplantation. World J. Surg. 1986; *10:* 369–380.

24 Nusslein H. G., Herbst M., Manger B. J., et al.: Total lymphoid irradiation in patients with refractory rheumatoid arthritis. Arthritis. Rheum. 1985; *28:* 1205–1210.

25 Hanly J. G., Hassan J., Moriarty M., et al.: Lymphoid irradiation in intractable rheumatoid arthritis. A double-blind, randomized study comparing 750-rad treatment with 2,000-rad treatment. Arthritis. Rheum. 1986; *29:* 16–25.

26 Brahn E., Helfgott S. M., Belli J. A., et al.: Total lymphoid irradiation therapy in refractory rheumatoid arthritis. Fifteen- to forty-month follow-up. Arthritis. Rheum. 1984; *27:* 481–488.

27 Ben-Chetrit E., Gross D. J., Braverman A., et al.: Total lymphoid irradiation in refractory systemic lupus erythematosus. Ann. Intern. Med. 1986; *105:* 58–60.

28 Cook S. D., Devereux C., Troiano R., et al.: Effect of total lymphoid irradiation in chronic progressive multiple sclerosis. Lancet. 1986; *i:* 1405–1409.
29 Rosenberg N. L., Lacy J. R., Kennaugh R. C., et al.: Treatment of refractory chronic demyelinating polyneuropathy with lymphoid irradiation. Muscle Nerve 1985; *8:* 223–232.

Richard T. Hoppe, MD, Department of Radiation Oncology,
Stanford University, Stanford, CA 94305 (USA)

Vaeth JM, Meyer JL (eds): Radiation Tolerance of Normal Tissues.
Front Radiat Ther Oncol. Basel, Karger, 1989, vol 23, pp 150–159

Normal-Tissue Effects of Irradiation for Kaposi's Sarcoma/AIDS[1]

Rodney Rodriguez[a,b], *James Fontanesi*[a,b], *John L. Meyer*[c], *Jerome Vaeth*[a], *Mark Rounsaville*[b], *Phil Vogt*[b,e]

[a] St. Mary's Hospital, San Francisco, Calif.;
[b] Veteran's Administration Hospital, Martinez, Calif.;
[c] St. Francis Memorial Hospital, San Francisco, Calif.;
[d] Children's Hospital, San Francisco, Calif.;
[e] University of California, Davis, Calif., USA

Introduction

By 1991, it is estimated that 270,000 patients will be diagnosed with acquired immune deficiency syndrome (AIDS) in the United States in accordance with the classification criteria of the Center for Disease Control, USA [24]. Approximately 15% of the cases will present with Kaposi's sarcoma (KS), and an additional 30% will develop KS during their disease course [9, 24]. With improved treatment of the opportunistic infections that are responsible for the majority of deaths and the use of antiviral agents, such as azidothymidine, a prolongation of survival has been observed [8] and may further increase the incidence of KS in AIDS patients.

Since the recognition of KS as part of the AIDS epidemic, several publications have analyzed the response of KS lesions to irradiation, often according to the dose of irradiation used [2–4, 12, 13, 20, 21, 23, 25]. In several of these series, there have been reports of unusually pronounced early normal-tissue reactions in skin (that were not previously noted in patients treated for classical KS) [11, 12, 14, 19] and in mucosal sites (that were atypical for the radiation doses and fractionation schedules used) [2–4, 12, 20, 23].

In this review, we report a retrospective analysis on 56 patients diagnosed with AIDS and treated with irradiation for KS at four San

Francisco Bay Area hospitals. We have determined normal-tissue responses in 182 treatment sites according to the daily and total radiation doses, number of treatment days, radiation type and energy, prior use of chemotherapy, and the presence of opportunistic infections.

Materials and Methods

The treatment records of all patients seen with the diagnosis of KS and AIDS and treated in the Departments of Radiation Oncology at St. Francis Memorial Hospital, Children's Hospital of San Francisco, St. Mary's Hospital of San Francisco, and the Veteran's Administration Medical Center, Martinez, were retrospectively reviewed. Clinical characteristics of these 56 patients are shown in table I. All patients were males in high-risk groups for exposure to human immunodeficiency virus and were treated for palliation of symptoms, primarily pain, bleeding or tumor bulk, and occasionally for cosmesis. Many patients had histories of opportunistic infections.

One hundred and eighty-two lesions were treated (table II) using radiation therapy delivered from low-energy X-ray units (60–122 kVp), a betatron generator (with the selection of 4, 6, or 8 MeV electrons), a ^{60}Co teletherapy unit, or a 4-MeV linear accelerator.

Response to treatment was evaluated one or more times per week during treatment and recorded into treatment records. Because retrospective review was anticipated by the participating physicians, they endeavored to be especially accurate in recording tumor response and normal-tissue toxicity. Mucosal toxicity was graded according to the RTOG classification, and skin toxicity was graded using a modification of the scoring system of Fowler et al. [8] (table III). Photography often was used to further document these effects. Both toxicities were graded prospectively in most cases and retrospectively in others.

Table I. Patient characteristics (n = 56; age range 24–54, mean 36 years)

White	51/56
Hispanic	3/56
Black	2/56
Homosexual	56/56
Intravenous drug users	1/56
Transfusion recipients	0/56
Previous opportunistic infections	
Pneumocystis pneumonia	25/56
Hepatitis	7/56
Cytomegalovirus	5/56
Mycobacterium	5/56
Gonorrhea	5/56
Syphilis	4/56
Toxoplasmosis	4/56
Herpes	4/56
Others	6/56

Table II. Treatment sites

Site	n
Mucosal	
Oral cavity	15
Oropharynx	4
Nasopharynx	1
Larynx	1
Paranasal sinus	1
Skin	
Penis	4
Face/neck	55
Upper extremities	20
Lower extremities	68
Torso	13

Table III. Mucosal and skin toxicities observed

RTOG classification of mucosal toxicity	
grade	description
0	no change over baseline
1	erythema, may experience pain not requiring analgesics
2	patchy mucositis which may produce inflammatory serosanguinous discharge, may have pain requiring analgesics
3	confluent fibrinous mucositis, may have pain requiring narcotics
4	ulceration, hemorrhage or necrosis
Early skin reactions occurring during or at the end of treatment (modification of Fowler's system)	
0	normal skin
1	erythema
2	dry desquamation
3	moist desquamation
4	necrosis
Late skin reactions occurring after treatment completed	
	hypopigmentation
	hyperpigmentation

Most patients returned to the treatment clinics for monthly evaluations after therapy, and scoring of tumor response and normal-tissue reaction was routinely emphasized at these visits. While intercurrent medical problems often interrupted long-term follow-up, all patients were seen after therapy, and most were followed for at least 3 months. For this review, all available information from hospital and medical office charts and tumor registries was used and was often supplemented by phone calls to the patients or their families.

Results

Mucosal Lesions

Twenty-two mucosal sites were treated with irradiation. Total doses ranged from 900 to 3,150 cGy with daily fractions ranging from 150 to 300 cGy. Eight sites developed scores <2, and fourteen sites developed scores ≥2. Tables IV and V show that development of mucosal toxicity with an RTOG score ≥2 did not appear to be related to the radiation energy or type, mean daily dose, or history of prior chemotherapy or of opportunistic infection. However, we did observe that mucosal sites developing scores ≥2 received treatment over a shorter period of time than those with scores ≤2. Analysis of treatments according to daily dose shows a clear trend toward increased reaction with larger daily fractions. Larger numbers of patients were not treated with fractions over 200 cGy because of this clear early trend. No correlation could be made between toxicity score and total dose used. Complete response rates observed at sites with scores <2 versus ≥2 were 38 and 50%, respectively, with partial response rates of 62 and 50%. No patient failed to achieve at least 50% objective tumor regression.

Two patients with grade 3 mucosal reactions consented to a biopsy of the treated area. Microscopic review showed infiltration by lymphohistiocytic inflammatory cells; neutrophils were occasionally seen. Some areas revealed epithelial cell degeneration, characterized by contracted eosinophilic cells with pyknotic nuclei. The supporting stroma demonstrated fibrosis and lymphohistiocytic infiltration with occasional plasma cells and eosinophils. None of these effects differed from radiation reactions occurring in non-AIDS patients.

Skin

One hundred sixty sites were irradiated for symptomatic KS involving the skin. Total doses ranged from 450 to 3,600 cGy (except for 1 patient who received one 180-cGy dose) with daily fraction sizes ranging from 65 to 400 cGy. Skin toxicity was graded by scoring effects during treatment or at the end of treatment. Thirty out of 160 (19%) sites developed reactions ≥2 during and 43 of 160 (27%) sites after treatment.

Comparing treatment parameters in patients with acute reaction scoring ≥2 to <2, there was no difference in radiation type or energy, mean daily dose, mean number of treatment days, mean total dose or prior chemotherapy, or opportunistic infection history (table VI, VII). Similar results were seen concerning the development of late reactions (table VIII). An unusual late reaction was the development of hypopigmentation in 12% of the patients. Eleven of 19 (58%) sites that developed

Table IV. Mucosal lesions – effect of the type of radiation energy, dose, previous chemotherapy, and history of opportunistic infections (mucosal lesions with RTOG score <2 vs. ≥2)

Score	Number of cases	Therapeutic units			Irradiation			Chemotherapy %	Opportunistic infections %
		superficial	^{60}Co/4 MeV	electrons	mean daily dose cGy	days	mean total dose cGY		
<2	8	14	79	7	191	22.8	2,175	7	29
≥2	14	13	88	0	188	13.6	1,640	0	38

Table V. Mucosal lesions – effect of daily dose and total dose on early reactions

Dose cGy	Cases	RTOG scores	Mean score	Score ≥2	
				n	%
Daily					
≤150	10	2, 0, 1, 3, 1	.7	3/10	30
	9	1, 3, 3, 1, 2			
151–200		3, 3, 1, 3, 3, 3, 1, 3, 3	2.5	7/9	78
201–300	0	–	–	–	
301–350	3	4, 2, 1	2.3	3/3	100
Total					
<999	1	1	1	0/1	
1,000–1,500	8	3, 2, 1, 3, 1, 3, 1, 0	1.75	4/8	
1,500–2,000	4	3, 3, 1, 1	2	2/4	
2,001–2,500	3	3, 3, 3	3	3/3	
2,501–3,000	2	3, 2	2.5	2/2	
≥3,001	4	4, 3, 1, 3	2.5	3/4	

Table VI. Skin lesions with early reactions – scores <2 vs. ≥2

Score	Number of cases	Therapeutic units			Irradiation			Chemotherapy %	Opportunistic infections %
		superficial	^{60}Co/4 MeV	electrons	mean daily dose cGy	days	mean total dose cGY		
<2	130	73	4	23	201	14	1,748	17	22
≥2	30	47	30	23	219	14.6	1,765	20	20

Table VII. Skin lesions without versus late reactions of hypopigmentation and hyperpigmentation

Late reaction	Number of cases	Therapeutic units			mean daily dose cGY	days	mean total dose cGY	Chemo-therapy %	Opportu-nistic infections %
		super-ficial	^{60}Co/4 MeV	elec-trons					
None	117	66	25	9	210	14	1,699	15	13
Hypo- and hyper-pigmentation	43	74	19	7	201	17	1,727	26	47

hypopigmentation had a previous history of chemotherapy treatment with Velban compared to 8% of the patients who did not have late skin reactions after Velban treatment.

Further analysis of acute and late reactions, with respect to toxicity versus total dose, failed to show an effect by total dose (table VIII). A trend toward the development of a high incidence of early reactions with scores ≥2 was observed with increasing daily fractions sizes (table IX, 5% with ≤150, 22 with 150–200, and 32% with 201–300).

Discussion

For decades, irradiation has been the mainstay of treatment for KS occurring in non-AIDS patients, and with the epidemic of AIDS the use of radiotherapy for KS has been continued. There is no difference evident in the pathological appearance by light microscopy of the 'epidemic' form of KS in comparison to its 'classical' form [5], and KS continues to be highly responsive to irradiation in the new clinical situation [6, 15, 25].

Several series have reported on the radiotherapeutic treatment of epidemic KS involving mucosal sites [4, 12, 13, 16, 17, 20, 21, 23], and several have reported unusual difficulties because of mucosal reactions after moderately low radiation doses [3, 4, 12, 20, 23, 27]. Cooper and Fried [3] reported on 5 patients with exaggerated mucosal toxicity. They speculated on causes, including the possible presence of subclinical infection or perhaps certain as yet undefined effects. In a subsequent communication [4], they describe four (4/4) patients who developed mucositis at relatively low doses (2,700 cGy treated at 300 cGy/fraction, 1,800 cGy treated at 300 cGy/fraction, 1,200 cGy treated at 200 cGy/fraction, and 750 cGy treated at 150 cGy/fraction). Watkins et al. [25], reporting on patients treated at the National Cancer Institute, also noted enhanced reactions in mucosal sites treated with irradiation: 7 of 8 patients receiv-

Table VIII. Skin lesions – effect of total dose on acute and late reactions

Total dose, cGy	Number of cases	Mean score	Score										Late reactions			
			0		1		2		≥3		≥2		hypopigmentation		hyperpigmentation	
			n	%	n	%	n	%	n	%	n	%	n	%	n	%
<999	12	0.75	8	67	1	8	1	8	2	17	3	25	3	25	0	0
1,000–1,500	42	0.8	21	50	11	26	10	24	0	0	10	24	2	5	3	7
1,501–2,000	54	0.85	21	39	24	44	6	11	3	6	9	17	9	17	10	19
2,001–2,500	28	0.6	15	54	10	35	3	11	0	0	3	11	3	11	6	21
2,501–3,000	19	1.0	9	47	5	26	1	5	4	22	5	27	1	6	0	0
≥3,001	5	0.8	1	20	4	80	0	0	0	0	0	0	0	0	4	80
Total	160	0.8	75		55		21		9				18		23	

Table IX. Skin lesions – effect of daily dose on acute and late reactions

Total dose, cGy	Number of cases	Mean score	Score										Late reactions			
			0		1		2		≥3		≥2		hypopigmentation		hyperpigmentation	
			n	%	n	%	n	%	n	%	n	%	n	%	n	%
≤150	29	0.8	15	51	13	44	1	5	0		1	5	15	51	12	41
151–200	93	0.9	32	34	41	44	15	16	5	6	20	22	15	16	12	13
201–300	34	0.1	15	44	8	24	7	21	4	11	11	32	2	6	5	15
301–350	0	0	0		0		0		0		0		0		0	
>351	4	0	4	100	0		0		0		0		0		0	

ing 1,200 cGy exhibited mucositis, and 4 required treatment interruption. No correlation could be made between the toxicity and OKT4 (helper) lymphocyte levels.

Our series of 22 patients confirms these earlier reports of pronounced mucosal reactions to irradiation of moderate dose. Patients experiencing mucosal reaction had a slightly higher total irradiation dose (2,175 vs. 1,640 cGy). However, fraction size, total treatment time, radiation type and energy, concurrent chemotherapy, and history of opportunistic infection failed to predict the development of reaction. Therefore, the most striking finding is the sporatic occurrence of the enhanced normal-tissue effect. Causative factors remain undefined, but are of great theoretical and practical interest for additional investigation.

It must be emphasized that all mucosal reactions have been transient and of brief duration; no permanent xerostomia or other late effects have been evident. Also, all patients have achieved partial or complete tumor response despite the restricted doses of irradiation used, providing meaningful palliative benefit. Because the mucosal reactions develop gradually, with little effect of the overall treatment time on the palliative response, we currently prefer to treat with the unusual fractionation schedule of 150 cGy, 4 days/week. Examination of patients after every other treatment has reduced treatment-related morbidity to a minimum. A treatment break of 1 week is given after 1,200 cGy, and a total dose of approximately 1,800 cGy is delivered. Based on our experience, we encourage the use of radiotherapy for symptomatic mucosal KS if treatment is administered with cautious fractionation programs and frequent examination of patients.

Our data concerning treatment of skin sites are not different from that reported in other series for epidemic KS [4, 12, 21]. Tumor response and consequent palliation of pain, bleeding, and tumor bulk were obtained in a very high percentage of patients with relatively low doses of irradiation. However, there has been a high incidence of radiation-induced hyperpigmentation or hypopigmentation and/or of residual tumor-induced tissue pigmentation following treatment. Therefore, cosmesis has been suboptimal in some cases, although improved from the pretreatment condition. Major tissue complications have been very uncommon.

References

1 Boylston, A. W.; Cook, H. T.; Francis, N. D.; Goldin, R. O.: Biopsy pathology of acquired immune deficiency syndrome (AIDS). J. clin. Path. *40:* 1–8 (1987).

2 Cooper, J. S.; Fried, P. R.; Laubenstein, L. J.: Initial observations of the effect of radiotherapy on epidemic Kaposi's sarcoma. J. Am. med. ASS. *252:* 934–935 (1984).

3 Cooper, J. S.; Fried, P. R.: Toxicity of oral radiotherapy in patients with acquired immune deficiency syndrome. Archs Otolar. Head Neck Surg. *113:* 327–328 (1987).

4 Cooper, J. S.; Fried, P. R.: Defining the role of radiation therapy in the management of epidemic Kaposi's sarcoma. Int. J. Radiat. Oncol. Biol. Phys. *13:* 35–39 (1987).

5 Dorfman, R. F.: Cutaneous and lymphatic Kaposi's sarcoma in Africa and the USA with observations on persistent lymphadenopathy in homosexual men at risk for the acquired immune deficiency syndrome. Front. Radiat. Ther. Onc., vol. 19, pp. 105–116 (Karger, Basel 1985).

6 El-Akkad, S.; Bull, C. A.; El-Senorussi, M. A., et al.: Kaposi's sarcoma and its management by radiotherapy. Archs Derm. *122:* 1396–1399 (1986).

7 Fischl, M. A.; Richman, D. O.; Griego, M. H., et al.: The efficacy of azidothymidine (AZT) in the treatment of patients with AIDS and AIDS-related complex. New Engl. J. Med. *317:* 187–191 (1987).

8 Fowler, J. F.; Morgan, R. L.; Silvester, J. A.; Bewley, D. K.; Turner, B. A.: Experiments with fractionated irradiation of the skin of pigs. Br. J. Radiol. *36:* 188–196 (1963).

9 Freidman-Kein, A. E.; Laubenstein, L. J.; Rubinstein, P., et al.: Disseminated Kaposi's sarcoma in homosexual men. Ann. intern. Med. *96:* 693–700 (1982).

10 Gottlieg, G. J.; Ackerman, A. B.: Kaposi's sarcoma: an extensively disseminated form in young homosexual men. Human Pathol. *13:* 882–892 (1982).

11 Hamilton, C. R.; Cummings, B. J.; Harwood, A. R.: Radiotherapy of Kaposi's sarcoma. Int. J. Radiat. Oncol. Biol. Phys. *12:* 1931–1935 (1986).

12 Harris, J. W.; Reed, T. A.: Kaposi's sarcoma in AIDS: the role of radiation therapy. Front. Radiat. Ther. Onc., vol. 19, pp. 126–132 (Karger, Basel 1985).

13 Hill, D. R.: The role of radiotherapy for epidemic Kaposi's sarcoma. Semin. Oncol. *14:* 19–22 (1987).

14 Holecek, M. J.; Harwood, A. R.: Radiotherapy of Kaposi's sarcoma. Cancer *41:* 1733–1738 (1978).

15 Lo, T. C. M.; Salzman, F. A.; Smedal, M. I.; Wright, K. A.: Radiotherapy for Kaposi's sarcoma. Cancer *45:* 684–687 (1980).

16 Morbid. Mortal. wkly Rep. *30:* 305–308 (1981).

17 Morbid. Mortal. wkly Rep. *31:* 507–514 (1982).

18 Morbid. Mortal. wkly Rep. *35:* 757–766 (1986).

19 Nisce, L. Z.; Safai, B.; Poussin-Rosillo, H.: Once weekly total and subtotal electron beam therapy for Kaposi's sarcoma. Cancer *47:* 640–644 (1981).

20 Nisce, L. Z.; Safai, B.: Radiation therapy of Kaposi's sarcoma in AIDS. Front. Radiat. Ther. Onc., vol. 19, pp. 133–137 (Karger, Basel 1985).

21 Nobler, M. P.; Leddy, M. E.; Huh, S. H.: The impact of palliative irradiation on the management of patients with acquired immune deficiency syndrome. J. clin. Oncol. *5:* 107–112 (1987).

22 Publ. Hlth. Rep., Wash. *101:* 459–466 (1986).

23 Real, F. X.; Krown, S. E.; Nisce, L. Z.; Oettgen, H. F.: Unexpected toxicity from radiation therapy in two patients with Kaposi's sarcoma receiving interferon. J. biol. Response Modif. *4:* 141–146 (1985).

24 Safai, B.; Johnson, K. G.; Myskowski, P. L., et al.: The natural history of Kaposi's sarcoma in the acquired immune deficiency syndrome. Ann. intern. Med. *103:* 744–750 (1985).

25 Watkins, S. B.; Findley, P.; Gelmann, E., et al.: Enhanced mucosal reactions in AIDS patients receiving oropharyngeal irradiation. Int. J. Radiat. Oncol. Biol. Phys. *13:* 1403–1408 (1987).
26 Welch, K.; Finkbeiner, W.; Alpers, C. E., et al.: Autopsy findings in the acquired immune deficiency syndrome. J. Am. med. Ass. *52:* 1152–1159 (1984).
27 Weshler, Z.; Loewinger, E.; Lowenthal, E.; Levinson, R.; Fuks, Z.: Megavoltage radiotherapy using water bolus in the treatment of Kaposi's sarcoma. Int. J. Radiat. Oncol. Biol. Phys. *12:* 2029–2032 (1986).

R. Rodriguez, MD, St. Mary's Hospital, San Francisco, CA 94143 (USA)

Vaeth JM, Meyer JL (eds): Radiation Tolerance of Normal Tissues.
Front Radiat Ther Oncol. Basel, Karger, 1989, vol 23, pp 160–161

Discussion

Dr. Yatvin: Dr. Eric Hall, in the studies you have done on transformation, in two of the drugs that you used, you had a decrease in transformation. Was heat, perhaps, inactivating those drugs? If you could mention what you thought what might account for that decrease in transformation? Does transformation occur when you remove the inhibitors that you had? In other words, you can prevent it? In the studies (with B-16 melanoma) that have been done, one can get them to grow, contact inhibited, but when you remove the inhibitor, they again act as a transformed cell.

Dr. Hall: The short answer is 'no' and 'yes'. So, I guess I should amplify a little. The answer to the first question is no, the heat is not inactivating the drug. The heat mixed with the drug produces significant increases in cytotoxicity, so the drug is not being inactivated. I think that is reasonably clear. The broader and longer question is what happens with these inhibitors of transformation. That is a very perceptive question and a complicated one to answer. Certainly, with many of these agents, one must keep the suppressing agent on for a significant period of time. These are all, of course, in vitro experiments. We are only talking about 6 weeks or so. With some of them you can add the inhibitor, and the expression of malignancy goes away. You take the inhibitor away, and you get a development of transformed focus again – with some, not with others. In an in vitro situation, what you might have happening is that if you can suppress the development of the clone of transformed cells at an early stage – stop it from ever growing to a point where it can take off – you can then permanently remove the inhibitor, and you don't get a re-expression afterwards of the tumor. But you are quite right, with some of these agents, not with all, in vitro, you can take them on and off and have the malignancy expressed or not expressed.

Dr. Gillette: Dr. Kinsella, when you first made the estimate of a 50-Gy tolerance dose for the aorta in beagles, you had an observation period of about 3 years. You have had longer observation after that. Perhaps you can comment on that.

We started our studies sometime after those of the National Cancer Institute and have just completed this past fall an observation period of 5 years of beagles given either intraoperative radiotherapy or a combination of IORT with a fractionated course of external beam irradiation or a fractionated course of XRT alone. What we have found is that a dose with a 50% probability of causing serious lesions in the aorta, and that included large thromboses and dissecting aneurysms, was 35 Gy with IORT alone and 27 Gy when given in combination with 50-Gy fractionated course given in 2-Gy fractions in 5 weeks. We have observed only one rupture of an aorta. That was at a higher dose of 47.5 Gy plus 50-Gy fractionated course. The dose that causes some pretty serious lesions in the aorta is lower than what was initially observed at the National Cancer Institute. I think we would agree with one of the final conclusions of Dr. Kinsella and his colleagues in that it does appear that doses of 15 or 20 Gy IORT seem to be reasonably well tolerated, even in combination with a 50-Gy fractionated course, but I do know that they have some longer observation periods.

Dr. Kinsella: We did follow those animals out 5 years and sacrificed them sometime in early 1987 and decided not to follow them any further. And certainly with every 6 months, having arteriograms and venacavograms, we didn't see any significant problems. Some dogs did develop focal narrowing. They didn't have any major problems. We didn't see any dissection of the aorta, and the histological changes were one of intimal or subintimal fibrosis but nothing major.

Vaeth JM, Meyer JL (eds): Radiation Tolerance of Normal Tissues.
Front Radiat Ther Oncol. Basel, Karger, 1989, vol 23, pp 162–176

Normal-Tissue Effects of Hyperthermia[1]

J. L. Meyer[a,b], *D. S. Kapp*[b]

[a]Department of Radiation Therapy, St. Francis Hospital, San Francisco, Calif.;
[b]Department of Radiation Oncology, Stanford University, Stanford, Calif., USA

Hyperthermia and Normal Tissues

Many biological and physical characteristics of normal tissues can influence both the delivery of hyperthermia treatment and the tissue responses to it: tissue-specific energy absorption characteristics, aspects of normal cell biology, human anatomy and normal-tissue physiology (especially the vascular response to hyperthermia), as well as a variety of clinical concerns can be important.

Biologically, we know that cellular thermal sensitivity can vary appreciably and sometimes unpredictably between different normal cell types [15]. In some cases, but certainly not all, tumors can be more heat sensitive than their normal-tissue counterparts. The tissue resting temperature before treatment, and the rate of heating during treatment, can influence thermal sensitivity [14] – of importance for near-surface tumors and for skin that can be initially cooler than deeper tissues. A prior thermal exposure (and certain other cellular 'stresses') can induce thermotolerance [15, 41]. The radiation history of the tissue may effect thermal sensitivity in some cases [3, 19, 28, 60], as well as vascular and metabolic changes during treatment which alter the cellular microenvironments. Further, pharmocologic influences can modify cell sensitivity to heat [15].

The physical characteristics of normal tissues influence and limit tumor heating in several important ways. The power that reaches and is absorbed in tumors is determined by the nature of the overlying normal tissue types, their thickness, and the orientation of their fascial planes to the energy sources. Fat distribution is especially important for certain electromagnetic methods and bone and air distribution for ultrasonic

[1]This work was supported in part by Grant No. CA-44665 from the National Cancer Institute.

ones. Blood flow can produce substantial temperature gradients between and within normal tissues and tumors, and blood flow rates can change during each treatment and over the several sessions of treatment [51]. The therapeutic objective, targeting of the treatment power into tumors with the maximal avoidance of normal tissues, sometimes can be aided by active normal-tissue cooling during treatment.

Clinically, the cardiovascular tolerance of patients and their tolerance of treatment-induced discomfort and other effects are often power limiting during treatment [24, 40, 52]. Such protective responses of the human body may add greater safety to the therapy, since medical constraints limit the number of tissue sites than can be invasively monitored by temperature sensors (although such monitoring is crucial).

All of these interrelations between hyperthermia and normal tissues constitute a range of effects at least as great, if not greater, as between irradiation and normal tissues. The combination of hyperthermia with irradiation creates even more complexity. Several reviews have summarized concerns about the effects of hyperthermia on normal tissues from the points of view of biology [11, 15, 18], pathology [8], and clinical oncology [23, 24, 37–39, 45]. Here we would like to make a few pertinent comments.

General Concepts

Normal tissue reactions usually develop earlier after hyperthermia than after irradiation, as Hume and Myers [20] have shown in a murine system evaluating skin reactions. Studies evaluating other normal tissues, including intestine [19], testis [17], kidney [7], and brain [33], also reveal this. Most probably this results from the multiple direct effects of heat on cell organelle structure and function, in addition to its effects on mitotic activity [15, 18]. In situations where reversible normal tissue reactions occur, they generally resolve earlier after hyperthermia than after irradiation, as Stone and Harding [54] and Hume [18] have shown in murine skin.

Evaluating the results from several experimental systems, Field and Morris [12] have summarized the relationship between the duration of treatment and the treatment temperature in achieving a given tissue effect. When temperatures above about 43 °C are used, each degree increase in temperature allows a decrease in the time of exposure by close to 50% for the same effect. A parallel observation is the fact that increasing temperature with the same duration of treatment steeply increases effect. Thus, there is a certain commonality in the 'time-temperature relationship' between systems which remains true despite the different end points used in these systems and the different specific temperatures and times required for these end points. These concepts have been incorporated into a thermal dose formulation that attempts to relate varying treatment temperatures to biologically equivalent ones at 43 °C [46].

Thermotolerance is an egalitarian finding that can greatly influence the heat responsiveness of both tumors and normal tissues and has been demonstrated in almost all cells and tissues evaluated [15]. Brief (15–30 min), low temperature (41.0 °C) exposures can induce thermotolerance in normal tissues and tumors within 1 hour [41]. Thermotolerance can affect the radiosensitization as well as the direct cytotoxic effects of hyperthermia and can persist to some extent for 5 days or longer [42, 57]. Clinical studies are now underway to evaluate the significance of these factors in human tumors and normal tissues, and early results indicate that they are also active phenomena here [1, 22].

In the clinic, hyperthermia usually will be employed in combination with irradiation, often in previously irradiated tissues. Will prior irradiation affect the hyperthermic enhancement of radiation effect? In several murine systems, thermal enhancement ratios based on experimental isoeffects have been calculated both for previously irradiated and for unirradiated tissues [18]. Prior irradiation appears to have little effect on enhancement ratios, either for early- or late-effect assay end points.

These and other small-animal (primarily murine) studies give valuable information about the relative sensitivities of normal tissues under varying conditions. To establish the specific temperature sensitivities of individual organ systems, large-animal studies have been undertaken to hopefully model human tissue responses, and additional information is now accumulating from several ongoing human clinical trials.

Tissue Responses to Hyperthermia

Skin

Hyperthermia Alone. The times and temperatures necessary to induce small, visible burns in the skin of pigs and human volunteers were comprehensively studied by Moritz and Henriques [43] 4 decades ago. At controlled temperatures, varying from 44 to 100 °C, circulating hot water was contacted to skin through an aperture of 25 mm for the pig and 7 mm for the human studies; exposure times varied from 1 to 7 h. (This method would likely result in a rapid fall-off of temperatures over the first 3–4 mm of tissue depth.) Treated sites were observed visually until the reactions had subsided, and histological verification of necrosis confirmed the visual appearance in a subgroup of sites.

Overall, the time-temperature exposures necessary to induce necrosis were very similar for pigs and humans and were reproducible at each exposure level. 'The lowest surface temperature that was responsible for cutaneous burning in these experiments was 44 °C and the time required to cause irreversible damage to epidermal cells at this temperature was approximately 6 h . . . and for each degree rise in surface temperature, between 44 and 51 °C, the time required to produce such injury was reduced by approximately one-half' [43].

In the humans, discomfort occurred during treatment with temperatures of 47.5–48.5 °C, but was experienced more by some subjects than by others. Burns sometimes followed treatments in which there was no discomfort, and vescicle formation did not always precede transepidermal necrosis. We will discuss our own clinical experience after considering the effect of hyperthermia on subcutaneous fat and muscle tissues, which also can be within the treatment fields with superficial hyperthermia methods.

Hyperthermia and Irradiation. Few controlled, quantitative investigations evaluating the enhancement of irradiation effect on specific tissues in large animals or humans have been reported. However, Hand et al. [16] evaluated the response of porcine skin to X-rays alone or in combination with microwave hyperthermia. Using waveguide applicators operating at 2,450 MHz, they delivered temperatures of 42 or 44 °C (monitored at the skin surface) for 90 min following each of one or three fractions of irradiation (giving total doses of 1,000–3,900 rad). Treated sites were visually monitored for 16 weeks by multiple observers who independently scored the evident damage on a graded scale. Average scores of the maximum evident damage showed therapeutic enhancement ratios of only 1.05–1.1, indicating that little enhancement of irradiation effect had occurred. Since these hyperthermia treatment temperatures are often used clinically, their results would be expected to parallel the human situation.

Mesenchymal Tissues: Fat and Skeletal Muscle

Workers at Stanford University have performed normal-tissue investigations in swine to attempt to identify and quantify the pathological changes in subcutaneous fat and skeletal muscle tissues [9, 35, 36]. A radiofrequency capacitive system was used to treat sections of the flanks of pigs, and initial studies showed that tissue temperatures were fairly

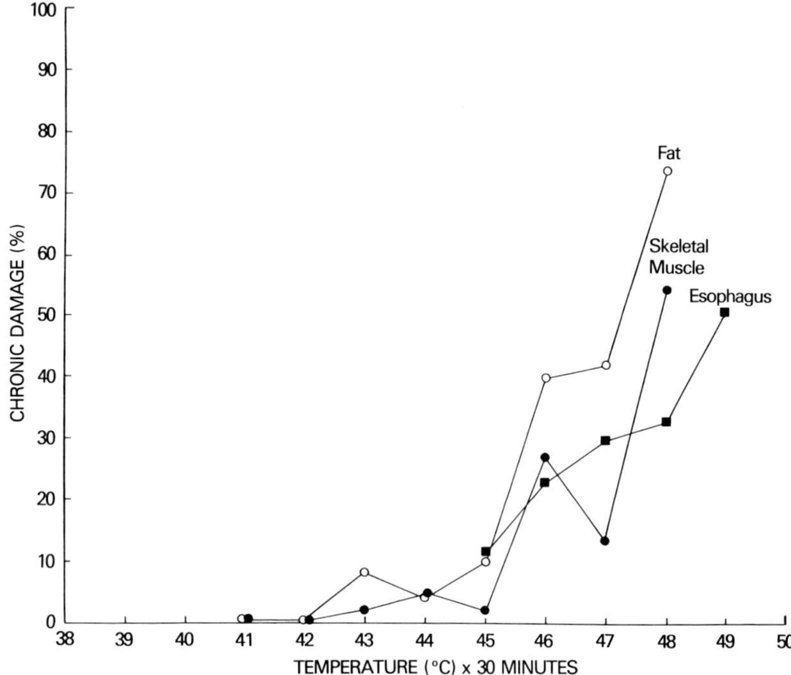

Fig. 1. Thermal sensitivity of three porcine normal tissues. Scoring systems were based on the histological changes identified by light microscopy which varied between the tissues. Scores are expressed as the percent of the maximum possible in each scoring system. From Martinez et al. [35] (fat, skeletal muscle) and Li et al. [29] (esophagus), with permission.

constant (±0.5 °C) across the treatment field at given power levels. Treatments were given at specific temperatures ranging from 41.0 to 48.0 °C, and all treatments were for 30 min.

Evaluation criteria were developed to grade the acute and chronic histologic changes identified. At 24 h after treatment, acute effects included edema, vascular damage, necrosis, and granulocytic infiltration. At 30 days, chronic effects included fibrosis, regeneration of myocytes, chronic diffuse mononuclear infiltration, foreign body giant cell reaction, diffuse granulocytic infiltration, and necrosis and abscess formation. The severity of each effect was assessed using a predetermined scoring system.

Acute tissue changes developed at and above 43 °C, but proved to be mostly transient in the range of 43–45 °C. Chronic tissue damage became increasingly pronounced above exposures of 45 °C and was severe in both fat and skeletal muscle tissues following 48 °C (fig. 1). A priming treatment of 43 °C for 30 min 4 h before challenge at higher temperatures substantially decreased the chronic thermal toxicity in both fat and muscle tissues, indicating that thermotolerance had been induced. Based on isoeffect levels in our grading system, this thermotolerance provided an advantage of about 2 °C in normal-tissue protection.

These results lend substantial support for attempting in clinical work to keep temperatures at or below 45 °C for 30 min. (For 60-min exposures, the time-temperature relationship mentioned above would suggest temperatures at or below 44 °C.) These results are specific for mesenchymal tissues; other tissues within the treatment field may be more heat sesitive. Also, these results concern previously untreated tissues, and prior irradiation has been shown in murine studies to affect normal-tissue sensitivity to hyperthermia [18]. Furthermore, the combination of hyperthermia and irradiation can increase the normal-tissue effects of both modalities, as has been observed in human trials by Arcangeli et al. [2] and Overgaard and Overgaard [44].

To our knowledge, our studies are the first to demonstrate thermotolerance in tissues of large animals. Thermotolerance in normal tissues could be useful clinically: a sublethal priming exposure to more superficial normal tissues could thermally protect them prior to high-temperature treatment to deeper lying tumors and thereby improve the therapeutic ratio.

Skin and Subcutaneous Tissues: Clinical Experience

A variety of methods are available for the treatment of superficial tumor volumes. At Stanford University, clinical work began utilizing planar ultrasound applicators operating at 1–3 MHz. More recently, we [24] have used primarily microwave devices (at 95–915 MHz) with spiral strip, horn, and waveguide types of design. The clinically useful penetration of these and other similarly designed applicators is limited to approximately 2–4 cm depth; however, with newer equipment (both microwave and ultrasound, surface treatment areas and, therefore, total treatment volumes have significantly increased in size. Technical and clinical aspects of treatment have been reviewed recently by us [24].

Our treatment objectives have been to bring tumors to at least 43–45 °C while maintaining normal superficial tissues ≤43.0 °C (more recently ≤43.5 °C). Complications have been classified, according to their time of occurrence, as acute (during treatment or within 24 h), subacute (24 h–30 days), or chronic (30 days and beyond).

Acute complications in 830 superficial treatment sessions have been predominantly during the treatment delivery. Patients made some men-

Table I. Reported toxicities of superficial hyperthermia

Authors	Number of courses	Toxicity	Incidence, %
U et al. [56]	53	superficial burn,	13
		deep burn	8
Corry et al. [6]	30	blistering	13
Marmor and Hahn [34]	52	superficial burn,	19
		ulceration	10
Perez et al. [45]	101	2nd- to 3rd-degree burns	6
Kapp et al. [24]	299	blistering,	10
		burn/normal-tissue ulcer,	2
		tumor ulcer,	6
		infection	1

tion of local pain, usually mild, during 48.8% of treatments. This was a much greater problem with ultrasound methods (79%) than with microwave methods (47%), presumably because of ultrasound wave reflection and absorption at soft tissue-bone interfaces causing stimulation of periosteal pain receptors. All other effects were rare (referred pain in 1.8%, other transient minor problems in 1.0% of the cases) [24].

This unwanted discomfort also compromises therapy, since power reduction is often required and results in decreased temperatures. This was much more of a problem during treatments with ultrasound (49% of treatments) than with microwave (23% of treatments). In sites receiving both microwave and ultrasound treatment (on different treatment days), average temperature distributions were lower with ultrasound by at least 1 °C [39].

Blisters and other minor subacute complications have been uncommon in our experience and in that of other investigators (table I), perhaps because power is reduced with the development of symptoms during treatment. Tumors can ulcerate after high-temperature treatment. However, only five ulcerations or burns have occurred in normal tissues, and other chronic complications have been uncommon. In obtaining this low rate of complications, 8–20 surface temperature sensors were monitored constantly through the treatment period, and all surface temperatures were maintained below 43.0–43.5 °C. Insofar as there was some heterogeneity of surface temperatures, most sites were actually less than 42.0 °C.

Two of our five normal-tissue ulcers/burns occurred in scars. In both cases, the monitored surface temperatures were 43 °C or less. However, temperatures measured from probes placed on the skin surface can differ from true intradermal temperatures in some cases: work in our clinic has shown that surface temperatures can underestimate those inside scars by 1–2 °C [unpubl. observations]. Clearly, greater caution must be exercised when treating fields containing scar tissues.

These patients typically have received daily radiation fractions of 180–200 rad immediately before hyperthermia. We have not observed any prominent enhancement of irradiation effect in normal tissues by hyperthermia, in agreement with many other investigators [37, 53]. Enhanced reactions have been noted when large radiation fractions have been used: when Arcangeli et al. [2] used 500-rad fractions, the rate of moist desquamation increased from 36% with radiation alone to 64% with combined therapy; however, this enhancement did not occur when they used smaller radiation fractions.

Overgaard and Overgaard [44] and Arcangeli et al. [2] have investigated the effect of introducing a time delay between irradiation and hyperthermia: 3–5 and 4 h, respectively. In both cases, both tumor response and skin reaction decreased with use of the delay. But in both cases, the decrease was greater for the skin reaction than for the tumor response. This may be a way of relatively protecting normal tissues when using large radiation fractions.

In studies using moderate radiation fraction sizes, the low rates of complications often have been achieved despite prior irradiation of the treatment site [37]. Preliminary data suggest that higher response rates to treatment with hyperthermia plus irradiation occur in tumors arising in previously irradiated fields compared to unirradiated ones [31].

Gastrointestinal Tract

Esophagus. Li et al. [29] have evaluated the effects of heat on the esophagus of swine using an intraluminal microwave applicator (operating at 434 MHz for acute-damage experiments and at 2,450 MHz for late-damage experiments). Treatment was given at 45–49 °C for 30 min, with temperatures monitored at the center of the applicator within the esophagus. In a subset of animals, temperatures were measured across the luminal wall; the temperature gradient across it increased from 2 to 4 °C, as the inner surface temperature increased from 45 to 48 °C. In biopsies taken 48 h after treatment, histological evaluation showed increasingly severe effects above 45 °C, and this was also true of biopsies taken 30 days after treatment. 43 °C for 30 min, given 4 h before, induced thermotolerance with a 2-°C benefit in normal-tissue protection – results very similar to those reported for fat and skeletal muscle (fig. 1).

Intestine. Li et al. [unpubl. commun.] have been performing similar experiments in the normal rectum of swine, and this tissue appears to be more sensitive to hyperthermia than the esophagus. Ger et al. [13] treated sections of canine large bowel by irrigation with water at 51 °C for 7 h and found that the mucosa showed remarkable potential for repair: treated areas showed substantial reepithelialization on histological examination 6–8 weeks after treatment. (This study did not report measurement of tissue temperatures, and this contact method would likely treat only a few millimeters of the inner bowel wall with these high temperatures.)

Several institutions have used the Annular Phased Array System (APAS; BSD Corp., Salt Lake City, Utah, USA), a 16-aperture radiative electromagnetic device (70–120 MHz) that encircles transverse areas of the patient [55]. Apertures radiate coherently toward the central axis, causing regional heating, and the power deposition characteristics are such that normal-tissue temperatures in the immediate area of the tumor are likely to be similar to the tumor temperatures monitored.

In work at Stanford [24] with this device, tumor temperatures averaged over the treatment period were 43.0 °C (maximum) and 40.8 °C (average) in 44 sessions for tumors of the deep pelvis. Despite the possibility of increased blood flow to normal tissues during treatment [51], it is possible that portions of large and small bowel, bladder, ureter, and urethra also achieved these temperatures. However, none of the treated patients had clinically evident complications in these tissues. In 1 case, the treated tumor ulcerated after therapy; in another, an infection developed – complications that were not specific to the normal tissues. Our results are similar to those reported by Sapozink et al. [52]. In 43 patients treated with the APAS, symptoms during treatment often were power limiting to the treatment. However, posttreatment complications were uncommon, and those few that did occur were often thought to be related to tumor necrosis rather than to direct normal-tissue toxicity. At Stanford, a small number of patients with abdominal and pelvic tumors were treated with a multitransducer ultrasound system, and few if any deep-tissue complications resulted despite maximum tumor temperatures averaging 42.2 °C [10, 24].

Liver. Prionas et al. [48] treated normal canine liver using a capacitive radiofrequency system operating at 0.5 MHz. The 30-min intraoperative treatments used temperatures of 43.0–47.5 °C. At 28 days after treatment, a variety of pathological changes were noted, and significant levels of damage could be seen after temperatures as low as 41 °C. A prior thermal exposure failed to protect against the effects of subsequent treatment. Ries et al. [50] used a radiofrequency interstitial method to treat canine liver at 44.0 °C for 40 min. Transient posttreatment elevations of hepatic enzymes were noted, and histological examination of the treated sites 4 weeks after treatment showed limited fibrosis, alterations in liver architecture, sinusoidal dilation, and ultrastructural changes. While further work is needed, these studies raise caution regarding the thermal sensitivity of the liver.

A limited amount of clinical information reinforces this concern: (1) In the period 1920–1940, iatrogenic fever therapy was used for a number of disorders and often induced systemic temperatures of 40.0–41.0 °C for several hours. Jaundice, hyperbilirubinemia, and autopsy evidence of hepatic damage were reported in some patients [26]. (2) Hepatic damage has been demonstrated in autopsy series that have studied individuals succumbing to heatstroke [25]. (3) It was shown [47] in early clinical trials using systemic hyperthermia for malignancy that temperatures above 42.0 °C were poorly tolerated, in particular causing clinically evident liver and brain damage. (4) Wills et al. [59] documented histologic changes in hepatic tissue from 3 patients who received therapeutic hyperthermia to >40 °C for 65, 125, and 495 min, respectively. (5) Systemic hyperthermia, with core temperatures of 41.8–42.0 °C for 2 h, has resulted in hepatic enzyme changes in the experience of Van der Zee et al. [58], as well as others [5, 27, 47].

Pancreas. In a preliminary communication, Ramey et al. [49] reported results of interstitial treatment of canine pancreas at 42–43 °C for 60 min. Amylase and lipase levels transiently increased, but returned to normal values within 7 days. However, histological evaluations revealed focal areas of inflammation and necrosis in the treated areas.

Genitourinary Tract

Bladder. Irrigation techniques for the treatment of superficial bladder malignancies have typically employed chemotherapy in the warmed perfusate, thereby obscuring the effect of the hyperthermia itself. However, Ludgate et al. [30] treated patients with hyperthermic irrigation alone at 44 °C. One-hour treatments did not induce cystoscopic changes or urinary symptoms in patients, but 3- to 4-hour treatments resulted in partial mucosal necrosis, chronic inflammation, and markedly reduced bladder capacity. Many patients became symptomatic with urinary frequency, and some required urinary diversion. Jacob et al. [21] obtained biopsies from 10 patients after receiving hyperthermic irrigation alone at

44 °C. One-hour treatments did not induce ultrastructural changes in biopsies taken immediately after therapy. However, 2-hour treatments resulted in definite changes in specimens taken 4 days later: structural alterations were apparent in multiple organelles and were prominent in mitochondria.

Nervous System

Britt et al. [32] evaluated hyperthermia effects on canine normal brain using an interstitial microwave antenna array system. After treatment for 50–70 min at temperatures of up to 47 °C, brains were removed immediately and histologically examined after fixation. Acute neuronal damage was evident after 42.0–42.5 °C. Neuronal cell lysis was evident at temperatures greater than 43 °C, and damage to the white matter was evident after 43.0–43.5 °C. These workers [4] also have performed investigations on normal brain in cats treated by ultrasonic methods and have obtained similar acute results and have extended their studies to chronic changes [33]: the brain appears to be one of the most thermally sensitive of tissues.

Future Studies

While clinical trials are now evaluating the responses of tumors to hyperthermia induced by a variety of approaches, many aspects of normal-tissue response to hyperthermia remain poorly defined. Of greatest concern, hyperthermia currently is combined with irradiation in most treatment programs, but the magnitude of thermal enhancement of irradiation effect remains largely unknown for most normal tissues [23]. Considerable interest exists in the combination of hyperthermia with chemotherapy, but few investigations have reported effects of combined chemotherapy and hyperthermia on normal tissues. The introduction of new applicators will bring unique power distributions with each, and comparative evaluations of normal tissue effects will be warranted. In many ways, further investigations on the normal tissue effects of hyperthermia will be key to evaluating the therapeutic gain that this modality can provide.

References

1 Anderson, R.L.; Kapp, D.S.; Woo, S.Y.; Rice, G.C.; Lee, K.J.; Hahn, G.M.: Predictive assays for tumor response to single and multiple fractions of hyperthermia. Recent results. Cancer Res. (in press).

2 Arcangeli, G.; Nervi, C.; Cividalli, A.; Lovisolo, G. A.: Problem of sequence and fractionation in the clinical application of combined heat and radiation. Cancer Res. *44:* suppl., pp. 4857–4863 (1984).

3 Baker, D. G.; Sager, H.; Constable, W.; Goodchild, N.: The response of previously irradiated skin to combinations of X-radiation and ultrasound-induced hyperthermia. Radiat. Res. *96:* 367–373 (1983).

4 Britt, R. H.; Lyons, B. E.; Pounds, D. W.; Prionas, S. D.: Feasibility of using ultrasound hyperthermia in the treatment of malignant brain tumors: tissue damage threshold and thermal dosimetry studies. Med. Instrum. J. *17:* 172–177 (1983).

5 Bull, J. M.; Lees, D.; Schuette, W.; Whang-Pang, J.; Smith, R.; Bynum, G.; Atkinson, E. R.; Gottdiener, J. S.; Gralnick, H. R.; Shawker, T. H.; DeVita, V. T.: Whole body hyperthermia: a phase I trial of a potential adjuvant to chemotherapy. Ann. intern. Med. *90:* 317–323 (1979).

6 Corry, P. M.; Barlogie, B.; Tilchen, E. J.; Armour, E. P.: Ultrasound-induced hyperthermia for the treatment of human superficial tumors. Int. J. Radiat. Oncol. Biol. Phys. *8:* 1225–1229 (1982).

7 Elkon, D.; Fechner, R. E.; Homzie, M. J.; Baker, D. G.; Constable, W. C.: Response of mouse kidney to hyperthermia. Archs. Pathol. Lab. Med. *104:* 153–158 (1980).

8 Fajardo, L. F.: Pathological effects of hyperthermia in normal tissues. Cancer Res. *44:* suppl., pp. 4826–4835 (1984).

9 Fajardo, L. F.; Meyer, J. L.; Meshorer, A.; Prionas, S.; Martinez, A.; Hahn, G. M.: Thermal injury and thermotolerance in mesenchymal tissues. Front. Radiat. Ther. Onc., vol. *18*, pp. 144–152 (Karger, Basel 1984).

10 Fessenden, P.; Lee, E. R.; Anderson, T.; Strohbehn, J. W; Meyer, J.; Samulski, T. V.; Marmor, J. B.: Experience with a multi-transducer ultrasound system for localized hyperthermia of deep tissues. IEEE Trans. biomed. Engng *31:* 126–135 (1984).

11 Field, S. B.: The response of normal tissues to hyperthermia alone or in combination with X-rays; in Streffer, van Beuningen, Dietzel, Rottinger, Robinson, Scherer, Seeber, Trott, Cancer therapy by hyperthermia and radiation (Urban & Schwarzenberg, Baltimore 1978).

12 Field, S. B.; Morris, C. C.: The relationship between heating time and temperature: its relevance to clinical hyperthermia. Radiother. Oncol. *1:* 179–186 (1983).

13 Ger, R.; Ravo, B.; Harris, M.; Waxman, M.; Addei, K. A.: Mucosal destruction and regeneration of the colon by local hyperthermia. Dis. Colon Rectum *29:* 177–181 (1986).

14 Gerner, E. W.; Culver, P. S.; Sim, D.: Functional dependencies of T, ΔT and dT/dt in temperature-induced cytotoxicity. Radiat. Res. *94:* 557 (1983).

15 Hahn, G. M.: *Hyperthermia and cancer* (Plenum Publishing, New York 1982).

16 Hand, J. W.; Hopewell, J. W.; Field, S. B.; Foster, J. L.: An investigation into the combined effects of X-irradiation and microwave heating on pig skin. Int. J. Radiat. Oncol. Biol. Phys. *6:* 59–66 (1980).

17 Hand, J. W.; Walker, H.; Hornsey, S.; Field, S. B.: Effects of hyperthermia on the mouse testis and its response to X-rays, as assayed by weight loss. Int. J. Radiat. Oncol. Biol. Phys. *35:* 521–528 (1979).

18 Hume, S. P.: Experimental studies of normal tissue response to hyperthermia given alone or combined with radiation; in Overgaard, Hyperthermic oncology, vol. 2 (Taylor & Francis, London 1985).

19 Hume, S. P.; Marigold, J. C. L.; Field, S. B.: The effect of local hyperthermia on the small intestine of the mouse. Br. J. Radiol. *52:* 657–662 (1979).

20 Hume, S. P.; Myers, R.: An unexpected effect of hyperthermia on the expression of X-ray damage in mouse skin. Radiat. Res. *97:* 186–199 (1984).

21 Jacob, J.; Hindmarsh, J. R.; Ludgate, C. M.; Chisholm, G. D.: Observations on the ultrastructure of human urothelium: the response of normal bladder of elderly subjects to hyperthermia. Urol. Res. *10:* 227–237 (1982).

22 Kapp, D. S.; Bagshaw, M. A.; Meyer, J. L.; Hahn, G. M.; Samulski, T. V.; Fessenden, P.; Lee, E. R.; Lohrbach, A. W.: Hyperthermia as an adjuvant to radiation in the treatment of superficial metastases: a randomized trial of 2 vs. 6 treatments (abstract) 34th Annu. Meet. Radiat. Res. Soc., vol. 24 (1986).

23 Kapp, D. S.: Areas of need for continued phase II testing in human patients; in Paliwal, Hetzel, Dewhirst, Biological, physical and clinical aspects of hyperthermia (American Institute for Physics, New York 1988).

24 Kapp, D. S.; Fessenden, P.; Samulski, T. V.; Bagshaw, M. A.; Cox, R. S.; Lee, E. R.; Lohrbach, A. W.; Meyer, J. L.; Prionas, S. D.: Stanford University Institutional Report: phase I evaluation of equipment for hyperthermia treatment of cancer. Int. J. Hyperthermia. *4:* 75–115 (1988).

25 Kew, M.; Bersohn, I.; Seftel, H.; Kent, G.: Liver damage in heatstroke. Am. J. Med. *49:* 192–202 (1970).

26 King, A. J.; Williams, S. I.; Nicol, C. S.: Hyperthermia in the treatment of resistant gonococcal and non-specific urethritis. Br. J. vener. Dis. *19:* 141–154 (1943).

27 Larkin, J. M.; Edwards, W. J.; Smith, D. E.; Clark, P. J.: Systemic thermotherapy: description of a method and physiologic tolerance in clinical subjects. Cancer *40:* 3155–3159 (1977).

28 Law, M. P.; Ahier, R. G.; Samaia, S.: Thermal enhancement ratio of radiation damage in previously irradiated skin. Br. J. Radiol. *58:* 161–167 (1985).

29 Li, D.-J.; Zhou, S.-L.; Qui, S.-L.; Qiao, S.-J.: Thermodamage, thermosensitivity and thermotolerance of normal swine oesophagus. Int. J. Hyperthermia *3:* 143–151 (1987).

30 Ludgate, C. M.; McLean, N.; Carswell, G. F.; Newsam, J. E.; Pettigrew, R. T.; Tulloch, W. S.: Hyperthermic perfusion of the distended urinary bladder in the management of recurrent transitional cell carcinoma. Br. J. Urol. *47:* 841–848 (1976).

31 Luk, K. H.; Pajak, T. F.; Perez, C. A.; Johnson, R. J.; Conner, N.; Dobbins, T.: Prognostic factors for tumor response after hyperthermia and radiation; in Overgaard, Hyperthermic oncology, vol. 1, summary papers (Taylor & Francis, London 1984).

32 Lyons, B. E.; Britt, R. H.; Strohbehn, J. W.: Localized hyperthermia in the treatment of malignant brain tumors using an interstitial microwave antenna array. IEEE Trans. biomed. Engng *31:* 53–62 (1984).

33 Lyons, B. E.; Obana, W. G.; Borcich, J. K.; Kleinman, R.; Singh, D.; Britt, R. H.: Chronic histopathological effects of ultrasonic hyperthermia on normal feline brain tissue. Radiat. Res. *106:* 234–251 (1986).

34 Marmor, J. B.; Hahn, G. M.: Combined radiation and hyperthermia in superficial human tumors. Cancer *46:* 1986–1991 (1980).

35 Martinez, A. A.; Meshorer, A.; Meyer, J. L.; Hahn, G. M.; Fajardo, L. F.; Prionas, S. D.: Thermal sensitivity and thermotolerance in normal porcine tissues. Cancer Res. *43:* 2072–2075 (1983).

36 Meshorer, A.; Prionas, S.; Fajardo, L. F.; Meyer, J. L.; Hahn, G. M.; Martinez, A. A.: The effects of hyperthermia on normal mesenchymal tissues. Application of a histologic grading system. Archs Pathol. Lab. Med. *107:* 328–334 (1983).

37 Meyer, J. L.: The clinical efficacy of localized hyperthermia. Cancer Res. *44:* suppl., pp. 4745–4751 (1984).

38 Meyer, J. L.: Clinical and technical considerations in planning a course of hyperther-

mia and irradiation. Front. Radiat. Ther. Onc. vol. *21*, pp. 107–121 (Karger, Basel 1987).
39 Meyer, J.; Kapp, D.; Bagshaw, M.; Samulski, T.; Fessenden, P.; Lee, E.: Complications from microwave and ultrasound hyperthermia: effect of treatment volume (Abstract). 34th Annu. Meet. Radiat. Res. Soc., vol. *24* (1986).
40 Meyer, J.; Kapp, D. S.; Fessenden, P.; Hahn, G. M.: Hyperthermic oncology: current biology, physics and clinical results; in Schönbaum, International encyclopedia of pharmocology and therapeutics (Pergamon Press, Oxford, in press).
41 Meyer, J. L.; Van Kersen, I.; Becker, B.; Hahn, G. M.: The importance of thermotolerance after 41.0 °C hyperthermia: *in vitro* and *in vivo* tumor and normal tissue investigations. Int. J. Radiat. Oncol. Biol. Phys. *11:* 973–981 (1985).
42 Meyer, J. L.; Van Kersen, I.; Hahn, G. M.: Tumor responses following multiple hyperthermia and X-ray treatments: role of thermotolerance at the cellular level. Cancer Res. *46:* 5691–5695 (1986).
43 Moritz, A. R.; Henriques, F. C.: Studies of thermal injury. II. The relative importance of time and surface temperature in the causation of cutaneous burns. Am. J. Path. *23:* 695–720 (1947).
44 Overgaard, J.; Overgaard, M.: A clinical trial evaluating the effect of simultaneous or sequential radiation and hyperthermia in the treatment of malignant melanoma; in Overgaard, Hyperthermic oncology, vol. 1 (Taylor & Francis, London 1984).
45 Perez, C. A.; Nussbaum, G.; Emami, B.; Von Gerichten, D.: Clinical results of irradiation combined with local hyperthermia. Cancer *52:* 1597–1603 (1983).
46 Perez, C. A.; Sapareto, S. A.: Thermal dose expression in clinical hyperthermia and correlation with tumor response/control. Cancer Res. *44:* suppl., pp. 4818–4825 (1984).
47 Pettigrew, R. T.: Cancer therapy by whole body heating; in Wizenberg, Robinson, Proc. Int. Symp. on Cancer Therapy by Hyperthermia and Radiation (American College of Radiology Press, Baltimore 1975).
48 Prionas, S. D.; Taylor, M. A.; Fajardo, L. F.; Kelly, N. I.; Nelsen, T. S.; Hahn, G. M.: Thermal sensitivity to single and double heat treatments in normal canine liver. Cancer Res. *45:* 4791–4797 (1985).
49 Ramey, R. L.; Milligan, A. J.; Merrick, H. W.: Evaluation of the tolerance of the canine pancreas to interstitial hyperthermia (Abstract). 35th Annu. Meet. Radiat. Res. Soc., vol., 38 (1987).
50 Ries, M. C.; Milligan, A. J.; Merrick, H. W.; Dobelbower, R. R.: Biochemical and cellular effects of radiofrequency induced interstitial hyperthermia on normal canine liver. Int. J. Radiat. Oncol. Biol. Phys. *14:* 529–536 (1988).
51 Samulski, T. V.; Valdagni, R.; Fessenden, P.; Kapp, D. S.: Correlations of thermal washout rate, steady state temperatures and tissue type in deep seated recurrent or metastatic tumors. Int. J. Radiat. Oncol. Biol. Phys. *13:* 907–916 (1987).
52 Sapozink, M. D.; Gibbs, F. A.; Egger, M. J.; Stewart, J. R.: Regional hyperthermia for clinically advanced deep-seated pelvic malignancy. Am J. clin. Oncol. *9:* 162–169 (1986).
53 Scott, R. S.; Johnson, R. J. R.; Story, K. V.; Clay, L.: Local hyperthermia in combination with definitive radiotherapy: increased tumor clearance, reduced recurrence rate in extended follow-up. Int. J. Radiat. Oncol. Biol. Phys. *10:* 2119–2123 (1984).
54 Stone, H. B.; Harding, R. P.: Reversible injury after mild hyperthermia. Int. J. Radiat. Oncol. Biol. Phys. *12:* 823–827 (1987).
55 Turner, P. F.: Regional hyperthermia with an annular phased array. IEEE Trans. Biomed. Engng *31:* 106–114 (1984).

56 U, R.; Noell, K. T.; Woodward, K. I.; Worde, B. T.; Fishburn, R. I.; Miller, L. S.: Microwave-induced hyperthermia in combination with radiotherapy of human malignant tumors. Cancer *45:* 638–646 (1980).
57 Urano, M.; Rice, L.; Kahn, J.; Sedlacek, R. S.: Studies on fractionated hyperthermia in experimental animal systems. I. The foot reaction after equal doses: heat resistance and repopulation. Int. J. Radiat. Oncol. Biol. Phys. *6:* 1519–1523 (1980).
58 Van der Zee, J.; Van Rhoon, G. C.; Wike-Hooley, J. L.; Faithfull, N. S.; Reinhold, H. S.: Whole-body hyperthermia in cancer therapy: a report of a phase I–II study. Eur. J. Cancer clin. Oncol. *19:* 1189–1200 (1983).
59 Wills, E. J.; Findlay, J. M.; McManus, J. P. A.: Effects of hyperthermia therapy on the liver. II. Morphological observations. J. clin. Path. *29:* 1–10 (1976).
60 Wondergem, J.; Haveman, J.: The response of previously irradiated mouse skin to heat alone or combined with irradiation: influence of thermotolerance. Int. J. Radiat. Biol. *44:* 539–552 (1983).

John L. Meyer, MD, Department of Radiation Therapy, St. Francis Memorial Hospital, PO Box 7726, San Francisco, CA 94120 (USA)

Vaeth JM, Meyer JL (eds): Radiation Tolerance of Normal Tissues.
Front Radiat Ther Oncol. Basel, Karger, 1989, vol 23, pp 177–184

Chemical Modifiers of Normal-Tissue Radiation Injury[1]

Theodore L. Phillips

Department of Radiation Oncology, University of California,
San Francisco, Calif., USA

Introduction

The degree of radiation injury which occurs to critical and secondary normal tissues during a course of curative treatment may be significantly modified by a number of chemical compounds. In some situations, the agents are being employed to enhance radiation response in the tumor, and normal-tissue injury modification is a deleterious side effect. In other situations, drugs are employed to suppress or reduce normal-tissue injury. This review will cover various agents which modify radiation response in normal tissue both favorably or unfavorably.

Four major types of chemical compounds have been employed in the clinic and studied in the laboratory that modify normal-tissue injury. These include hypoxic cell sensitizers, halogenated pyrimidines, sulfhydryl-containing radioprotectors, and cytotoxic chemotherapy. This presentation will briefly review the laboratory results for each class of compounds as measured by normal-tissue injury. Available clinical trial results will then be presented to indicate the degree of injury to normal tissue which may be expected or the degree of reduction of injury in the case of radioprotectors. The emphasis will be placed on controlled clinical trials with concomitant irradiation.

[1]This work was supported in part by National Cancer Institute Grant No. CA24139 (RTOG) and Office of Health and Environmental Research, USDOE, Contract No. DE-AC03-76-SFO1012.

Hypoxic Cell Sensitizers

Hypoxic cell sensitizers were developed as tumor-specific enhancers of radiation damage because of the perceived presence of hypoxic cells only in tumors. There is significant evidence that some normal tissues also contain at least a small percentage of hypoxic cells. This evidence is quite clear for the skin, but there are also suggestive data for brain, spinal cord, liver, and other organs. The fraction of hypoxic cells is generally quite small compared to that found in tumors and not normally influential on response in normal tissues at conventional fraction sizes. When large fractions are given, however, the effect of hypoxic cells can sometimes be detected. Enhancement in the range of 1.2 has been described for skin irradiated with single doses after treatment with large doses of misonidazole [15, 16]. Some reports have shown the opposite effect in the gut.

In clinical trials, misonidazole was employed at significantly lower doses than in a number of the single-dose mouse experiments. Thus, no enhanced radiation effect on normal tissue was observed in any of the phase II studies or in any of the seven phase III studies conducted by the Radiation Therapy Oncology Group (RTOG) [17]. Some other effects were noted, however, which may have been due to an interaction of the toxicity of the drug with radiation effects and organ damage caused by tumor.

In both the misonidazole brain metastasis randomized trial [11] and the misonidazole glioma study [10] of the RTOG, there was decreased survival in patients receiving misonidazole when the entire randomized patient group was considered. When patients with favorable prognostic indicators, in particular no distant metastases and high Karnofsky scores, are considered, these differences disappear. It seems possible that the central nervous system toxicity associated with misonidazole has interacted with the injury caused by both the tumor and the radiation to the brain and has shortened the survival time in patients with poor prognosis. This kind of effect should not be seen with the newer generation of agents that do not cross the blood-brain barrier.

In the RTOG randomized trial for carcinoma of the cervix published recently by Leibel et al. [8], there was an apparent increased rate of tumor failure and decreased survival in the arm receiving misonidazole. In this situation, i was given as a daily dose during external beam radiotherapy of 400 mg/m^2. This difference did not reach statistical significance. The effect may be due to chance, although it is reasonable to consider that there may be a suppression of the immune response or other factors leading to an increased local and metastatic failure rate.

The RTOG is now conducting a trial of SR 2508, the third-generation hypoxic cell sensitizer, for treatment of head and neck cancer. The University of California at San Francisco has participated in this study as well as in the first-phase study which was unrandomized. We have observed a modest decrease in mucosal reactions in patients receiving SR 2508 as compared to our historical controls [Phillips, personal commun.].

Halogenated Pyrimidines

Halogenated pyrimidines have been developed because of their potential for differential sensitization of tumor and normal tissue. The differential depends not on the presence of hypoxic cells, but an increased cell turnover rate in the tumor compared to surrounding irradiated normal tissue. In order for there to be a successful enhancement of the therapeutic ratio, there must be a greater percentage of tumor cells than normal cells in cycle. Those cells must also incorporate sufficient halogenated pyrimidine for significant sensitization. In the initial evaluation of bromodeoxyuridine (BUdR) as a sensitizer, Bagshaw and Doggett [1] employed patients with head and neck cancer. They found significant sensitization with intra-arterial BUdR of the oral mucosa on the side of placement of the catheter in the common carotid. In a small randomized trial, there was no apparent increase in control or survival in the group receiving BUdR. Thus, the apparent enhancement of normal tissue to the same degree as the tumor obviated any potential advantage. Other sites would appear more advantageous. These include the central nervous system where there is quite slow turnover in endothelium and oligodendroglia [4]. Labeling indices have varied from a few to as high as 50% in brain metastases and in the intermediate range for anaplastic gliomas and glioblastoma multiforme. Earlier trials [9] with BUdR in tumors of the central nervous system and in sarcomas of the bone did not report any enhanced normal-tissue damage and did claim increased tumor response.

BUdR has been evaluated in a number of mouse experiments in which skin reaction was graded [2]. The enhanced response of normal skin was quantitated with a dose-modifying factor (DMF) score of 1.1–1.2.

In a recent evaluation of BUdR given intravenously at our institution, we have noted some increased skin reaction in the irradiated field, but not to the extent that is dose limiting [14]. Similar effects were seen at the National Cancer Institute [6]. In a phase I evaluation of intravenous iododeoxyuridine at the National Cancer Institute, some mild enhancement of skin response and intestinal response was observed as well as direct toxicity in bone marrow and the liver [5].

It appears that enhanced reaction to radiation in normal tissue with halogenated pyrimidines would be a limiting factor in the treatment of head and neck cancer and probably gastrointestinal malignancies. On the other hand, the treatment of central nervous system tumors, sarcomas, and probably peripheral lung carcinomas would be possible, and one would expect a differential effect.

Sulfhydryl Radioprotectors

Since the discovery in the 1940s that sulfhydryl-containing compounds would protect mammalian tissue against ionizing radiation, the potential for such protection to improve radiotherapy has been explored. Initially, it was found that chemicals such as cysteamine would protect tumor and normal tissues equally, and, thus, no therapeutic gain could be predicted. In the late 1960s, Yuhas and Storer [18] reported that thiophosphate-type sulfhydryl compounds did differentially protect normal tissue and tumor. The best of these compounds, WR 2721, protected a wide range of normal tissues and did not protect most tested solid tumors.

A large series of studies was undertaken by a number of investigators which showed that there was protection against both acute and late effects of radiation [12]. The DMF ranges from as high as 3 for bone marrow to 1.2 for acute radiation pneumonitis. Generally, no protection could be shown of the central nervous system and of most solid tumors.

Explanations of the differential protection include pharmacologic distribution of the drug which is excluded from the central nervous system and from tumors because of its very low partition coefficient and its very poor lipid solubility. In addition, there is some evidence that the drug is actively concentrated in normal tissues. Finally, sulfhydryl radioprotectors are far less effective against hypoxic as compared to aerated cells and, thus, would be expected to protect normal tissue differentially at higher radiation doses.

Human trials have been carried out in Japan and in the United States [7]. The Japanese trials with a relatively low dose, i.e., 100 mg/patient/day, were reported to show protection of the oral mucosa and the salivary glands. No difference in tumor response was noted in these head and neck patients. Trials in the USA have consisted of a phase I evaluation of single-dose WR 2721 in radiotherapy patients, and a second phase I study with multiple-dose WR 2721 in radiotherapy patients has been completed. The maximum tolerated doses were established as 740 mg/m^2 in a single dose and 350 mg/m^2 in multiple doses 5 days/week. Currently active US studies involve hemibody irradiation for palliation of metastases with WR 2721 and pelvic irradiation for advanced malignancies.

Cytotoxic Chemotherapy

Since the early 1960s, it has been recognized that some cancer chemotherapy drugs are major enhancers of radiation damage in normal tissues. The drugs may be classified into three groups: (1) general enhancers of radiation response in essentially every tissue; (2) drugs that cause additive damage in specific tissues; and (3) drugs for which there is little interaction [3, 13].

Only a small number of drugs fall into the first category, the major example being actinomycin D. It apparently inhibits repair of sublethal damage and causes enhanced response, primarily with fractionated radiotherapy. Adriamycin has also been an enhancer, although it appears to do this only in certain tissues such as the heart and, perhaps, the gastrointestinal tract. Most other agents act in an additive fashion in tissue in which they themselves cause direct normal-tissue injury. There are numerous examples of this, including bleomycin in the lungs, cisplatin in the kidneys, adriamycin in the heart, and cyclophosphamide in the bladder.

Other compounds such as cyclophosphamide show little interaction with radiation in most tissues because of their lack of effect in those tissues. On the other hand, cyclophosphamide does damage the pulmonary vasculature, and additive interaction can be shown. We have conducted a series of single-dose radiation experiments in the LAF-1 mouse administering maximum tolerated chemotherapy 2 h prior to irradiation.

Pulmonary lethality which involves whole-lung irradiation and measurement of death between 100 and 160 days was used to evaluate interaction in the lung. Results of these experiments are shown in table I. The first column includes the dose-effect factors (DEF), i.e., the ratio of the dose for the effect without drug divided by the dose for the same effect with drug. It can be seen that the DEF, the ratio of dose without drug to dose with drug to achieve the same effect, values are greater than 1.00 for adriamycin, bleomycin, cisplatin, cytoxin, melphalan, and methotrexate. The values are statistically significant, as shown by the upper and lower confidence limits for adriamycin, bleomycin, cisplatin, cytoxin, and methotrexate. These data make it clear that single doses of actinomycin D have little effect, whereas, prior work by ourselves and others indicates, fractionated irradiation and actinomycin D has a major effect.

Table I. Pulmonary DEF values (LD50/60 days)

Drug	DEF values	Confidence limit	
		lower	upper
Actinomycin	0.98	0.85	1.09
Adriamycin	1.31	1.09	1.57
BCNU	0.78	0.67	0.91
Bleomycin	1.16	1.01	1.35
Cisplatin	1.22	1.08	1.38
Cytoxan	2.05	1.56	2.68
5-Fluorouracil	0.98	0.85	1.09
Melphalan	1.05	0.94	1.17
Methotrexate	1.61	1.30	2.00
Nitrogen mustard	0.97	0.83	1.13
Vincristine	0.91	0.82	1.01

Table II. Esphogeal DEF values (LD50/28 days)

Drug	DEF values	Confidence limit	
		lower	upper
Actinomycin	1.20	0.17	1.63
BCNU	1.37	1.19	1.75
Bleomycin	1.02	0.56	2.06
Cisplatin	1.68	1.25	2.49
Cytoxan	1.10	0.92	1.47
Methotrexate	5.57	0.04	770.20
Vincristine	1.17	0.77	2.10

Table III. Renal DEF values (LD50/360 days)

Drug	DEF values	Confidence limit	
		lower	upper
Actinomycin	1.03	0.85	1.37
Adriamycin	1.93	1.16	3.22
BCNU	1.42	0.67	3.09
Bleomycin	3.18	0.46	22.94
Cisplatinum	1.37	0.37	5.12
Cytoxan	1.76	1.19	2.71
5-Fluorouracil	1.04	0.80	1.39
Methotrexate	1.27	0.49	3.29
Melphalan	1.01	0.83	1.28
Nitrogen mustard	1.14	0.91	1.49
Vincristine	1.11	0.70	1.83

Esophageal DEF values are shown in table II. It can be seen that significant enhancement occurred with BCNU, cisplatin, and methotrexate. These studies were performed with esophageal lethality end point which measures death within 28 days after thoracic irradiation.

The third series of studies is shown in table III, in which the renal LD_{50} at 360 days was used as the end point. Significantly elevated DEF values occurred for adriamycin and cyclophosphamide. Additional drugs showed an elevation of the LD_{50}, but, because of wide scatter in the response, these were not statistically significant at the 5% level. The confidence limits shown in tables I–III are the 95% confidence limits.

Many clinical reviews have catalogued the enhanced response seen with various cytotoxic agents. In general, it can be stated that enhanced acute response will occur with any agent that affects the mucosa or skin such as bleomycin, 5-fluorouracil, or methotrexate. Enhanced late damage is seen with many of these agents as well, although it is not radiotherapy dose limiting.

References

1 Bagshaw, M.A.; Doggett, R.L.S.; Smith, K.C., et al.: Intra-arterial 5-bromodeoxyuridine and X-ray therapy. Radiology 1967;99:886–894.

2 Brown, J.M.; Goffinet, D.R.; Cleaver, J.E., et al.: Preferential radiosensitization of mouse sarcoma relative to normal skin by chronic intra-arterial infusion of halogenated pyrimidine analogs. J. Natl. Cancer Inst. 1971;47:75–89.

3 Fu, K.K.: Biological basis for the interaction of chemotherapeutic agents and radiation therapy. Cancer 1985;55:2123–2130.

4 Hoshino, T.; Sano, K.: Radiosensitization of malignant brain tumors with bromouridine (thymidine analogue). Acta. Radiol. (Ther. Phys. Biol.) 1969;8:15–26.

5 Kinsella, T.J.; Russo, A.; Mitchell, J.B., et al.: A phase I study of intravenous iododeoxyuridine as a clinical radiosensitizer. Int. J. Radiat. Oncol. Biol. Phys. 1985;11:1941–1946.

6 Kinsella, T.J.; Mitchell, J.B.; Russo, A., et al.: Continuous intravenous infusions of bromodeoxyuridine as a clinical radiosensitizer. J. Clin. Oncol. 1984;2:1144–1150.

7 Kligerman, M.M.; Glover, D.F.; Turrisi, A.T., et al.: Toxicity of WR-2721 administered at single and multiple doses. Int. J. Radiat. Oncol. Biol. Phys. 1984;10:1772–1776.

8 Leibel, S.; Bauer, M.; Phillips, T., et al.: Radiotherapy with or without misonidazole for patients with stage IIIB or IVA squamous cell carcinoma of the uterine cervix: A Radiation Therapy Oncology Group randomized trial. Int. J. Radiat. Oncol. Biol. Phys. 1985;11(suppl 1):127.

9 Martinez, A.; Goffinet, D.R.; Donaldson, S.S., et al.: Intra-arterial infusion of radiosensitizer (BUdR) combined with hypofractionated irradiation and chemotherapy for primary treatment of osteogenic sarcoma. Int. J. Radiat. Oncol. Biol. Phys. 1985;11:123–128.

10 Nelson, J.S.; Diener-West, M.; Schoenfeld, D., et al.: A randomized comparison of

misonidazole sensitized radiotherapy plus BCNU and radiotherapy plus BCNU for treatment of malignant glioma after surgery: A final report of an RTOG study. Int. J. Radiat. Oncol. Biol. Phys. 1986;12:1793–1800.
11 Phillips, T. L.; Diener, M. D.; Wasserman, T. H., et al.: Hypofractionated radiotherapy with or without misonidazole for the treatment of brain metastases. Int. J. Radiat. Oncol. Biol. Phys. 1984;10:145–146.
12 Phillips, T. L.; Kane, L. J.; Ultey, J. F.: Radioprotection of tumor and normal tissues by thiophosphate compounds. Cancer 1973;32:528–535.
13 Phillips, T. L.; Wharam, M. D.; Margolis, L. W.: Modification of radiation injury to normal tissues by chemotherapeutic agents. Cancer 1975;35:1678–1684.
14 Phuphanich, S.; Levin, E. M.; Levin, V. A.: Phase I study of intravenous bromodeoxyuridine used concomitantly with radiation therapy in patients with primary malignant brain tumors. Int. J. Radiat. Oncol. Biol. Phys. 1984;10:1769–1772.
15 Stone, H. B.; Withers, H. R.: Tumors and normal tissue response to metronidazole and irradiation in mice. Radiology 1974;113:441–444.
16 Stone, H. B.: Personal commun.
17 Wasserman, T. H.; Stetz, J. A.; Phillips, T. L.: Radiation Therapy Oncology Group clinical trials with misonidazole. Cancer 1981;47:2382–2390.
18 Yuhas, J. M.; Storer, J. B.: Differential chemoprotection of normal and malignant tissues. J. Natl. Cancer Inst. 1969;42:231–335.

T. L. Phillips, MD, Department of Radiation Oncology, University of California, San Francisco, CA 94143 (USA)

Vaeth JM, Meyer JL (eds): Radiation Tolerance of Normal Tissues.
Front Radiat Ther Oncol. Basel, Karger, 1989, vol 23, pp 185–193

Normal-Tissue Tolerance to Fast-Neutron Teletherapy

R. G. Parker, C. M. Burnison, Ahmad Sadeghi

Department of Radiation Therapy, University of California,
San Francisco, Calif., USA

The success of any therapeutic method rests on a satisfactory therapeutic ratio. Inasmuch as the investigation of fast-neutron teletherapy was discontinued of nearly 2 decades because of observation of serious long-term sequelae [1], current investigators have placed a high priority on the study of normal-tissue effects.

Consequently, many studies of normal-tissue responses in animals preceded revived clinical interest. Since the initiation of clinical applications in England in the 1960s and in the US in the 1970s, acute and long-term sequelae have been carefully recorded. A series of dose-searching studies to establish normal-tissue tolerances antedated the current phase III protocol studies in the USA.

Physical and Biological Differences between Photon and Fast-Neutron Irradiation

Currently available, clinically usable beams of fast neutrons generated by high-energy cyclotrons have dose distribution profiles in tissue similar to those of photons from ^{60}Co teletherapy units or from 4- to 6-MeV linear accelerators [2]. Neutrons, which have masses similar to protons, but are unchanged, interact with atomic nuclei rather than with orbital electrons to produce recoil protons, alpha particles, heavy nuclear fragments, and gamma rays. The kinetic energy released per unit mass of the absorber by interactions with neutrons is proportional to the hydrogen content of the absorber. Thus, in tissues of high hydrogen content this interaction may be responsible for 90–95% of the heavy (2,000 times the mass of an electron) recoil protons formed [3]. This situation is very different than that following photon interactions with the orbital electrons of tissue atoms and translates into a relatively larger dose in fat and smaller doses in tissues of high atomic number, such as bone, for neutrons compared to photons. Kinetic energy released per unit mass ratios for neutrons in tissues other than fat and bone range from 0.94 to 1.07 [3].

Another physical difference of clinical interest is the reintroduction of the build-up process of recoil protons by the use of lead filtration in the neutron beam. This allows the maintenance of skin sparing despite the use of bolus on the skin surface [4].

There are several radiobiologic bases for differences in the acute and long-term effects of fast neutrons and photons in normal tissues. Cellular responses, both in tumors and normal tissues, are less dependent on the presence of oxygen at the time of irradiation with neutrons than with photons. Thus, poorly oxygenated normal tissues, such as cartilage, might be relatively more susceptible to neutrons than to photons. However, the few reports of damage to laryngeal or costal cartilages by the several thousand patients treated have been explainable by high total doses.

The avascular lens seems unusually sensitive to fast-neutron irradiation. In studies in laboratory animals, a relative biological effectiveness (RBE) as high as 10 for high doses and 50 for small doses has been reported for the development of cataracts [5].

Slow or inadequate cell cycle redistribution is less protective against neutrons than photons. A relative lack of redistribution of target cells for late normal-tissue injury could contribute to the high RBE values recorded for slowly responding normal tissues [6, 8].

As reflected in postirradiation cell survival curves, the 'shoulder' associated with photon irradiation implies multihit cell-killing phenomena and the capacity for repair of damage, while the lack of such a 'shoulder' after neutron irradiation implies single-hit cell killing and a lack or impairment of the capacity for repair of damage. This could translate as a higher RBE neutrons/X-rays for late effects than for acute effects, if the target cells for late effects in normal tissues accumulate and repair substantial amounts of sublethal injury [9].

Thus, the dissociation of RBE neutrons/X-rays values for acute and late effects reflects the differences between responses to photons and a lack of such differences after neutron irradiation [8]. If the acute effects produced by neutrons and photons are equalized, the late effects will be greater following neutrons. If the late effects are equalized, the acute effects will be less after photon irradiation.

Fast-Neutron Therapy Sequelae

These physical and radiobiological differences between the effects of fast-neutron and photon irradiation have been reflected in clinical applications.

CNS and Peripheral Nerve Tolerance

Early trials of fast-neutron irradiation of glioblastoma multiforme resulted in some encouraging tumor responses [10], but these studies were abandoned because no differences were detected between total doses required to eliminate tumor and total doses causing unacceptable damage to normal brain. In a later report [11], although in 14 of 15 patients the tumor was replaced by coagulation necrosis following a total dose of 1,550–1,800 cGy of neutrons in three increments of 150 cGy weekly, there was unacceptable extensive gliosis and demyelination of normal brain [12]. Twenty-five of 36 patients remained neurologically stable until 1–2 months prior to death, when slow mental deterioration, unresponsive to steroids, was noted. In a later randomized study [13], although a local boost of 1,500 cGy of neutrons after 5,000 cGy of photons destroyed most tumors, no survival benefit was noted compared to complete treatment with photons.

In early studies of fast-neutron irradiation of cancers arising in the head and neck, several instances of damage of the cervical spinal cord were reported [14–16]. This resulted in a current arbitrary total dose limitation of about 1,000 cGy of neutrons. This limit approximates a previously suggested RBE neutrons/photons of 5.2 based on irradiation of rat spinal cords using 16-MeV neutrons [17].

Recently, several patients have complained of unilateral discomfort in the distribution of the sacral nerve, appearing during the 2nd week of treatment, symptomatically responding to adrenal steroids, and then completely disappearing within a few weeks [18, 19]. The etiology has not been documented.

Eye

As in conventional photon radiation therapy, the eye is excluded from the neutron treatment volume whenever possible. In addition, the short survival of many of the patients treated for advanced cancers of the head and neck has curtailed evidence of long-term effects. Thus, although a high RBE for cataracts in experimental animals has been reported [5], and many early workers studying neutrons developed cataracts [20], this risk has not proved 'clinically important' to date. In a study of 93 eyes receiving a range of doses of neutrons [21], 11 developed cataracts, usually diagnosed between 7 and 12 months after treatment. Acute and long-term effects elsewhere in the eye were considered comparable to those expected after photon irradiation.

Head and Neck

In a recent RTOG report on 330 patients treated for cancers arising in the head and neck [22], it was noted that the frequency of life-threatening or fatal late normal-tissue toxicity was twice as frequent (20%) for patients treated with low-energy (15 MeV d-Be) as with high-energy (50 MeV p-Be) accelerators (9%). Although adjustments were made for variations in the RBE values for various energy beams, corrections were not possible for the very different depth-dose profiles of the different beams. Inasmuch as many of the current data on normal tissue effects have resulted from the use of generators of low or intermediate energies, the frequency and severity of long-term effects should be reduced by the current use of high-energy accelerators.

Skin

The intensity of skin reactions seemingly has been greater in patients treated with neutrons than in those treated conventionally. These differences relate to less 'skin sparing' of the neutron beams based on physical absorption characteristics, to the frequent need for large fields to treat large tumors, and perhaps indirectly to greater absorption of neutrons in subcutaneous fat. In a study on pig skin [23], for a given acute response, the late effects were greater following neutron irradiation than after gamma irradiation, and late responses to neutrons were not altered by reducing daily doses to less than 200 cGy.

Soft Tissues

In the early US clinical trials, fibrosis in the soft tissues of the neck following neutron irradiation seemed more severe than expected following conventional photon irradiation [24]. This was attributed, in large part, to a 10–15% increase in absorption of neutron energy in subcutaneous fat [25]. In a report of the M. D. Anderson-TAMVEC randomized clinical trial [26], when two neutron and three photon fractions were used weekly, there was no increase in complications in the soft tissues of the neck compared to the group irradiated with photons. In a study of 22 patients irradiated only with neutrons for cancers arising in the head and neck [27], 8 had detectable subcutaneous fibrosis. In 4 patients with severe change, the neck mobility was limited. All significant reactions occurred in those receiving more than 22 Gy. No untoward long-term reactions were noted when the total dose was less than 20 Gy.

In 38 patients having major surgery before or after fast-neutron therapy of advanced head and neck cancers, 37% suffered major complications [28]. The frequency of complications varied, depending on whether surgery was prior to irradiation (0/12), planned and accomplished shortly after irradiation (4/5), or done for attempted salvage after irradiation failure (10/21).

Pelvis

In 128 patients with extensive intrapelvic cancers, life-threatening or fatal complications were noted in 4% of those treated with high-energy cyclotrons and in 37–50% of those treated with low- or intermediate-energy cyclotrons, even though the total neutron doses were higher in the former group [29].

Inasmuch as encouraging results have been reported for the neutron irradiation of patients with adenocarcinoma of the prostate, stages C and D1, recent reports of severe rectal reactions resulting in three colostomies amongst 10 patients treated in a randomized trial at the M. D. Anderson Hospital [30] and two colostomies amongst 31 patients treated at the University of California at Los Angeles with 20.4 Gy in 12 increments over 4 weeks have been a cause of concern. However, such severe reactions have not been noted in 63 patients irradiated in Seattle [31] and in only 1 of 87 patients treated in Chicago [32]. An additional treatment arm of 1,800 cGy in 12 increments of 150 cGy over 4 weeks will be tested.

Although the higher rates of late complications following neutron irradiation compared to photon irradiation, such as reduced bladder capacity and pelvic fibrosis, can be attributed to the use of low-energy neutron beams [33, 34], a lack of apparent superiority of tumor clearance has, at least momentarily, discouraged further trials of patients with bladder cancers [35].

Although in an early report [36] 4 of 43 patients receiving two increments of fast neutrons and three increments of photons weekly for locally advanced carcinoma of the cervix developed major bowel complications, this frequency was no greater than that of the control photon treatment group. A trial using only fast-neutron beams from isocentric, high-energy cyclotrons has been discontinued because of poor patient entry into the study.

Abdomen

Potential radiobiological advantages of fast neutrons over photons and a few early favorable reports [37, 38] spawned hope that local tumor control and survival could be improved for patients with locally advanced cancers of the pancreas. In an RTOG study [39] designed to deliver doses equivalent to 6,400 cGy of photons at 180- to 200-cGy increments to the tumor without exceeding 5,000 cGy to the bowel outside the target volume, 4,000 cGy to the spinal cord, or 3,500 cGy to the liver, no advantage was found for treatment with fast neutrons alone or with neutrons plus photons. Of 15 patients treated with neutrons alone, 3 had moderate to severe reactions in the stomach and small bowel. The development of long-term sequelae was limited by a median survival of 5.6 months. Based on a study of 24 dogs receiving fast-neutron irradiation to total doses of 2,250 cGy or more, while islet cells expressed no damage, there was degeneration and necrosis of acinar cells and hemorrhages, erosions, ulcerations, and fibrosis in stomach and duodenum [40].

Thorax

Improved local control with high-dose photon radiation therapy for patients with non-small-cell lung cancer has been favorably reflected in long-term, although not median, survival [41]. Consequently, a trial of fast-neutron treatment seemed appropriate. In an early study [42] at autopsy, tumor control was more frequent in those patients irradiated with 6.2-MeV neutrons plus photons than in those treated conventionally with photons. About the same time, 4 of 18 patients with Pancoast tumors survived for more than 2 years (mean survival 11.5 months), while none of 5 patients treated with photons live that long (mean survival 4.2 months) [43]. In these and other studies [44], low-energy, fixed beams of neutrons were used. Severe toxicities, including subcutaneous fibrosis, pneumonitis, pulmonary fibrosis, and myelitis, as well as rib fracture were reported in 31% of those treated with neutrons, in 15% of those treated with neutrons plus photons, and in 5.4% of those treated with photons [44]. Inasmuch as more accurate delivery of beams to smaller volumes has become possible with the introduction of high-energy, isocentric generators, the frequency of complications should be reduced.

Summary and Conclusions

The potential for serious long term sequelae following fast neutron teletherapy, initially noted by Stone, has prompted careful study of irradiated animals and patients.

Fast neutrons and photons have different physical and radiobiological characteristics which can be bases for differencs in acute and long term sequelae. There is greater absorption of neutrons than photons in fat, related to the high hydrogen content, and less absorption in bone, related to a higher atomic number, for neutrons compared to photons. Neutron-induced responses in cells and tissues are less affected than responses to photons by hypoxia, cell age and repair.

The high relative biological effectiveness of neutrons in the brain and spinal cord has deterred treatment of malignant tumors arising in brain, despite effective tumor cell killing, and has prompted intricate planning of treatment for head and neck cancers, so as to avoid the spinal cord.

While the treatment of locally advanced (stages C, D1) adenocarcinomas of the prostate with fast neutrons has been encouraging, serious long term rectal reactions, resulting in colostomies in 5 patients, are a cause of concern.

No advantage for neutrons over photons has been defined within acceptable bowel tolerance for the irradiation of carcinomas of the pancreas.

While local control of non-small cell lung cancers may prove to be better for fast neutrons than for photons, pneumonitis, and fibrosis of the lung will require the treatment of limited tissue volumes.

The clinical exploitation of apparently more effective tumor cell killing by neutrons than photons for cancers of the salivary glands, prostate, soft tissues and bone, will require the irradiation of small volumes in order to limit serious long term sequelae.

References

1 Stone, R. S.: Neutron therapy and specific ionization. AJR 1948; *59:* 771–785.

2 Smith, A. R.; Almond, P. R.; Smathers, J. B., et al.: Dosimetric properties of the fast neutron therapy beams at TAMVEC. Radiology 1974; *113:* 187–193.

3 Bewley, D. K.: Fast neutron beams for therapy; in Ebert, M.; Howard, A.; (eds): Curr. Top. Radiat. Res. Amsterdam, North-Holland, 1970, vol. VI, pp. 251–292. Amsterdam.

4 Smathers, J. B.: Personal commun, 1986.

5 Bateman, J. L.; Bond, V. P.: Lens opacification in mice exposed to fast neutrons. Radiat. Res. 1967; 7 (suppl): 239–249.

6 Hussey, D. H.; Jardine, J. H.; Raulston, G. L., et al.: 50-$MeV_d \rightarrow Be$ neutrons: A comparison of normal tissue tolerance in animals with clinical observations in patients. Int. J. Radiat. Oncol. Biol. Phys. 1982; *8:* 2083–2088.

7 Ornitz, R. D.; Bradley, E. W.; Mossman, K. L., et al.: Clinical observations of early and late normal tissue injury in patients receiving fast neutron irradiation. Int. J. Radiat. Oncol. Biol. Phys. 1980; *6:* 273–279.

8 Withers, H. R.; Thames, H. D.; Peters, L. J.: Biological bases for high RBE values for late effects of neutron irradiation. Int. J. Radiat. Oncol. Biol. Phys. 1982; *8:* 2071–2076.

9 Withers, H. R.: Neutron radiobiology and clinical consequences. Strahlentherapie 1985; *161:* 739–745.

10 Parker, R. G.; Berry, H. C.; Gerdes, A. J., et al.: Fast neutron therapy of glioblastoma multiforme. AJR 1976; *127:* 331–335.
11 Laramore, G. E.; Griffin, T. W.; Gerdes, A. J., et al.: Fast neutron and mixed (neutron/photon) beam teletherapy for grades III and IV astrocytomas. Cancer 1978; *42:* 96–103.
12 Shaw, C. M.: Sumi, S. M.; Alvord, E. C., et al.: Fast neutron irradiation of glioblastoma multiforme. Neurosurgery 1978; *49:* 1–12.
13 Griffin, T. W.; Davis, R.; Laramore, G., et al.: Fast neutron radiation therapy for glioblastoma multiforme. Results of an RTOG study. Am. J. Clin. Oncol. 1983; *6:* 661–667.
14 Maor, M. H.; Hussey, D. H.; Barkley, H. T., et al.: Neutron therapy for head and neck cancer: A final report of the MDAH-TAMVEC pilot studies. Int. J. Radiat. Oncol. Biol. Phys. 1983; *9:* 1255–1260.
15 Duncan, W.; Orr, J. A.; Arnott, S. J., et al.: Fast neutron therapy for squamous cell carcinoma in the head and neck: Results of a randomized trial. Int. J. Radiat. Oncol. Biol. Phys. 1987; *13:* 171–178.
16 Laramore, G. E.; Griffin, T. W.; Tesh, D W., et al.: Phase I pilot study of fast neutron teletherapy for advanced carcinomas of the head and neck. Cancer 1983; *51:* 192–199.
17 Hornsey, S.; Morris, C. C.; Myers, R., et al.: Relative biological effectiveness for damage to the central nervous system by neutrons. Int. J. Radiat. Oncol. Biol. Phys. 1981; *7:* 185–189.
18 Laramore, G.: Personal commun., 1988.
19 Parker, R. G.; Burnison, C. M., et al.: Peripheral nerve responses to neutron irradiation, in preparation.
20 Abelson, P. H.; Kruger, P. G.: Cyclotron-induced radiation cataracts. Science 1949; *110:* 655–657.
21 Roth, J.; Brown, N.; Catterall, M., et al.: Effects of fast neutrons on the eye. Br. J. Ophthalmol. 1976; *60:* 236–244.
22 Griffin, T.; Pajak, T.; Laramore, G., et al.: Analysis of neutron radiotherapy complications. Bull Cancer (Paris) 1986; *73:* 582–586.
23 Withers, H. R.; Flow, B. L.; Huchton, J. L., et al.: Effect of dose fractionation on early and late skin responses to γ-rays and neutrons. Int. J. Radiat. Oncol. Biol. Phys. 1977; *3:* 227–233.
24 Parker, R. G.; Berry, H. C., et al.: Preliminary clinical results from U.S. fast neutron teletherapy studies. Cancer 1977; *40:* 1434–1438.
25 Catterall: Observations on the reactions of normal and malignant tissues to a standard dose of neutrons; in Barendsen, G. E.; Broese, J.; Breur, K. (eds): High LET, Radiations in Clinical Radiotherapy. New York, Pergamon Press, 1979, pp 11–15.
26 Maor, M. H.; Hussey, D H.; Barkley, H. T., et al.: Neutron therapy for head and neck cancer. II. Further follow-up on the M. D. Anderson-TAMVEC randomized clinical trial. Int. J. Radiat. Oncol. Biol. Phys. 1983; *9:* 1261–1265.
27 Cohen, L.; Hendrickson, F., et al.: Late reactions and complications in patients treated with high energy neutrons p (66 MeV) Be (49 MeV). Int. J. Radiat. Oncol. Biol. Phys. 1981; *7:* 179–184.
28 Griffin, T. W.; Weisberger, E. C.; Laramore, G. E., et al.: Complications of combined surgery and neutron radiation therapy in patients with advanced carcinoma of the head and neck. Radiology 1979; *132:* 177–178.
29 Russell, K. J.; Laramore, G. E.; Krall, J. M., et al.: Eight years experience with neutron radiotherapy in the treatment of stages C and D prostate cancer: Updated results of the RTOG 7704 randomized clinical trial. Prostate 1987; *11:* 183–193.

30 Maor, M. H.: Personal commun., 1988.
31 Laramore, G.: Personal commun., 1988.
32 Hendrickson, F.: Personal commun., 1988.
33 Duncan, W.; Williams, J. R., et al.: An analysis of the radiation related morbidity observed in a randomized trial of neutron therapy for bladder cancer. Int. J. Radiat. Oncol. Biol. Phys. 1986; *12:* 2085–2092.
34 Catterall, M.; Bewley, D. K.: A randomized comparison of photons and 15 MeV neutrons for the treatments of carcinoma of the bladder (letter). Br. J. Radiol. 1986; *59:* 185.
35 Russell, K. J.; Laramore, G. E.; Griffin, T. W.: Fast neutron radiotherapy for the treatment of carcinoma of the urinary bladder: A review of clinical trials, in press.
36 Morales, P.; Hussey, D. H.; Maor, M. H., et al.: Preliminary report of the M. D. Anderson Hospital randomized trial of neutron and photon irradiation for locally advanced carcinoma of the uterine cervix. Int. J. Radiat. Oncol. Biol. Phys. 1981; *7:* 1533–1540.
37 Al-Abdulla A. S. M.; Hussey, D. H.; Olson, M. H., et al.: Experience with fast neutron therapy for unresectable carcinoma of the pancreas. Int. J. Radiat. Oncol. Biol. Phys. 1981; *7:* 165–172.
38 Cohen, L.; Woodruff, K. H., et al.: Response of pancreatic cancer to local irradiation with high energy neutrons. Cancer 1985; *56:* 1235–1241.
39 Thomas, F. J.; Krall, J., et al.: Evaluation of neutron irradiation of pancreatic cancer. Results of a randomized RTOG clinical trial, in press.
40 Zook, B. C.; Bradley, E. W.; Casarett, G. W., et al.: Pathologic effects of fractionated fast neutrons of photons on the pancreas, pylorus and duodenum of dogs. Int. J. Radiat. Oncol. Biol. Phys. 1983; *9:* 1493–1504.
41 Perez, C. A.; Stanley, K., et al.: A prospective randomized study of various irradiation doses and fractionation schedules in the treatment of inoperable, non small-cell carcinoma of the lung: Preliminary report by the RTOG. Cancer 1980; *45:* 2744–2753.
42 Eichhorn, J. H.; Lessel, A.; Matschke, S.: Comparison between neutron therapy and ^{60}Co gamma ray therapy of bronchial, gastric and esophageal carcinomata. Eur. J. Cancer. 1974; *10:* 361–364.
43 Sawada, K.; Fukuma, S., et al.: Clinical experience in patients with Pancoast's tumor treated by fast neutron radiotherapy. Gan No Rinsho 1983; *7:* 111–114.
44 Laramore, G. E.; Bauer, M., et al.: Fast neutron and mixed beam radiotherapy for inoperable non-small cell carcinoma of the lung: Results of an RTOG randomized study. Am. J. Clin. Oncol. 1986; *9:* 233–243

Robert G. Parker, MD, Department of Radiation Therapy, University of California, San Francisco, CA 94143 (USA)

Vaeth JM, Meyer JL (eds): Radiation Tolerance of Normal Tissues.
Front Radiat Ther Oncol. Basel, Karger, 1989, vol 23, pp 194–201

Normal-Tissue Tolerance in Brachytherapy

Bernard Pierquin, Jean-Jacques Mazeron, Laval Grimard, Ginette Marinello

Centre Hospitalo-Universitaire Henri-Mondor, Créteil, France

In this paper the use of brachytherapy is considered solely in the context of low-dose rate continuous irradiation. By this we mean the delivery of a maximum dose (60–70 Gy) in a relatively short period of time: a few days. This time-dose relationship constitutes, in our minds, the essential characteristics of this technique of radiotherapy. In simple terms, brachytherapy will deliver '60 Gy within 6 days', while fractionated irradiation delivers '60 Gy in 6 weeks'. It is well known that, within normal tissue tolerance (late effects), a high dose cannot be given over a short period, unless it is delivered continuously or semi-continuously at a low-dose rate. The question is whether or not this improves the therapeutic ratio by increasing tumor control and decreasing radiation sequelae. The radiobiologists cannot unequivocally answer this question [3–6, 13, 14]. Their experimental results on the oxygen enhancement ratio, sublethal or potentially lethal damage repair, and G2 block are evasive and contradictory. No experimental model comes close to the clinical situations encountered by the radiation oncologist. It is only from clinical data that we can observe different biological effects and draw a few practical conclusions.

We will first describe briefly the technical and dosimetric aspects of brachytherapy as practised in Paris [11] and then present our results in the context of clinical tolerance levels. We use ^{192}Ir sources consisting of continuous wires sheathed in platinum. They are available in diameters of 0.3 and 0.5 mm for interstitial implant and gynecologic plesiotherapy, respectively. We rely entirely on an afterloading approach to reduce radiation exposure to the operators and optimize the implant design through an accurate placement of needles, guide gutters, nylon tubes, and other instruments. Our recent publication [11] covers this field of radiotherapy with complete descriptions of the techniques and basic concepts of dosimetry for interstitial brachytherapy in the Paris System and for plesiotherapy in the Créteil System. Briefly, the dose distribution in the Paris

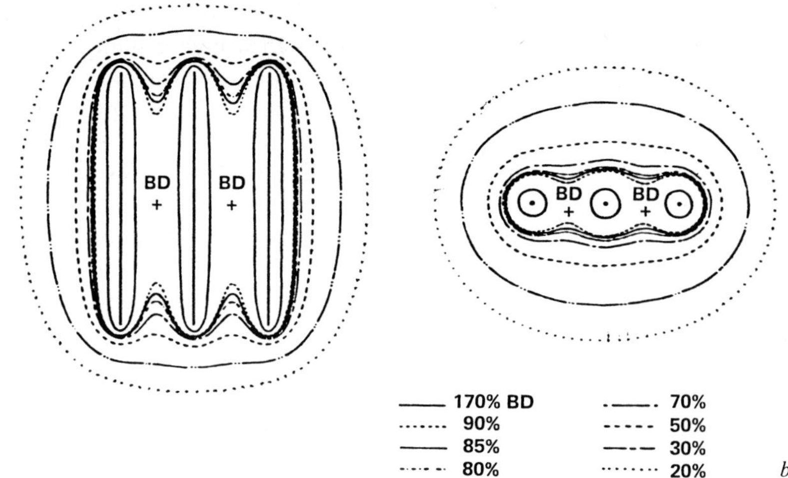

Fig. 1. Distribution of the dose at the plane of the sources *(a)* and at the central plane *(b)* for a pattern consisting of three coplanar lines each 6 cm long and spaced at 1.8 cm. The values of the isodose curves are expressed as a percentage of the basal dose rate *(BD)*.

System is based on the following three principles: (1) radiation lines must be rectilinear, parallel, and arranged so that their centers are located in the same plane; (2) the linear activity along each radioactive line must be uniform and identical for all lines, and (3) adjacent radioactive lines must be equidistant from each other – for large tumors the sources in adjacent planes form either equilateral triangles or squares such that the principle of equidistant lines is still observed.

The minimum dose rate inside the pattern is calculated in the central plane and defined as the basal dose rate. The tumor dose is prescribed at the reference isodose fixed at 85% of the basal dose rate (fig. 1). The volume of tissue surrounding a radioactive line, which receives a dose equal to or greater than twice the reference dose (tumor dose), is defined as the hyperdose sleeve. This volume is related to spacing between lines. Tissue necrosis is observed for sleeve diameters exceeding 10 mm. This diameter depends upon the length of the active lines and the spacing between these lines. A diameter of 10 mm corresponds more or less to 8–10 cm of length and 2–2.2 cm of spacing. This is the reason why it is practical to recommend spacing between 1 and 2 cm and to follow a recommended upper limit of spacing for each site. With large spacing (15 mm), radiosclerotic phenomena or necrosis are observed which are not identically tolerated by all tissues and structures. Recommended upper limits of spacing for each site must be defined. We should point out that the dose in the center of the target volume is about 15% higher than the tumor dose which is prescribed at the reference isodose. This must be considered in all assessments of radiation effects in brachytherapy.

As a first approximation, in comparison with standard fractionated irradiation, the tolerance of normal tissue is equivalent for the same given dose. The acute effects will vary in time and intensity, depending upon the tissue involved. For example, while the skin manifestations at 60–70 Gy are mild and appear 15 days after the 1 day of implantation, consisting of erythema and dry desquamation, the mucosa reacts intensely on the 11th day with severe radiation mucositis and thick fibrinous exudate. Interestingly, the same phenomenon is seen at low-dose rate external irradiation [10]. The late effects consist of radiation fibrosis, skin atrophy, and telangiectasia. We see telangiectasia covering the hyperdose sleeves when the implant is superficial. Although telangiectasia represents a cosmetic sequela, overall skin tolerance is satisfactory, with necrosis seen only after 100 Gy. The mucosa cannot tolerate such a high dose, with some necrosis observed at 70 Gy.

Endocurietherapy delivers a high dose over a short period of time, and tolerance is linked to the volume. For any given dose of radiation, the tolerance will decrease with larger volume. This concept is widely accepted and comes from the radium era, when implantations were limited to small volumes. However, results from three sources of clinical data do not support this hypothesis. First, long experience with the modern practice of brachytherapy using flexible iridium wire and treating large tumors does not correlate complications with target-volume sizes. Second, a long history of gynecologic plesiotherapy indicates a favorable therapeutic ratio, although the pear-shaped isodose encompasses a large area, giving at least 60 Gy to the uterus, the cervix, and the upper third of the vagina, with 120 Gy in the cervix. Finally, the secondary evidence, with regard to brachytherapy, from patients treated with low-dose rate telecobalttherapy at Henri-Mondor [10–12] does not support this hypothesis. In summary, the volume in brachytherapy is not the explanation, but an element of the complex function of dose rate and volume-dose factors influencing normal tissue tolerance.

Does the time to deliver the dose in brachytherapy have an impact on local control and tolerance of normal tissue? In 1973 we published our results of patients treated with ^{192}Ir to a reference dose of 70 Gy [2, 9]. Our conclusions were as follows: 'The different linear activities of ^{192}Ir wires, which we have used for implantation, together with our system of dosimetry, have resulted in a three-fold variation in the total time over which our standard tumor dose has been delivered to the 263 cases here assessed, which have been treated exclusively by interstitial therapy. Necrosis and recurrence rates have been related to overall treatment time for squamous carcinomas of the skin, lip, penis, anterior tongue, and floor of the mouth. It is found, though without enough cases for statistical proof, that overall treatment time may vary from 3 to 9 days without apparent effect upon either necrosis rate or recurrence rate. We conclude that adjustments to overall time which have sometimes been suggested to compensate for such a supposed biological effect are unnecessary, and may even sometimes result in underdosage of the tumor' [9]. From this work our impression was that an isoeffect plateau exists at a low-dose rate (<1 Gy/h). There was no significant difference between a very low-dose rate (<0.6 Gy/h), where 9–10 days were required to deliver the dose, and a higher rate (≥0.6 Gy/h), where the same dose was given over a period of 3–4 days. We did not know the limits of this plateau, but the logical reasoning was that necrosis would be seen more often in implantations of short duration (<3 days) and that tumor recurrence would occur more commonly in protracted implants (>10 days). During that same period Awwad et al. [1] came to similar conclusions using a different method. They looked at 20 patients with tumors of the mobile tongue treated with radium needles according to the rules of Patterson and Parker [8]. Overall, there were recurrences. Among the 20 patients, there were 6 patients in whom 60 Gy would have been given in less than 5 days, and, therefore, the dose was reduced to less than 60 Gy. Five of the 7 recurrences occurred in these 6 patients. Awwad et al. [1] concluded that the dose for tumor control should not be reduced because of a higher dose rate in brachytherapy. Obviously, they could not comment on normal tissue tolerance.

Accumulated data from endocurietherapy and low-dose rate telecobalttherapy have improved the conclusions drawn 15 years ago. With regard to endocurietherapy, Mazeron et al. [7] have just completed a retrospective analysis of 168 patients treated in Créteil for T_1 and T_2 epidermal carcinomas of the mobile tongue. The relationship of dose and dose rate with local control and tissue necrosis is more complex than it appeared in 1973. For analysis the doses received were grouped into two categories: 60 and 65–70 Gy. The dose rates were also combined into two groups: 0.3 to <0.6 and ≥0.6–1.0 Gy/h. The results are shown in table I. We note that while at 60 Gy there are no differences in terms of complications or normal tissue tolerance with regard to the dose rate, there is a significantly higher relapse rate in patients treated at 0.3–0.6 Gy/h (34% vs. 9%). For patients receiving a tumor dose of 65–70 Gy, the dose rate does not influence local control, but has an impact on normal tissue tolerance with 29% of tissue necrosis at ≥0.6–1.0 Gy/h in comparison with

Table I. Treatment of T_1 and T_2 epidermal carcinomas of the mobile tongue

Low-dose rate, Gy/h			
<0.6		>0.6	
60 Gy	70 Gy	60 Gy	70 Gy
Recurrence			
11/32 (34%)	4/46 (9%)	2/23 (9%)	3/51 (6%)
Necrosis			
1/21 (5%)	5/41 (12%)	2/20 (10%)	14/48 (29%)

12% at 0.3 to <0.6 Gy/H. This analysis indicates that the isoeffect plateau below 1 Gy/h is not uniform as previously thought, with different radiobiological effects from 0.3 to 0.9 Gy/h expressed by different normal tissue tolerance and/or tumor control for the same given dose. It is only from clinical data that such findings are meaningful. Finally, in the context of this analysis, the therapeutic ratio is optimal at 60 Gy for a dose rate above 0.6 Gy/h and at 70 Gy below this dose rate (fig. 2).

We will now present some data on low-dose rate telecobalt radiotherapy as it relates to our understanding of normal tissue tolerance in brachytherapy. Seventeen years ago, we began this technique aiming to mimic the time-dose relationship employed in curietherapy. This was done to determine whether the improved normal tissue tolerance [3, 4, 6, 13, 14], and increased tumor sensitivity [5] observed in radiobiological experiments with these dose rates could be exploited at a clinical level [10, 12].

With regard to low-dose rate telecobalt therapy in cancer of the oropharynx, we noted that: 'It is important to underline the very clear correlation between the dose rate and the risk of necrosis. There appears to be a phenomenon in low-dose rate radiotherapy. Under the conditions of our radiation protocol, an upper limit of dose rate is situated around 1.5 Gy/h, beyond which the risk of necrosis is high. Indeed, the 3 patients irradiated at rates greater than 1.5 Gy/h have all developed significant necrosis in healthy tissue within the target volume (in both soft tissue and bone). Two have died of necrosis (1 patient having received a dose rate of 1.8 Gy/h, the other 1.7 Gy/h), and the third is in a precarious state with a necrosis, which still has not healed after more than 2 years (dose rate of 1.7 Gy/h; fig. 3).

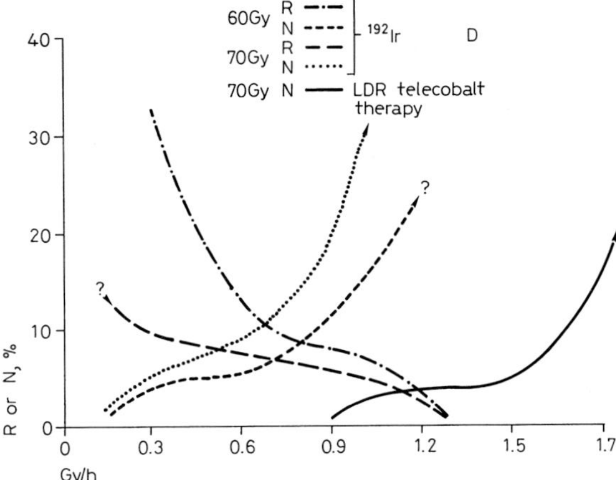

Fig. 2. Treatment of mobile tongue cancer. R = Recurrence; N = necrosis; LDR = low-dose rate.

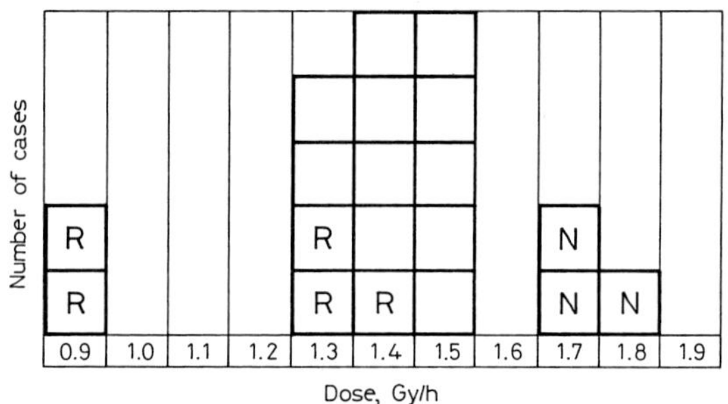

Fig. 3. Distribution of patients as a function of dose rate. R = Recurrence; N = necrosis. Squares without designation represent nonevident disease.

On the other hand, none of the patients irradiated at rates of 1.5 Gy/h or less have developed necrosis in epithelium, muscle or bone. This finding correlates well with observations made during the course of irradiation. Whenever a dose rate of 1.5 Gy/h was exceeded, a marked increase in the severity of skin reactions was observed which is in marked contrast to the remarkable cutaneous tolerance to low-dose rate radiotherapy which we have observed at rates of less than 1.5 Gy/h. There is, therefore, a sudden change at dose rates from 1.5 Gy/h onward which seems to impose an upper limit to the more desirable radiobiological effect of low-dose rate radiotherapy (fig. 4), [10].

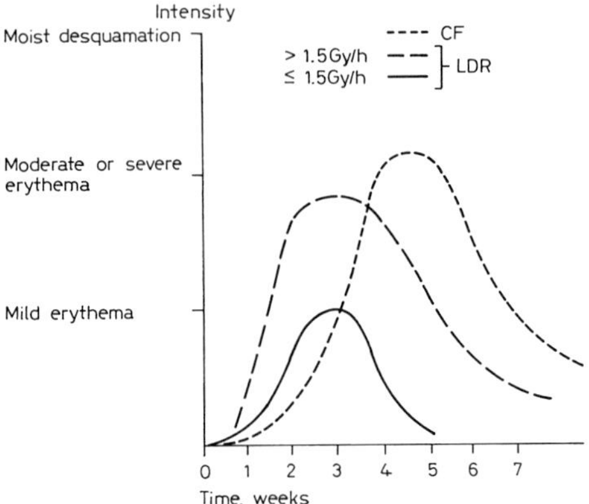

Fig. 4. Skin reaction as a function of technique. CF = Classical fractionation; LDR = low dose rate.

The upper limit of 1.5 Gy/h for low-dose rate telecobalt therapy is also found in breast irradiation, especially for the acute skin reaction. During the last 2 years, we have started to compare low-dose rate telecobalt therapy (45 Gy: 5 fractions, within 5 days, 7 h/day) with standard telecobalt-therapy (45 Gy: 25 fractions within 5 weeks) in patients with large breast cancers. At low-dose rate, the acute skin reactions are minimal except over the midline where a vertical band, a few centimeters wide, presents severe dermatitis 2 weeks after irradiation. This skin reaction occurs exactly where the dose rate is close to or above 1.5 Gy/h. It is too early to comment on late sequelae in low-dose rate telecobalt therapy in breast cancer.

Needless to say, the radiobiological phenomena encountered in brachytherapy and low-dose rate telecobalttherapy cannot be completely similar, as the two techniques have some basic differences. While the former irradiates continuously at a lower dose rate, the latter irradiates 7 h/day at slightly higher dose rates, allowing ample time for sublethal damage repair between fractions.

In conclusion, the isoeffect plateau (or slow progression) up to 1.5 Gy/h, occurring in low-dose rate telecobalttherapy has a much lower threshold in brachytherapy. The upper limit of this isoeffect plateau is unknown, but is probably around 1 Gy/h. In a large series of patients treated exclusively by endocurietherapy for T_1 and T_2 carcinomas of the mobile tongue, dose rate effects were studied at or below 1 Gy/h. The normal tissue tolerance differed above and below 0.6 Gy/h for a tumor dose of 65–70 Gy. This supports the concept of a nonuniform isoeffect plateau from 0.3 to 0.9 Gy/h, (fig. 2). As we accumulate more clinical data on normal tissue tolerance in brachytherapy, our understanding of the complex function of dose rate and volume-dose factors will enable us to improve our patients' care.

References

1 Awwad, H. K.; Burgers, J. M. V.; Marcuse, H. L.: The influence of tumor dose specification on the early clinical results of interstitial tongue implants. Radiology *110:* 177–182 (1974).

2 Burgers, J. M. V.; Awwad, H. K.; Van der Laarse, R.: Relation between local cure and dose-time volume factors in interstitial implants. Int. J. Radiat. Oncol. Biol. Phys. *11:* 715–723 (1985).

3 Hall, E. J.; Bedford, J. S.; Oliver, R.: Extreme hypoxia: its effect on the survival of mammalian cells irradiated at high and low dose rates. Br. J. Radiol. *39:* 302–307 (1966).

4 Hall, E. J.: Radiation dose-rate: a factor of importance in radiobiology and radiotherapy. Br. J. Radiol. *45:* 81–97 (1972).

5 Kal, H. B.; Barendsen, G. W.: Effects of continuous irradiation at the low dose rate on a rat rhabdomyosarcoma. Br. J. Radiol. *45:* 279–283 (1972).

6 Kal, H. B.; Sissingh, H. A.: Effectiveness of continuous low dose rate gamma irradiation on rat skin. Br. J. Radiol. *47:* 673–678 (1974).

7 Mazeron, J. J.; Grimard, L.; Marinello, G.; Pierquin, B.: Dose time factor in low dose rate brachytherapy of epidermoids carcinomas of the mobile tongue (Abstract). ESTRO 7th Annual Meeting, p. 232 (1988).

8 Patterson, R.; Parker, H.: A dosage system for gamma-ray therapy. Br. J. Radiol. *7:* 592–601 (1934).

9 Pierquin, B.; Chassagne, D.; Baillet, F.; Paine, C. H.: Clinical observations of the time factor in interstitial radiotherapy using iridium-192. Clin. Radiol. *24:* 506–509 (1973).

10 Pierquin, B.; Calitchi, E.; Mazeron, J. J.; Le Bourgeois J. P.; Leung, S.: A comparison between low dose rate radiotherapy and conventionally fractionated irradiation in moderately extensive cancers of the oropharynx Int. J. Radiat. Oncol. Biol. Phys. *11:* 431–439 (1985).

11 Pierquin, B.; Wilson, J. F.; Chassagne, D.: Modern Brachytherapy (Masson, New York 1987).

12 Pierquin, B.; Calitchi, E.; Mazeron, J. J.; Le Bourgeois, J. P.; Leung, S.: Update on low dose rate irradiation for cancers of the oropharynx – May 1986. Int. J. Radiat. Oncol. Biol. Phys. *13:* 259–261 (1987).

13 Steel, G. G.; Down, J. D.; Peacock, J. H.; Stephens, T. C.: Dose rate effects and the repair of radiation damage. Radiother. Oncol. *5:* 321–331 (1986).

14 Wambersie, A.; Stienon-Smoes, M. R.; Octave-Prignot, M.; Dutreix, J.: Effect of dose-rate on intestinal tolerance in mice. Implications in radiotherapy. Br. J. Radiol. *52:* 153–155 (1979).

Bernard Pierquin, MD, Centre Hospitalo-Universitaire Henri-Mondor,
F-9410 Créteil (France)

Vaeth JM, Meyer JL (eds): Radiation Tolerance of Normal Tissues.
Front Radiat Ther Oncol. Basel, Karger, 1989, vol 23, pp 202–214

Normal Tissue Tolerance to Intraoperative Radiation Therapy
Experimental and Clinical Studies

Timothy J. Kinsella[a], *William F. Sindelar*[b]

[a]Department of Human Oncology, University of Wisconsin School of Medicine, Madison, Wisc.;
[b]Surgery Branch, National Cancer Institute, Bethesda, Md., USA

Introduction

Intraoperative radiotherapy (IORT) is an area of renewed clinical interest in the treatment of locally advanced tumors of the abdomen, pelvis, retroperitoneum, and, possibly, the mediastinum. The strategy of IORT is quite simple. It involves the use of a large dose of radiation delivered, at the time of surgical exploration, to a tumor or tumor bed and potential areas of locoregional spread. The use of IORT may improve the therapeutic ratio of tumor control to normal tissue toxicity for two major reasons. First, the extent of the tumor can be more precisely defined at surgery and directly irradiated. Second, all or part of sensitive normal tissues or organs may be excluded from the treatment volume by operative mobilization, customized lead shielding, and/or the selection of appropriate electron beam energies. In theory, these are definite advantages compared to conventional external beam irradiation where the tumor (or target) volume can be difficult to define, even with contrast computerized tomography scanning, and where the total radiation dose is often limited by the tolerance of adjacent normal tissues incidentally incorporated within the external beam treatment volume.

The concept of IORT is similar in some aspects to the use of interstitial or intracavitary irradiation where a large dose can be delivered to a specified tumor volume with relative sparing of adjacent tissue. IORT may have an advantage over brachytherapy techniques by providing a more homogenous dose distribution especially to large volumes (>5 cm), although the dose rate used for IORT (usually 200–1,000 cGy/min) may be less biologically advantageous. The idea for IORT is not new. Finisterer [1] in 1915 described a technique of 'eventration' treatment which combined laparotomy and intraoperative orthovoltage irradiation to a locally advanced gastric carcinoma. Two decades later, Eloesser [2], from the Stanford University reported short-term local control with acceptable normal tissue toxicity in 4 of 6 patients with locally advanced gastrointestinal cancers using low-energy X-rays at exploration. Although there were a few small clinical series using IORT in the 1940s and 1950s, technical limitations of X-ray equipment and energy retarded further development of IORT.

The recent era of IORT began in the 1960s, and its development is credited to Abe and Takahashi [3] at Kyoto University in Japan. In general, their approach to IORT has involved gross surgical resection followed by delivery of 2,000–4,000 cGy to the tumor bed using high-energy electrons generated by a betatron. When resection is not possible, higher doses of irradiation are delivered to the intact tumor at exploration and often combined with external beam irradiation. At present, over 3,000 patients have been treated with IORT in Japan. Approximately 30 Japanese institutions are now involved in IORT.

More recently, several US centers have initiated clinical trials using IORT with some promising preliminary results [4]. Approximately 1,000 patients have been treated at five US centers using various combinations of IORT external beam irradiation, and surgery. Investigators at Howard University and the National Cancer Institute use IORT in a manner similar to the Japanese, giving high doses (≥2,000 cGy) of electrons to the tumor bed and areas of locoregional spread following gross surgical resection. The general approach to IORT at Massachusetts General Hospital, Mayo Clinic, and Joint Center for Radiation Therapy is to combine conventional fractionated external beam irradiation (4,500–5,000 cGy) with an IORT boost (1,500–2,000 cGy) using high-energy electrons (Massachusetts General Hospital and Mayo) or 300-Kv x-rays (Joint Center for Radiation Therapy). A number of other US institutions have started to use IORT, and the Radiation Therapy Oncology Group has developed several ongoing clinical trials.

Information on normal tissue tolerance to large single doses of irradiation as used in IORT is quite limited. Clearly, a first principle of IORT is to exclude as many normal tissues as possible from the radiation beam. However, the practical clinical use of IORT necessitates the inclusion of some adjacent normal tissues, and it is necessary to establish tolerance limits applicable to IORT for tissues such as major blood vessels and nerves that are not normally dose limiting with conventional radiotherapy.

Reliable information on an IORT dose-tumor response relationship is also lacking in contrast to data for conventionally fractionated external beam therapy where a dose of 4,500–5,000 cGy over 5 weeks is considered adequate to provide high levels of control of microscopic residual disease following gross surgical resection of most solid tumors. For gross residual or unresectable disease, higher doses of fractionated irradiation (6,000–7,500 cGy over 7–10 weeks) may control small tumors (< 5cm), but are often ineffective in permanently controlling larger tumors. A second goal of the clinical IORT studies will be to establish 'equivalent' IORT dose guidelines for use alone or combined with external beam therapy. While it has been estimated that an IORT dose equivalent factor may be two or three times less than an external beam dose with conventional fractionation, this factor is based on an extrapolation from experimental tumor data. Carefully controlled clinical trials are needed to study the validity of this estimated IORT dose equivalent factor, taking into account issues of local-regional tumor control and normal tissue toxicity. This paper summarizes the available experimental and clinical data on normal tissue effects.

Experimental Normal Tissue Studies with IORT

The initial experimental work on normal tissue tolerance to IORT was performed by Abe and Arakawa [5] who subjected dogs to laparotomy and intraoperative single-dose irradiation. They determined that the major retroperitoneal blood vessels could be irradiated with no significant acute toxicity, but that hollow viscera such as the gastrointestinal tract had to be excluded from the radiation field. While this study established the early clinical guidelines for use of IORT in Japan, a comprehensive study of both acute and late radiation effects on normal tissues in abdomen and retroperitoneum was not undertaken until approximately 9 years ago, when investigators at the National Cancer Institute and elsewhere began a series of experimental studies using adult American foxhounds to assess normal tissue tolerance to large single doses of IORT. These large animals were necessary to allow for careful adequate surgical exposure and placement of IORT cones for field sizes comparable to those used in human studies. Several recent reports have addressed the findings of some of these normal-tissue studies in detail [6–12].

A major concern in the use of IORT to treat tumors which involve the retroperitoneum has been potential acute and late radiation damage to *major blood vessels*. Since these blood vessels are relatively fixed structures and often are contiguous with the tumor, establishing their tolerance is central to the clinical application of IORT. Fortunately, it appears that major blood vessels will maintain their structural integrity with long-term follow-up (up to 5 years), even following doses as high as 5,000 cGy. Histological studies have shown few histopathological changes in these vessels treated to 3,000 cGy or below. Above 3,000 cGy, subintimal and medial fibrosis are evident within 1 year following IORT in both aorta and vena cava, and loss of elastic elements in the walls of large arteries can be observed. Hyalinization of the walls of large veins has not resulted in significant narrowing or occlusion. Additionally, premature atherosclerosis has not been observed.

As expected, the bowel does not tolerate the large doses used in IORT. Within months following a dose of 2,000 cGy, an irradiated segment of *small intestine* developed mucosal ulceration and atrophy, fibrosis of the muscularis, and loss of coordinated peristalsis. With higher doses delivered to a segment of functional small intestine, the gross and microscopic changes were more marked and resulted in obstruction or perforation. However, in a surgically bypassed defunctionalized loop of small intestine, structural integrity was maintained following IORT doses up to 4,500 cGy. Irradiation of the *large intestine* showed similar histopathological changes with obstruction developing after 2,000–3,000 cGy and perforation after 4,500 cGy. Clearly, it appears that the bowel is a dose-limiting structure for IORT, and in the clinical setting functional bowel must be excluded from the IORT field.

The tolerance of *liver and bile duct* to IORT is important to study, since IORT may have clinical application for some locally advancing upper abdominal tumors. Todoroki [13] treated the liver hilum of rabbits and reported hepatic parenchymal atrophy and necrosis as well as marked biliary fibrosis using a single dose of >3,000 cGy. At the National Cancer Institute, irradiation of the extrahepatic bile duct in dogs resulted in fibrosis with eventual stenosis at all doses over 2,000 cGy [6]. Secondary changes of biliary cirrhosis were evident within a few months of developing significant bile duct stenosis.

The tolerance of the *genitourinary tract* to IORT has also been studied using the experimental dog model [7, 12]. The kidney showed changes of parenchymal atrophy and necrosis with doses of >2,000 cGy. A ureter tolerated a dose of 2,000 cGy, but fibrosis and progressive obstruction developed following >3,000 cGy. The bladder wall maintained structural integrity up to 5,000 cGy, although contraction resulted in ureterovesical junction narrowing or obstruction in some dogs receiving >3,000 cGy [12]. From these studies, it appears necessary to exclude the ureter from an IORT field, especially if the dose exceeds 2,000 cGy. While part of a kidney may be included within an IORT field, a nephrectomy is recommended if it is necessary to include an entire kidney. Final-

Table I. Summary of single-dose IORT toxicity to normal intact structures in a large animal model (American foxhound) with follow-up to 5 years (based on National Cancer Institute studies)

Organ or tissue	Maximum dose without severe complications cGy	Comments and findings
Aorta	5,000	patency to 5,000 cGy; fibrosis over 3,000 cGy
Vena cava	5,000	patency to 5,000 cGy; fibrosis over 3,000 cGy
Intestine (functional)	2,000	ulceration, fibrosis, and stenosis over 2,000 cGy
Intestine (defunctionalized)	4,500	intact to 4,500 cGy; fibrosis over 2,000 cGy
Bile duct	2,000	Fibrosis and stenosis over 2,000 cGy
Kidney	2,000	hyalinization necrosis over 2,000 cGy
Ureter	3,000	fibrosis and stenosis over 3,000 cGy
Nerve	2,000	fibrosis and fiber loss over 2,500 cGy; paralysis over 4,000 cGy
Bladder	2,500	stenosis of the ureterovesical junction over 2,500 cGy, bladder mucosa intact up to 4,000 cGy

ly, irradiation of part of the bladder wall seems reasonable, especially if it does not include the ureterovesical junction.

Peripheral nerves are uncommonly injured with conventional fractionated external irradiation. However, a preliminary analysis of a clinical IORT study of retroperitoneal sarcomas revealed that some patients developed severe pain with evidence of motor and/or sensory changes in the distribution of an irradiated nerve within 6–8 months of IORT [10, 14]. Non-invasive studies on these patients could not differentiate between nerve entrapment (perineural fibrosis) or direct nerve injury. An experimental dog study involving irradiation of the femoral and sciatic nerve documented dose-related leg paresis with a threshold for clinical nerve injury as low as 2,500 cGy [10]. Histological study of the irradiated nerves in these dogs reveals primary nerve injury manifest as loss of nerve fibers without evidence of vascular occlusion or thrombosis.

A summary of the maximum tolerable IORT dose to intact normal tissues without significant clinical complications with follow-up to 5 years based on the National Cancer Institute studies is shown in table I. More recently, the tolerance of mediastinal structures to IORT has been studied by National Cancer Institute investigators, but follow-up is limited to between 1 and 2 years [11, 15]. Based on the limited follow-up, it

Table II. Pathologic changes in canine mediastinal and thoracic viscera following intraoperative radiotherapy (2,000, 3,000, or 4,000 cGy) with follow-up to 1 year

Irradiated organ or tissue	Pathologic changes
Lung	Peribronchial and perivascular chronic inflammation > 3,000 cGy acutely; late pleural plaques, pulmonary fibrosis, consolidation at all doses
Esophagus	minimal changes at 2,000 cGy; mild chronic inflammation with occasional instances of severe focal mucosal ulceration > 3,000 cGy
Trachea	minimal changes at 2,000 cGy; mild chronic inflammation with occasional instances of submucosal fibrosis and severe mucosal ulceration > 3,000 cGy
Major blood vessels	medial and adventitial fibrosis and obliterative endarteritis of vasa vasorum at all doses
Atrium	obliterative endarteritis of microvasculature; instances of severe coagulative necrosis with chronic inflammation at all doses
Phrenic nerve	minimal changes at all doses

appears that intact mediastinal structures tolerate IORT doses of 2,000 cGy without significant complications (table II).

In addition to assessing the tolerance of intact normal tissues, it is of equal importance to determine the tolerance of *surgically manipulated normal tissues* to IORT. When IORT is used following surgical resection, it is often necessary to irradiate surgically manipulated tissues (e.g., vascular anastomoses, bypassed intestine) which lie within or immediately adjacent to the tumor bed. Some experimental studies evaluating the tolerance of surgically manipulated tissues have been reported.

The tolerance of *arterial anastomoses* was studied by transecting the abdominal aorta and performing an end-to-end anastomoses followed by immediate IORT [9]. The anastomoses healed adequately following doses up to 4,500 cGy, although progressive histological changes of subintimal and medial fibrosis were evident at doses >3,000 cGy. The fibrosis resulted in stricture at the anastomosis site in some dogs, occasionally progressing to total occlusion. However, clinical arterial insufficiency has not been observed in these dogs followed for up to 5 years because of the development of collateral vessels.

In similar fashion, the tolerance of *gastrointestinal suture lines* and *biliary-enteric anastomoses* were studied [8, 9]. The suture line of a defunctionalized Roux-en-Y intestinal loop remained intact, although, after longer follow-up, the irradiated bowel showed progressive fibrosis and

Table III. Summary of single-dose IORT toxicity to surgically manipulated tissues in a large-animal model (American foxhound) based on National Cancer Institute studies

Surgically manipulated tissues	Maximum Dose without severe complications cGy	Comments and findings
Aortic suture line	4,500	intact to 4,500 cGy; fibrosis and stenosis over 2,000 cGy, sometimes producing late occlusion at > 2 years
Intestinal suture line	4,500	intact to 4,500 cGy; fibrosis and stenosis over 2,000 cGy
Biliary suture line	2,000	suture line disruption at 2,000 cGy
Bronchial stump	4,000	intact to 4,000 cGy; only mild fibrosis at 1 year

narrowing. Applying this approach to the anastomosis between transected bile duct and a defunctionalized loop of small bowel resulted in failure to heal the anastomosis with the lowest dose of 2,000 cGy.

Finally, a canine model of pulmonary resection and IORT was investigated recently [16]. Following penumonectomy, bronchial stump dehiscence was not observed with doses up to 4,000 cGy with follow-up to 1 year. A summary of the tolerance of surgically manipulated tissue in the dog to IORT is presented in table III.

The results of these experimental studies on intact and surgically manipulated normal tissues have served as a general framework for the clinical application of IORT. Longer follow-up on some of these studies is needed. Additional work on normal tissue tolerance to a combination of external beam fractionated irradiation and single-dose IORT is needed also.

Normal Tissue Tolerance to IORT–Clinical Studies

The clinical studies of IORT both in Japan and in the USA have concentrated on locally advanced malignancies of abdomen, pelvis, and retroperitoneum. While over 3,000 patients have been treated in Japan and approximately 1,000 in the USA, conclusive data on the benefit of IORT are still lacking. Preliminary results indicate that it is technically feasible to use IORT alone or combined with a major surgical procedure, and acute morbidity is quite acceptable [3, 4, 8, 17, 18]. However, most phase-III trials at the National Cancer Institute and elsewhere are still too early to determine whether IORT alone or combined with external beam radiation is clearly superior to conventional therapy in terms of local control and normal tissue toxicity.

An accurate analysis of normal tissue toxicity in human clinical trials is of utmost importance. The overall IORT-related complication rate in the first 85 patients treated at the National Cancer Institute was 20%, considered quite acceptable in a population of advanced disease patients [19] (see table IV). For purposes of analysis, the complications were scored on the basis of anatomic location of the tumor. Complications were scored on the basis of anatomic location of the tumor. Complications occurring during the IORT procedure and during the early post-treatment period (<6 months) were relatively infrequent, but were severe in 4 of 7 patients. Late complications developed in 11 patients: upper gastrointestinal hemorrhage from duodenal ulceration was common in patients treated for unresectable pancreatic cancer, and motor-sensory neuropathies were seen among patients having IORT to major nerve trunks in pelvis or retroperitoneum. We concluded that IORT is associated with definite complications, and possible IORT toxicity must be considered in evaluating the potential treatment benefit for each patient.

An assessment of clinical complications of IORT combined with external beam irradiation in locally advanced rectal cancer has been published by Tepper et al. [17, 20] from the Massachusetts General Hospital. In an attempt to improve local control in patients with gross residual or unresectable rectal carcinoma, these investigators used a combined modality approach consisting of pre- or postoperative external beam irradiation (5,000 cGy), surgery, and an IORT 'boost' of 1,000–1,500 cGy, depending on the surgical findings. Fifty-one patients completed the entire treatment, including 29 patients with primary unresectable rectal cancer and 22 patients with recurrent rectal cancer. A detailed analysis of complications showed that approximately 25% of the patients had significant soft-tissue complications, being somewhat higher in patients treated for recurrent tumors (40% complication rate) compared to patients with primary tumors (15%). Although the overall complication rate was comparable to a historical control population treated with surgery and external beam irradiation, pelvic pain in the absence of apparent recurrent tumor was reported in 3 patients treated for recurrent tumors who received IORT.

The initial report of pelvic pain believed related to an IORT-related neuropathy of the lumbo-sacral plexus was described by investigators at the National Caners Institute [10]. Of the 5 patients described in this

Table IV. Summary of IORT-related normal tissue complications in the first 85 patients treated at the National Cancer Institute

Category	Total number of patients	Operative mortality	Patients with compli-cations	IORT-related complications		
				During procedure	Early (before 6 months)	Late (after 6 months)
Upper abdomen	44	8	7	2 (1 vascular)	2 (fistula)	3 (gastrointestinal bleeding)
Lower abdomen and pelvis	7	0	1	0	0	1 (neuropathy)
Retroperitoneum	24	1	6	0	3 (1 skin burn, 2 pseudocyst)	4 (1 vertebral fracture, 3 neuropathy)
Pelvic girdle and extremities	10	0	3	0	0	3 (1 necrosis sacrum, 2 neuropathy)
Total	85	9 (11%)	17 (20%)	2 (2%)	5 (6%)	11 (13%)

original report, 3 patients had retroperitoneal sarcomas and were treated as part of a randomized prospective trial of adjuvant radiation therapy following gross resection. In a recent update of this study, which compared high-dose external beam irradiation (5,000–5,500 cGy) versus IORT (2,000 cGy) and low-dose external beam irradiation (3,500 cGy) [14], 1 additional patient (total or 4 of 15 IORT patients) developed lumbosacral neuropathy as a late complication compared to only 1 of 20 patients receiving conventional fractionated radiation therapy (actually occurring during the immediate postoperative period prior to initiation of radiation therapy). The IORT-related neuropathy occurred 6–9 months following treatment and manifested as moderate to severe pain associated with a mixed motor-sensory nerve deficit. Two of these 4 patients were tested by electromyography and nerve conduction studies and showed reductions in motor unit activity in the affected muscle as well as in velocity and amplitude of the affected nerve action potential. All 4 IORT patients showed a gradual recovery of function and decrease in pain over several months with conservative medical management, including analgesics for pain control and physical therapy.

This randomized prospective trial of IORT in resectable adult retroperitoneal sarcomas is the first published report detailing treatment

Table V. Treatment complications in the prospective randomized study of adjuvant radiation therapy in adult retroperitoneal soft-tissue sarcomas

Category	Total	IORT arm	Control arm
Number of patients	35	15	20
Number with complications	22	10	12
Percent with complications	65	67	60
Complications			
Treatment death	2	1	1
Hemorrhage	2	1	1
Cardiopulmonary	2	1	1
Sepsis-abscess	6	1	5
Fistula	6	0	6*
Acute enteritis	14	1	12*
Chronic enteritis	8	2	7*
Intestinal obstruction	5	1	4
Ureteral obstruction	4	2	2
Vascular insufficiency	2	1	1
Neuropathy	5	4	1
Myelosuppression	4	1	3
Nephritis	0	0	0
Other	2	1	1

*$p > 0.05$.

complications compared to a control group receiving standard fractionated external beam irradiation [14] (see table V). Overall, treatment complications occurred in 63% of patients with no difference in frequency between the IORT and control arms. Two treatment deaths occurred; 1 IORT patient died of a pulmonary embolus, and 1 control patient died prior to receiving any external beam irradiation of hemorrhagic and septic complications of a gastrointestinal fistula. Radiation enteritis was a common complication. Severe acute, but transient, enteritis occurring during postoperative external beam irradiation, and requiring a radiation treatment break of more than 10 days, developed in 12 of the 20 patients receiving high-dose conventional radiotherapy, but only in 1 of 15 patients receiving combined IORT and low-dose external beam irradiation. Late radiation enteritis, developing months (usually >6 months) after treatment and resulting in intractable abdominal pain and/or intestinal obstruction, occurred in 7 patients receiving high-dose radiotherapy and in 2 patients receiving IORT low-dose radiation. Both acute and late radiation enteritis occurred significantly more often in the control group

($p_2 < 0.05$). Additionally, gastrointestinal fistulae developed postoperatively in 6 control patients, significantly more frequently than in IORT patients who developed no fistulous complications ($p_2 < 0.05$).

Other complications that occurred with similar frequency in the IORT and control groups included infections, ureteral obstruction, gastrointestinal hemorrhage, cardiopulmonary complications, and vascular insufficiency. Four of the 6 patients receiving chemotherapy developed dose-limiting myelosuppression with early termination of the planned course of chemotherapy. Hematologic toxicity occurred in 3 control patients and in 1 IORT patient. No renal complications were seen.

In addition to assessment of clinical complications, the National Cancer Institute group has also published a report of pathological tissue changes following IORT [21]. Ninety patients with a variety of advanced-stage malignancies were treated with surgical resection, when feasible, and with intraoperative radiotherapy. Certain patients received additional external beam radiotherapy. During clinical follow-up, 45 patients died. In 22 patients (49% of deaths), detailed autopsy was performed between 1 and 18 months after treatment, with special attention directed towards assessing radiation damage to various tissues. Histological changes related to irradiation were generally manifested as fibrosis. Mild fibrotic changes in retroperitoneal soft tissues and mild hypocellularity in vertebral bone marrow were consistently present in patients treated for pancreatic carcinoma, gastric carcinoma, and retroperitoneal or pelvic sarcomas. Fibrosis of the soft tissues of the porta hepatis without narrowing of the bile duct was present in patients treated for pancreatic or gastric cancer. Perineural fibrosis was present in retroperitoneal and pelvic nerve trunks in patients treated for abdominal or pelvic sarcomas and in patients treated for unresectable carcinoma of the pancreas. Significant radiation-related changes were generally not observed in major blood vessels, intestine, or ureter. Intact irradiated primary tumors consistently displayed necrosis.

This autopsy study demonstrates that radiation-related histopathologic changes do occur following IORT and external beam treatment. The changes observed in patients are similar to the changes seen in our previously reported series of dogs treated with IORT. The human autopsy study suggests that the dog is a valid experimental model to study tissue effects of radiation and is a legitimate means of experimentally establishing dose guidelines for clinical IORT protocols. The current study is limited to a small number of patients having a limited disease spectrum. As experience with IORT accumulates, and postmortem analyses are performed on more patients, a broader picture of the spectrum of radiation-related histopathologic tissue changes should emerge.

Since the clinical use of IORT is continually increasing in the United States, Japan, and elsewhere, it is very important that a standardized set of guidelines regarding toxicity is established. Between 1983 and 1986, an IORT working group was funded by the National Cancer Institute to establish quality control parameters for the use and evaluation of IORT. A detailed outline for grading acute and late effects of IORT has been published and should be used in all subsequent clinical reports of IORT [22].

References

1 Finsterer, H.: Zur Therapie inoperabler Magen- und Darmkarzinome mit Freliegung und nachfolgender Röntgenbestrahlung. Strahlentherapie *6:* 205–213 (1915).

2 Eloesser, L.: The treatment of some abdominal cancers by irradiation through the abdomen combined with cautery excision. Ann, Surg. *106:* 645–652 (1937).

3 Abe, M.; Takahashi, M.: Intraoperative radiotherapy: the Japanese experience. Int. J. Radiat. Oncol. Biol. Phys. *7:* 863–868 (1981).

4 Kinsella, T. J.; Sindelar, W. F.: Intraoperative radiation therapy; *in* Devita, Hellman, Rosenberg, Principles and practice of oncology; 2nd ed., pp. 2293–2304 (Lippincott, Philadelphia 1985).

5 Abe, M.; Arakawa, M.: Fundamental studies on surgical irradiation. Histological and hematological changes following irradiation during laparotomy of dogs. Jap. Soc. Cancer Ther. *2:* 271–278 (1967).

6 Sindelar, W. F.; Tepper, J.; Travis, E. L.: Tolerance of bile duct to intraoperative irradiation. Surgery *92:* 533–540 (1982).

7 Sindelar, W. F.; Tepper, J.; Travis, E. L.; Terrill, R.: Tolerance of retroperitoneal structures to intraoperative radiation. Ann Surg *196:* 601–608 (1982).

8 Sindelar, W. F.; Kinsella, T. J.; Tepper, J.: Experimental and clinical studies with intraoperative radiotherapy. Surgery Gynec. Obstet. *157:* 205–219 (1983).

9 Tepper, J. E.; Sindelar, W.; Travis, E. L.: Tolerance of canine anastomoses to intraoperative radiation therapy. Int. J. Radiat. Oncol. Biol. Phys. *9:* 987–991 (1983).

10 Kinsella, T. J.; Sindelar, W. F.; DeLuca, A. M.: Tolerance of peripheral nerve to intraoperative radiotherapy (IORT): clinical and experimental studies. Int. J. Radiat. Oncol. Biol. Phys. *11:* 1941–1946 (1985).

11 Barnes, M.; Pass, H.; DeLuca, A.; Sindelar, W.; Kinsella, T. J.: Response of the mediastinal and thoracic viscera of the dog to intraoperative radiation therapy. Int. J. Radiat. Oncol. Biol. Phys. *13:* 371–378 (1987).

12 Kinsella, T. J.; Sindelar, W. F.; DeLuca, A. M.: Tolerance of the canine bladder to intraoperative radiotherapy: an experimental study. Int. J. Radiat. Oncol. Biol. Phys. *14:* 939–946 (1988).

13 Todoroki, T.: The late effects of single massive irradiation with electrons of the liver hilum in rabbits. Jap. J. gastroent. Surg. *11:* 169–177 (1978).

14 Kinsella, T. J.; Sindelar, W. F.; Lack, E.; Glatstein, E.; Rosenberg, S. A.: Preliminary results of a randomized study of adjuvant radiation therapy in resectable adult retroperitoneal soft tissue sarcomas. J. clin. Oncol. *6:* 18–25 (1988).

15 Sindelar W. F.; Hoekstra, H. J.; Kinsella, T. J.: Tolerance of canine esophagus to intraoperative electron beam radiotherapy. Int. J. Radiat. Oncol. Biol. Phys. *15:* 663–670 (1988).

16 Pass, H. I.; Sindelar, W. F.; Kinsella, T. J.; Delivery of intraoperative radiation therapy after pneumonectomy: experimental observations and early clinical results. Ann. thor. Surg. *44:* 14–20 (1987).
17 Tepper, J. E.; Gunderson, L. L.; Orlow, E.: Complications of intraoperative radiation therapy. Int. J. Radiat. Oncol. Biol. Phys. *10:* 1831–1839 (1984).
18 Sindelar, W. F.; Hoekstra, H. J.; Kinsella, T. J.: Surgical approaches and techniques in intraoperative radiotherapy for intra-abdominal, retroperitoneal, and pelvic neoplasms. Surgery *163:* 247–256 (1988).
19 Sindelar, W. F.; Kinsella, T. J.; Hoekstra, H. J.; Tochner, Z.; Smith, R.; Glatstein, E.: Treatment complications in intraoperative radiotherapy. Int. J. Radiat. Oncol. Biol. Phys. *11:* suppl, pp. 117–118 (1985).
20 Tepper, J. E.; Cohen, A.; Wood, W. C.; Gunderson, L.: Intraoperative electron beam radiotherapy in the treatment of unresectable rectal cancer. Archs Surg *121:* 421–423 (1986).
21 Sindelar, W. F.; Hoekstra, H.; Restredo, C.; Kinsella, T. J.: Pathological tissue changes following intraoperative radiotherapy. Am. J. clin. Oncol. *9:* 504–509 (1986).
22 Tepper, J. E.; Gunderson, L. L.; Goldson, A. L.; Kinsella, T. J.; Shipley, W. U.; Sindelar, W. F.; Wood, W. C.; Martin, J. K.: Quality control parameters of intraoperative radiation therapy. Int. J. Radiat. Oncol. Biol. Phys. *12:* 1687–1695 (1986).

Timothy J. Kinsella, MD, Department of Human Oncology,
University of Wisconsin School of Medicine, Madison, WI 53792 (USA)

Vaeth JM, Meyer JL (eds): Radiation Tolerance of Normal Tissues.
Front Radiat Ther Oncol. Basel, Karger, 1989, vol 23, pp 215–220

Normal-Tissue Tolerance or Skin, Cartilage, and Bone

Robert G. Parker, Donald Karon[1]

Department of Radiation Therapy, University of California, Los Angeles, Calif., USA

The tolerances of skin, cartilage, and bone always have and continue to influence the therapeutic applications of ionizing radiations.

Skin

Initially, skin tolerance was a limiting factor in all applications from low-energy teletherapy generators. This led to the development of techniques exploiting multiple portals of entry and the use of radium in surface applications and teletherapy units. Although the introduction of megavoltage teletherapy units has minimized the importance of skin tolerance, this organ remains a subject for the study of radiation responses.

In general, the late effects of irradiation that we are interested in were really acute effects. Although they are uncomfortable, the acute reactions are really not a major factor once you get the patient through the events. Once the late effects of skin irradiation start, they progress, they are irreversible, and often they are very regrettable.

The basic pathophysiology in early and late effects in skin is a disruption, temporary or permanent, of the basoregenerative layer. That relates to the severity of the insult, but for the most part, what one does is predictable, and these changes go through a range of intensity. There are many factors involved. One factor which tends to be overlooked is the increment size. If one looks at all those radiobiological formulas that have monopolized our literature for years, this was not properly dealt with. There was the first and landmark article by Strandquist who, for the first

[1]For a detailed bibliography on this subject, we refer the reader to the paper by R. G. Parker and G. Juillard; in Vaeth, J. M.; Meyer, J. L. (eds): Time, Dose and Fractionation in the Radiation Therapy of Cancer. Front Radiat. Ther. Oncel. Basel, Karger, 1988, vol 22, pp. 53–61.

time, related dose and time. On his historic graph everything runs in a straight line with equal slope. We know now that is incorrect, but this was a monumental contribution at that time. Carl von Essen who was a fellow resident of mine (as was Jerry Vaeth) made a major advance by pointing out that, amongst other things, the slope is not equal for different effects. As the lesions get larger, one moves out on the abscissa towards longer overall treatment time in order to get tumor kill with acceptable complications. What we would like to deal with is a proportionality of early to late effects. In a recent symposium, Lester Peters pointed out that if you do things that change in the direction of increasing the acute reaction, you have a built – in safety factor as you may quit early and, therefore, save the patients a catastrophy. However, if you go in the other direction and do things to the standard application which is 200 rad a day, 5 days a week for 4–6 weeks, you have fallen into a trap. If you match acute reactions going in this direction with large-dose fractions, you have fallen into a very serious trap. This is not a new phenomenon and was noted in the literature but largely ignored, i.e., that late changes are related to dose fractions and size. In the radiobiology literature, Withers points out that even though the acute reaction was greater for total higher doses well fractionated, the late reactions were less. Studying the human skin, irradiated for breast cancer, if one equalizes the acute erythema reaction, the acute erythema with multiple doses of less than 200 cGy with one or two larger doses, over the years the changes will separate and become increasingly more severe for the pattern with large-dose fractions. This information can be extrapolated to other sites such as spinal cord and intestinal tract. This is not really a new information. It has just been overlooked again and again. An old study reported by a dermatologist pointed out that if one treats with 1,000 cGy × 4 compared with 300 cGy × 15, there is a disparity in long-term effects – in this case necrosis – with the larger fractions.

Cartilage

For many years, the myth of the intolerance of cartilage to radiation therapy influenced clinical management. Years after burial of this myth, resurrections are promoted by the unknowing.

The effects of irradiation on cartilage have been known for many years. There is really not much evidence that is new. For 20 years, we have known that one can treat to cancercidal doses over intact cartilage without damaging the cartilage. One can get into trouble treating over cartilage under certain circumstances. Unfortunately, those circumstances are present for the length of the patient's life, so whatever one does up front in treating over presumably healthy cartilage, the patient lives with tissue damage forever. One can reactivate a deleterious process anytime during the patient's life, particularly with trauma and consequent infection. There are some studies that I have intermittantly reported over the years, and while not earth shaking, there are very few data on this subject. Namely, if one incidentally irradiated the pinna while one is treating something else of interest – head and neck tumors – there is no problem if one goes to total dose levels of 6,000–6,500 cGy, with fractionated increments. If one treats epitheliomas, one can have problems that are very predictable if the cartilage is exposed and infected. The cartilages most at risk in practice are the cartilages of the larynx. The dose-response curve is very steep. Fletcher, early on, reported that if one makes only a slight increase in the dose over the same period of time, the complication frequency is going to increase. One can treat even over tumor-invaded cartilage and have no treatment-related complications.

Bone

Although the introduction of megavoltage generators has resulted in the lessening of absorption of radiations in bone, the potential for serious problems still exists. These primarily are risks of mandibular necrosis in the treatment of head and neck cancers and growth suppression in youngsters.

Many of you are treating immediately postoperatively hip replacement patients in an effort to suppress hypertrophic bone growth. We have irradiated patients with various treatment patterns, starting with a total of 2,000 cGy and less. We have not seen any problems with delayed wound healing or healing of the orthopedic site. Osteonecrosis of the mandible is still an issue that concerns us all. We have seen only 2 of these in 10 years at the University of California, Los Angeles, Calif., USA, in a fairly busy head and neck clinic, and I do not think we are overlooking many of them. We are avoiding the problem by intense supportive management. Every patient, including patients with Hodgkin's Disease who have any chance of change in salivation, e.g., patients being irradiated to the oral cavity, sees the oral surgeons/dentists prior to any radiation treatment. This has absolutely revolutionized the management of head and neck cancer as far as minimizing bone complications.

Costal necrosis has again become an issue with more aggressive radiation treatment of cancer of the breast. In early studies some 4 cases with rib damage were reported in a breast preservation series from several centers on the East Coast. I think that still happens, but, hopefully, it is rarely recognized in our institution. Femoral neck fracture, an issue that had about 2% incidence when I was in training, has essentially disappeared from the literature as a complication of radiation therapy. It is almost anecdotal.

Much more difficult to measure is, 'What do we do to growing bone?' Although pediatric radiotherapy is not a large proportion in most radiotherapy practices, it certainly is an important one. The radiation changes in growing bone are clearly related to the intensity of the dose. The changes increase with increasing intervals and are very closely related to the age of the patient at the time of the irradiation. The first article was written by Newhauser who defined the problems in bone growth secondary to irradiation. At that point in time he reported on only 22 patients treated with orthovoltage equipment. The dosimetry was completely unacceptable by today's standards, but the conclusions were correct, i.e., there are certain doses which do not express themselves as long-term problems. Rubin (Ann Arbor Group) pointed out that even physically uniform irradiation of the verebrae does not always prevent scoliosis, perhaps in part because of muscle damage on the tumor side. At the same time, Vaeth and Levitt described in the literature that there indeed is a close dose-response curve. As did Rubin, they described the bone changes related to dose and age of patient. Probert reported that with doses below 2,500 cGy, there were very few changes in children irradiated after the age of 6 years. Changes were noted mostly in youngsters irradiated below the age of 6. When the dose was increased to 3,500 cGy or greater, changes were much more marked. In the group of ages up to 6 years at the time of irradiation, there were easily recognizable bone changes. Historically, we have missed many of these growth changes by not measuring the sitting height. These changes are all in the vertebral column. Probert did not see any difference using megavoltage radiations when it was normalized for actual dose absorbed. Total-body irradiation is not innocuous, even though it can be lifesaving. The group in Seattle, based on 142 patients who have been followed for at least more than 3 years, found that if one changed the application from one dose of around 10 Gy to a fractionation of 2 Gy × 6 or 7, 3 years later, the average height was 8 cm more in the fractionated group. Thus, total-body irradiation causes many changes, including suppression of bony growth.

Many years ago, I reviewed every reported case of malignant tumor in irradiated bone and found some curious things. In many instances, the bone was not documented as normal prior to the treatment, and while tumors that were claimed to be radiation induced had to be in irradiated bone, sometimes they were not. Often the tumor was not histologically documented and merely implied by radiography. Sometimes, there was no latency period which would not allow ruling out concurrent disease.

When one is treating normal bones to high doses, how often is this a risk for radiation injury? Some data from San Francisco indicate that in patients that live 5 years or longer and received doses high enough to control cancer, the risk is only a fraction of 1%.

Conclusion

At this point in time, the relationship between the radiation insult and the consequent measurable damage in skin, cartilage, and bone is reasonably well defined. There is not much present research activity in these fields. The deleterious influence of large-dose increments for many tissues, including skin, has been carefully defined. Healthy adult cartilage tolerates irradiation treatment, no matter what the plastic surgeons say! Problems related to irradiation of mature bone have decreased in frequency and consequence, as radiotherapy itself has become more sophisticated and the radiotherapists themselves have become better trained. Problems related to radiation-induced arrest of bone development persist in a few very specific clinical situations and, at this time, must be accepted as a price for curative treatment.

References

1 Montague, E. D.; Schell, S. R.; Romsdahl, M. D.; Ames, F. C.: Conservation surgery and irradiation in the treatment of breast cancer; in Vaeth, Hyperthermia and radiation therapy/chemotherapy in the treatment of cancer. Front. Radiat. Ther. Onc., vol. 18 (Karger, Basel 1982).

2 Neuhauser, E. B. D.; Wittenborg, M. H.; Berman, C. Z.; Cohen, J.: Irradiation effects of roentgen therapy on the growing spine. Radiology *59:* 637–650 (1952).

3 Parker, R. G.: Tolerance of mature bone and cartilage in clinical radiation therapy; in Vaeth, Radiation effect and tolerance: normal tissue. Front. Radiat. Ther. Onc., vol. 6 (Karger, Basel 1972).

4 Paterson, R.: Treatment of malignant disease by radium and X-rays (Williams & Wilkins, Baltimore 1948).

5 Peters, L. J.: Contributions of the keynote discussant; in Fletcher, Nervi, Withers, Biological bases and clinical implications of tumor radioresistance, pp. 205–207 (Masson, New York 1983).

6 Phillips, T. L.; Sheline, G. E.: Bone sarcomas following radiation therapy. Radiology *81:* 992–996 (1963).

7 Probert, J. C.; Parker, B. R.; Kaplan, H. S.: Growth retardation in children after megavoltage irradiation of the spine. Cancer *32:* 634–639 (1973).

8 Sanders, J. E.; Pritchard, S., et al.: Growth and development following marrow transplantation for leukemia. Blood *68:* 1129–1135 (1986).

9 Strandquist, M.: Studien über die kumulative Wirkung der Röntgenstrahlen bei Fraktionierung. Acta radiol. *73:* suppl., pp. 1–300 (1944).

10 Traenkle, H. L.; Mulay, D.: Further observations on late radiation necrosis following therapy of skin cancer. Archs Derm. *81:* 908–913 (1960).

11 Turesson, I.; Notter, G.: The influence of fraction size in radiotherapy on the late normal tissue reaction. 1. Comparison of the effects of daily and once-a-week fractionation on human skin. Int. J. Radiat. Oncol. Biol. Phys. *10:* 593–598 (1984).

12 Vaeth, J. M.; Levitt, S. H.; Jones, M. D.; Holfretter, C.: Effects of radiation therapy in survivors of Wilm's tumor. Radiology *79:* 560–567 (1962).

13 Von Essen, C. F.: A spatial model of time-dose-area relationships in radiation therapy. Radiology *81:* 881–883 (1963).

14 Whitehouse, W. W.; Lampe, I.: Osseous damage in irradiation of renal tumors in infancy and childhood. Am. J. Roentg. *70:* 721–729 (1953).

15 Withers, H. R.; Thames, H. D.; Flow, B. L.; Mason, K. A.; Hussey, D. H.: The relationship of acute to late skin injury in 2 and 5 fractions/week γ-ray therapy. Int. J. Radiat. Oncol. Biol. Phys. *4:* 595–601 (1978).

Robert G. Parker, MD, Department of Radiation Oncology and Jonsson Comprehensive Cancer Center, University of California,
Los Angeles, CA 90024 (USA)

Vaeth JM, Meyer JL (eds): Radiation Tolerance of Normal Tissues.
Front Radiat Ther Oncol. Basel, Karger, 1989, vol 23, pp 221–237

Effect of Radiation on Normal Tissues in the Head and Neck

Bone, Cartilage, and Soft Tissue

Rodney R. Million, James T. Parsons, William M. Mendenhall

Department of Radiation Oncology, University of Florida College of Medicine, Gainesville, Fla., USA

Introduction

The analysis of the risks of radiation-induced injury to normal and abnormal tissues is best reviewed by the clinical settings in which irradiation is applied. It is not possible to generalize about cartilage, bone, or soft-tissue injury, since the risks differ with different anatomical situations, the biological dose applied, and other variables.

Radiation Effects on the Larynx

Adult cartilage at first has no blood vessels or lymphatics and contains mostly interstitial substance with very few cells of low mitotic activity. The thyroid, cricoid, and arytenoid cartilages, however, become progressively calcified and then ossified with aging and develop a blood supply and a typical central marrow cavity. The fate of calcified cartilage is almost always resorption followed by ossification. The ossification occurs earlier and more completely in men. At the time when most high-dose irradiation is aimed at the larynx, calcification with progression to ossification is already present in men and to a lesser extent in women. The epiglottis, which is primarily elastic cartilage, only occasionally shows a small plaque of calcification [10].

Keene et al. [8] studied chondronecrosis and osteomyelitis by whole-organ serial sectioning of 265 larynges with squamous cell carcinoma. Nearly all operations were for primary therapy or recurrence after radical radiation therapy. Two hundred and sixteen patients had been irradiated, and 49 patients had laryngectomy only.

A histological diagnosis of chondronecrosis was defined as 'cartilaginous components devoid of perichondrium and bathed in purulent exudate'. A histological diagnosis of osteomyelitis was defined as 'necrotic bone present (devitalized with empty lacunae) or marrow spaces containing acute inflammatory exudate'.

Significant chondronecrosis or osteonecrosis was frequently seen in combination with the presence of cancer and occurred in 27% of irradiated patients and in 24% of nonirradiated patients. There were six necroses following high-dose radiation therapy in patients with no tumor in the specimen. The arytenoids were necrotic in 3 cases, the thyroid alae in 3, the cricoid in 2, and the hyoid bone in 1. Five of the cases had T_{2-3} supraglottic larynx lesions, and 1 had a T_3 glottic lesion.

Incidental Irradiation of Normal Larynx

It is our practice to exclude the normal larynx from high-dose incidental irradiation. However, when treating carcinomas of the posterior pharyngeal wall or pyriform sinus, and the uncommon postcricoid and cervical esophagus carcinomas, it is impossible to exclude the posterior two thirds of the larynx for at least part of the treatment, and in many situations parts of the larynx receive a dose equivalent to the tumor dose. We have not observed clinical necrosis of the normal laryngeal skeleton with doses equivalent to 6,500–7,000 cGy in 6.5–8 weeks, 5 fractions/week, 1 fraction/day, nor with 7,440–7,920 cGy in 6.5–7 weeks, 120 cGy/fraction, 2 fractions/day, 5 days/week, with a 4- to 6-hour interval between fractions. In these cases, the anterior one third of the larynx is usually shielded from the portal from the beginning. One instance of osteochondronecrosis was observed at autopsy after 8,160 cGy, 120 cGy twice-a-day fractionation, was given to a T_4N_1 posterior pharyngeal wall lesion [25].

Irradiation of the Larynx Involved by Cancer

Squamous Cell Carcinoma of the Glottic Larynx

T_{1-2}: Treatment plans for T_{1-2} squamous cell carcinoma of the vocal cords encompass the thyroid, cricoid, and the arytenoid cartilages and approximately 2 cm of the infrahyoid epiglottis. The lateral portal sizes range from 4×4 to 6×6 cm. The dose to the arytenoids and posterior cricoid may be lower than or the same as the tumor dose, depending on the placement of the borders, weighting of the wedges, field arrange-

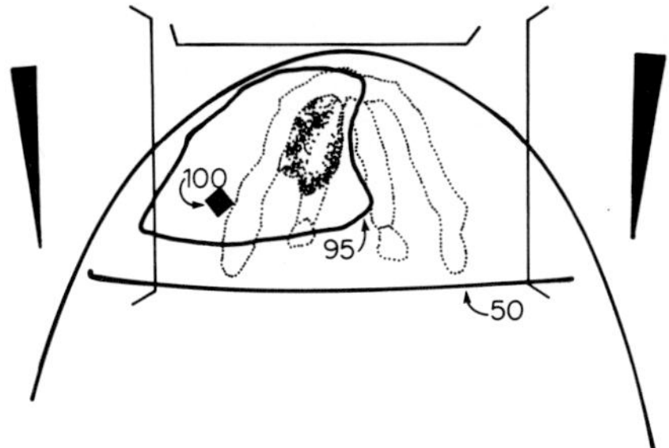

Fig. 1. Normalized isodose distribution for three-portal technique. The lateral wedged portals (4 × 4 cm) are each weighted 1.0, and the anterior portal (3.5 × 3.5 to 4 × 4 cm) is weighted 0.1 or 0.2. The maximum dose is shifted to the left side at a depth of 1 cm. The maximum dose is 5% greater than the tumor dose. This arrangement slightly reduces the high-dose volume and is the plan most often used within the past 5 years. The anterior portal is treated at the end of the treatment series after the lateral portals are completed. [From ref. 23, p. 341.]

ments, and so forth. Parts of the thyroid cartilage and the cricoid receive a dose 2–5% greater than the tumor when a three-field technique is used (fig. 1).

A recent analysis of 303 patients with T_{1-2} vocal cord cancer with a minimum 2-year follow-up (82% with a minimum 5-year follow-up) treated with ^{60}Co or 2-MV X-rays identified only 1 patient who had clinical and CT diagnosis of an osteochondronecrosis (fig. 2) [16].

An additional 4 moderate to severe soft-tissue complications were identified, only 1 of which required a total laryngectomy. Analyses of complications related to T stage, total dose, and dose per fraction are shown in table I and figure 3. The single example of osteochondronecrosis (fig. 2) occurred at a high dose of 6,750 cGy, 225 cGy/fraction, 5 fractions/week, given for a large T_2 lesion [16]. The dose for T_{1-2} lesions treated with 1 fraction/day, 225 cGy/fraction, is now limited to 6,525 cGy. The relationship of osteochondronecrosis to the dose per fraction and total tumor dose for T_{1-2} vocal cord carcinoma for four series is shown in table II [22].

T_3: Harwood et al. [5] reviewed 112 patients treated by radiation therapy between 1963 and 1977 with three basic schemes: 5,000 cGy in 24–26 fractions, 5,000 cGy in 20 fractions, and 5,500 cGy in 24 fractions. A single case of laryngeal necrosis was observed after 5,500 cGy in 24 fractions, 229 cGy/fraction. The necrosis healed without requiring a laryngectomy.

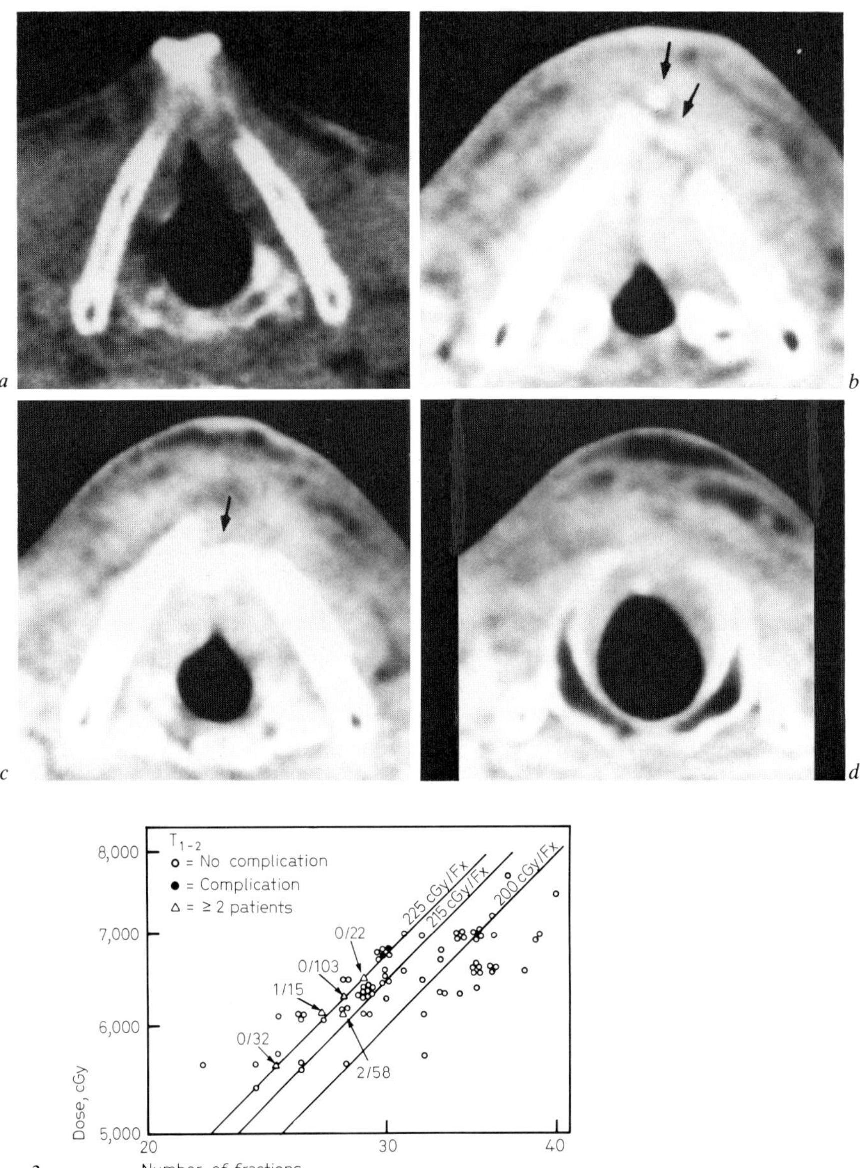

Fig. 2. A 62-year-old man presented with a squamous cell carcinoma of the anterior half of both vocal cords with involvement of the anterior commissure and about 3 mm of subglottic extension. The mobility was normal. The left ventricle was found to be involved with tumor on pathologic examination of the biopsy specimen. *a* The CT at the level of the vocal cords shows ossified thyroid and cricoid cartilage. The thyroid cartilage is either

Table I. Incidence of moderately severe and severe complications: 303 patients with T_{1-2} squamous cell carcinoma of the glottic larynx (number of complications/number of patients treated) [from ref. 16, table 5][a]

Total dose cGy	Dose per fraction, cGy					
	T_1		T_2		total	
	225–255[b]	185–224	225–245[c]	175–224	225–255	175–224
>7,000	no data	no data	no data	0/3	no data	0/3
6,700–7,000	no data	0/2	2/7 (29%)	0/12	2/7 (29%)	0/14
6,000–6,600	0/86	1/58 (1.7%)	1/61 (1.6%)	1/34 (2.9%)	1/147 (0.7%)	2/92 (2.2%)
5,400–5,700	0/36	0/2	no data	0/2	0/36	0/4

[a] Patients treated with once-a-day fractionation.
[b] Only 1 patient was treated at >235 cGy/fraction.
[c] Only 1 patient was treated at >235 cGy/fraction.

incompletely ossified anteriorly or possibly invaded by tumor (clinical stage T_2N_0). The patient was treated with radiation therapy consisting of 6,750 cGy in 30 fractions with a three-field technique. Approximately 8 months after treatment he developed 1+ arytenoid edema. At 1 year he reported a sore throat, right-ear pain, and increasing hoarseness for 1 month. Examination showed 1+ edema, but no evidence of recurrence. During the next 2 years he reported persistent hoarseness and continued to have 1+ edema. Approximately 3 years after treatment, the patient had sudden onset of swelling of the anterior neck, hoarseness, coughing, and dysphagia. The skin of the anterior neck was erythematous over the thyroid cartilage, and there was mild pain on palpation of the thyroid cartilage. There was 2+ laryngeal edema, but no stridor. The vocal cords were not easily visible, but seemed to move. No obvious cancer was noted, and no neck nodes were palpable. *b* The CT at the level of vocal cords shows a diffuse edema of the false vocal cords. The airway is narrowed. There is thickening of the tissues anterior to the larynx. The thyroid cartilage shows at least two bony sequestra (arrows). The arytenoids are normal. *c* The CT at the level of true vocal cords shows bilateral laryngeal edema. There is fragmentation and displacement of the thyroid cartilage (arrow). *d* The CT at the level of the cricoid shows normal appearance of cricoid. There is edema in the anterior subglottic area. The CT diagnosis included (1) necrosis of the laryngeal skeleton and (2) cannot exclude recurrence. Direct laryngoscopy was done; no tumor was seen, and biopsies were negative. The treatment consisted of antibiotics, and the symptoms had subsided by 6 weeks. At 3 months there was subcutaneous induration anterior to the thyroid cartilage, and the left thyroid ala bulged outward. Cords were normal, but the mucosa showed high-dose effects. The patient was free of disease at 5 years with a functioning larynx.

Fig. 3. T_{1-2} squamous cell carcinoma of the glottic larynx: incidence of moderately severe and severe complications as a function of dose and number of treatment fractions (Fx). The lines are not isoeffect lines and are for reference only. A circle indicates a single patient; a triangle denotes 2 or more patients. The number of patients represented by each triangle is given (number sustaining a moderately severe or severe complication over the number treated, with the arrow pointing to triangle). [From ref. 16, fig. 3.]

Table II. Osteochondronecrosis following irradiation for T_{1-2} vocal cord carcinoma [modified from ref. 23, p. 184]

Study	Primary site	Tumor dose cGy/number of weeks	Fraction size, cGy[a]	Number of patients	% with necrosis
University of Florida [16]	glottis (T_1)	5,400–7,000/4.5–7	180–255	184	0
	glottis (T_2)	as above	as above	119	0.08
Princess Margaret Hospital [7]	glottis (T_1)	5,500/5	210–230	378	0
Rush Presbyterian-St. Lukes [9]	glottis (T_{1-2})	6,500/5–5.5	225–250	146	0.7
Penrose [2]	glottis (T_{1-2})	6,100–6,600/3.5–4	approx-imately 300	16	6

[a] Fraction size standardized at 225 cGy after 1977.

Mendenhall et al. [13] and Parsons et al. [25] reviewed the University of Florida experience for 19 patients treated by 1 fraction/day and 14 patients treated by 2 fractions/day. One necrosis occurred following 7,680 cGy (twice-a-day fractionation) in a patient with a T_3N_0 cancer of the true vocal cord. The necrosis was believed to have been precipitated by biopsy. Six weeks following irradiation, the patient underwent direct laryngoscopy, and although the surgeon saw no evidence of tumor recurrence or substantial edema, eight deep biopsies were obtained. The patient's larynx was never free of edema thereafter, and total laryngectomy was required 5 months later. Neither the laryngeal biopsies nor the pathological specimens showed tumor. The patient remained free of disease at 5 years.

Squamous Cell Carcinoma of the Supraglottic Larynx

The risk of necrosis for four series of supraglottic larynx carcinomas treated by radiation therapy is shown in table III. The rate of necrosis is generally higher for supraglottic larynx carcinoma compared with vocal cord carcinomas. Necrosis is related to higher total dose, higher dose per fraction, and advancing tumor stage.

Squamous Cell Carcinoma of the Pyriform Sinus

The larynx receives a high dose of irradiation when a carcinoma of the pyriform sinus is treated for cure. In early lesions the anterior one

Table III. Relationship of osteochondronecrosis to stage, dose per fraction, and total tumor dose for squamous cell carcinoma of the supraglottic larynx

Study	Stage	Dose/number of weeks	Dose per fraction	Number of patients	% with necrosis
Virginia Medical Center [27]	I–IV	6,000 cGy/5–6		83	0
University of Florida [29]	I–IV	6,000–7,500 cGy/6–8	180–200	76	2.6[a]
	II–IV	7,000–7,680 cGy/6–6.5	120 twice daily	25	0
Princess Margaret Hospital [6]	T_{1-2}	5,000 cGy/4	250	410	1[b]
M.D. Anderson Hospital[c] [26]	T_{1-2}	1,700–2,100 ret (NSD)[d]	varied	48	4
	T_{3-4}	as above	varied	31	10

[a] Permanent tracheostomy required in 2 patients.
[b] T_1 (2 cases), T_2 (1 case), T_4 (1 case).
[c] Necroses occurred at doses equivalent to 6,700 cGy in 6 weeks (3 cases), 6,850 cGy in 30 fractions in 6 weeks (1 case), 2,100 ret (1 case).
[d] NSD dose equivalents: 1,700 ret = 5,800 cGy in 30 fractions over 6 weeks; 1,800 ret = 6,150 cGy in 30 fractions over 6 weeks; 2,000 ret = 6,850 cGy in 30 fractions over 6 weeks; 1,950 ret = 7,000 cGy in 35 fractions over 7 weeks; 1,900 ret = 6,500 cGy in 30 fractions over 6 weeks.

fourth of the larynx is shielded at the University of Florida. The larynx is often involved by the pyriform sinus cancer, except in a small lesion confined to the anterior or lateral wall. Mendenhall et al. [14] reported on 50 patients treated for cure. Two cases of osteochondronecrosis developed which required a permanent tracheostomy in 1 and total laryngectomy in the other. Both necroses occurred in stage IV patients after 7,000 cGy in 7 weeks.

Chondronecrosis and Bone Necrosis

Nose

Incidental Irradiation of the Nasal Cartilages and Nasal Bones

In treating cancers of the nasal cavity and paranasal sinuses, the normal nasal alar cartilages, nasal septum, and nasal bones frequently receive 7,000 cGy in 7–8 weeks; at the University of Florida, no chondronecrosis has been observed in this patient group.

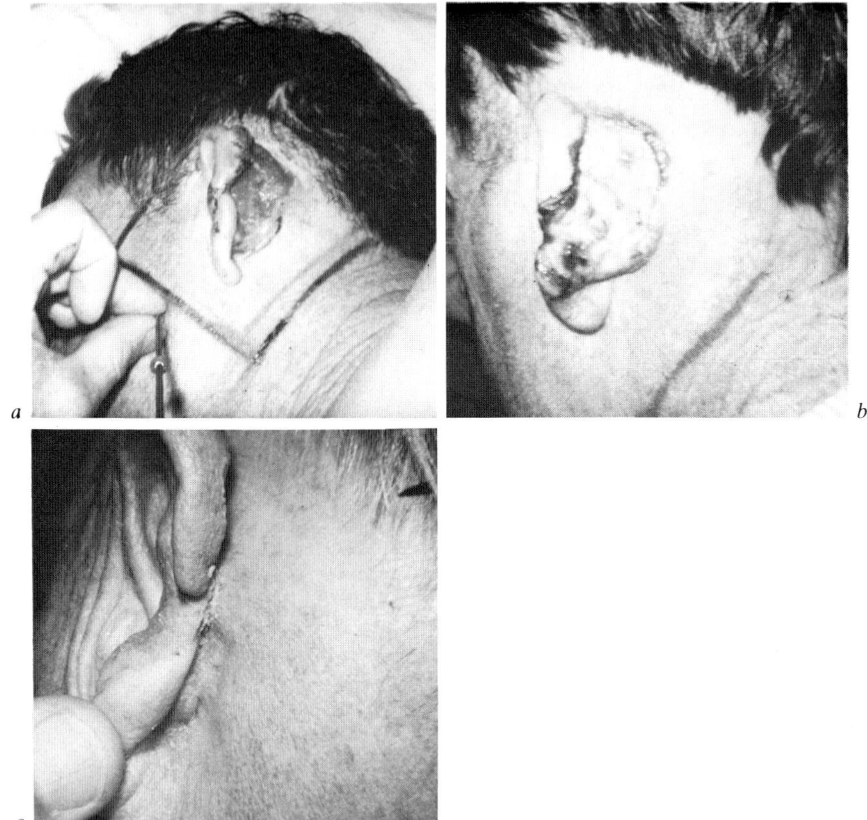

Fig. 4. a Squamous cell carcinoma of the left ear with cartilage invasion (the patient was blind in the right eye). The treatment plan is 6,500 cGy/7.5 weeks, ^{60}Co, with beeswax bolus, three-field technique. Superior and inferior portals angled 60° with wedges and a straight lateral open field (0°). *b* Appearance at 4,000 cGy. *c* There was no evidence of disease at 5.5 years. [From ref. 17, p. 500, fig. 26–24A, F, G.]

Irradiation of Cancers Approximating or Invading Nasal Cartilages or Nasal Bones

Carcinomas of the Nasal Vestibule. Carcinomas of the nasal vestibule frequently invade and perforate the nasal septum and the alar cartilages. Mendenhall et al. [12] reviewed 22 patients with squamous cell carcinoma of the nasal vestibule treated by radiation therapy. Eleven were stage T_4

(cartilage invasion). Fourteen were treated entirely or in part by interstitial radium needle implants, with needles inserted through cartilage and in some cases through the nasal bone. There were no cartilage or bone necroses. Some patients develop a soft-tissue ulcer during the postirradiation period and have some mild pain and tenderness. These ulcers heal with conservative treatment and are not thought to represent cartilage necrosis.

Wong et al. [30] reported the Princess Margaret Hospital experience for 56 patients with squamous cell carcinoma of the nasal vestibule. Eleven had cartilage invasion, and 3 had bone and cartilage invasion. No cartilage necroses developed. Two patients developed maxillary osteonecrosis.

Baris et al. [1] treated 22 patients with interstitial iridium implant, alone or combined with external-beam irradiation. Major complications were not seen.

Skin Cancers Involving the Nose. Skin cancers on the nose are often treated with high-dose irradiation. Even when such lesions invade cartilage, necrosis is rare after well-fractionated therapy [4].

External Ear

Incidental Irradiation of the Ear

All or part of the normal pinna is incidentally irradiated for parotid tumors, temporal bone lesions, and certain brain tumors. Cartilage necrosis has not been observed.

Irradiation of Skin Cancer Invading the Ear

Parker and Wildermuth [21] reviewed 38 patients with carcinoma of the pinna; 10 had cartilage invasion. There were no examples of chondronecrosis. Martin and Martin [11] and del Regato and Vuksanovic [4] reported similar results.

We have not observed cartilage necrosis despite giving high doses to advanced lesions with cartilage invasion [15]. A patient with an advanced squamous cell carcinoma of skin, invading and destroying cartilage, is shown in figure 4.

Bone Exposure/Osteoradionecrosis of Mandible/Maxilla

While there is a direct effect of radiation on bone itself, most bone, including the mandible, will tolerate rather high doses of radiation without serious problems as long as the tissues overlying the bone remain intact, and the bone is not subjected to excessive stress or trauma. Although occasional patients develop mandibular necroses beneath normal-appearing mucous membranes, 95% of necroses are associated with soft-tissue necrosis. Compared with the maxilla, the gingiva of the mandible has a rather tenuous blood supply. The mucosal covering is thin and constantly traumatized (by eating and dentures, for example). Once mandibular necrosis occurs, it is difficult to obtain healing. Necroses of the maxilla occur less often and heal more easily.

If the area of exposure is less than 1 cm, actual necrosis of the underlying bone and sequestration may not occur or may be minimal; roentgenograms appear normal. Small exposures generally heal spontaneously after a period of weeks to months. On the other hand, if the bone exposure enlarges and persists for a long period, bone necrosis followed by sequestration may occur. A segment of mandible or, rarely, maxilla is exposed, with a dead-appearing bone. Histologically, true osteoradionecrosis is characterized by damage to the cellular elements of bone, as well as vascular changes. The marrow space is infiltrated by inflammatory cells and loose connective tissue [19]. Such bone may become infected, after which the infectious, necrotic process may extend for a considerable distance in the involved bone. Roentgenograms show an irregular lytic defect that frequently extends beyond the clinically apparent area of destruction. Very severe necroses may lead to orofacial fistulas and pathologic fractures.

Most bone problems first appear 3–12 months after irradiation, but there is some risk for many years, especially if the patient undergoes dental extractions at some time in the future.

The mylohyoid ridge, which is normally prominent and covered by a thin gingival mucosa, and the anterior arch of the mandible are favorite sites of bone exposure. Posterior exposures, at the angle or ascending ramus of the mandible, sites that are well covered by muscle, are rare. If posterior necrosis does occur, it may result in severe infection and trismus [3].

Although the patient who has been edentulous for many years is still at risk of developing mandibular necrosis, his overall risk is less than in the dentulous patient. According to a number of practitioners with a great deal of clinical experience, patients who have undergone extractions just prior to irradiation are not at increased risk, if healing is adequate before irradiation is begun [18–20]. If the patient has teeth, radiation caries that develops in teeth that were within the field of irradiation may instigate a secondary radiation necrosis, particularly if it later becomes necessary to extract these teeth. Necrosis is most likely following extraction of mandibular teeth; although there may be some delay in healing following maxillary extractions, necroses are infrequent. Radiation caries in teeth that are outside the field of irradiation does not predispose to osteoradionecrosis, since the bone at these sites has not received high-dose irradiation; healing is usually normal after extraction.

Occasional patients have unerupted teeth in the molar area when they present for treatment. If well covered, these teeth usually cause no problem during the postirradiation period. If a tooth is partially erupted, it should generally be extracted if high-dose irradiation is anticipated [20]. In actual practice, most partially erupted third molars occur in younger patients whose tumors, usually lymphomas, require lesser doses of irradiation, so that postirradiation surgery can be accomplished at a later date with little risk. Impacted third molars encompassed by bone are not extracted prior to irradiation. However, if the impacted molar communicates with the adjacent molar socket or is not entirely surrounded by bone, extraction may be recommended by some dentists. When the resulting bone defect is large, a prolonged period of healing may be required.

Destruction of tissue by tumor increases the likelihood of necrosis; patients whose tumors involve the gingiva are at increased risk for bone exposure following irradiation. Patients who continue to smoke and drink after irradiation are also at increased risk. High doses, large treatment volumes, large fractions, and probably the addition of radical neck dissection, all place the patient at a greater risk. Patients whose treatment includes an interstitial implant are also more likely to develop necroses. Of 315 patients who received irradiation for carcinomas of the oral cavity/oropharynx at the University of Florida between September 1964 and August 1976, approximately 5% of the 198 patients whose treatment was by external-beam irradiation alone developed bone necrosis of mild or moderate severity (*i.e.*, healed spontaneously within less than 6 months or greater than 6 months, respectively); 1% developed severe osteoradionecrosis requiring mandibular resection. Of 117 patients whose treatment consisted of external-beam irradiation plus a radium implant, the rate of development of mild or moderately severe necrosis was 18%. Severe necrosis occurred in 3% [24].

Accelerated hyperfractionation, 120 cGy twice a day, has been used in 60 patients with T_{2-4} oropharyngeal carcinomas. Table IV shows the total risk of complications (including bone and soft-tissue necroses) according to dose. All moderately severe and severe injuries followed total doses of 7,920 cGy or more. One patient with a T_3N_2A carcinoma of the tonsillar fossa had a mandibular necrosis. Although the mandibular necrosis might possibly have been managed adequately by conservative

Table IV. Twice-a-day fractionation: complications according to dose in 60 patients who received definitive irradiation for T_{2-4} carcinomas of the oropharynx [from ref. 25, table 8][a]

Dose cGy	Number of Patients	Complications		
		mild	moderate	severe
≤7,440	15	1	0	0
7,680	14	1	0	0
7,920	9	2	0	2[b]
8,160	3	0	1	0
7,440–8,160 + 1,000–1,500 radium	19	5	1	0

University of Florida data; patients treated 3/78–4/84; minimum follow-up of 2 years.
[a] 120 cGy/fraction, two fractions per day, 4 h between fractions.
[b] Severe complications: 1 permanent gastrostomy, 1 mandibular necrosis.

means, the surgeon elected to perform a mandibulectomy 7 months after irradiation. Nineteen patients were managed by external beam, 7,440–8,160 cGy, plus a boost implant to a small volume in the tongue or tongue and tonsil. The incidence of serious complications has been surprisingly low with these dose levels.

Temporal Bone Necrosis

Osteoradionecrosis of the temporal bone is an unusual complication that may occur after high-dose irradiation of carcinomas of the middle ear, auditory canal, or mastoid. Incidental irradiation of the normal external auditory canal and temporal bone (*e.g.*, in the treatment of the nasopharynx or parotid tumors) rarely produces necrosis. In 1976, Wang and Doppke [28] reported seven bone necroses in patients who were irradiated postoperatively for ear tumors. Patients typically developed pain, nausea, vertigo, and ataxia. Clinical findings are those of chronic infection (*i.e.*, otitis media, mastoiditis, foul discharge from the ear canal) and exposed, devitalized bone. Fistulization may lead to meningitis or brain abscess.

Temporal bone necrosis is usually related to technical factors in the treatment. Total dose and fraction size are important; the complications in the patients treated by Wang and Doppke [28] all occurred after temporal bone doses calculated to be greater than or equal to 7,600 cGy at 200 cGy/fraction with megavoltage apparatus. At the University of Florida there has been 1 case that occurred after 6,850 cGy in 32 fractions (215 cGy/fraction) delivered to a parotid tumor. Osteonecrosis following irradiation of chemodectomas of the temporal bone structures has occurred in 1 patient at the University of Florida. The patient received 4,200 cGy to treat a postsurgical recurrent lesion and required revision mastoidectomy to remove a bony sequestrum 10 years after successful irradiation.

Soft-Tissue Necrosis

Atrophy of the mucosa and its supporting stroma, reduced tissue vascularity, and tissue destruction by tumor, all predispose the patient to soft-tissue necrosis. The risk of necrosis is increased by continued use of alcohol and tobacco.

The vast majority of soft-tissue necroses occur within 2 years after treatment. However, soft-tissue necrosis in association with bone exposure may occur at any time. Following interstitial therapy, the majority of necroses appear within 5–8 months.

Soft-tissue necroses are most common following irradiation of lesions within the oral cavity or oropharynx; they are unusual after treatment of cancers of the nasopharynx, hypopharynx, and larynx. Following successful irradiation of cancers of the posterior pharyngeal wall, an occasional patient is noted to have persistent soft-tissue ulceration at the site of tissue destruction by the neoplasm. Necrosis is related to fraction size, total dose, volume, and use of interstitial treatment. Of 315 patients with squamous cell cancers of the oral cavity/oropharynx who received radical irradiation at the University of Florida between 1964 and 1976, mild (spontaneously healed within 6 months) or moderately severe (spontaneously healed, but required longer than 6 months) soft-tissue necroses were observed in approximately 10% of the patients following external-beam irradiation alone and in approximately 20% of those who received a combination of external-beam and interstitial irradiation; severe soft-tissue necroses (requiring an operation or prolonged hospitalization) were rare, occurring in 1 (0.5%) of 198 patients treated by external-beam therapy alone and in 1 (1%) of 117 patients after external-beam plus interstitial irradiation [24].

Table IV shows the risks for all complications (including bone and soft tissue) for 60 patients treated with 120 cGy twice a day.

Radiation Effects on the Skin and Subcutaneous Tissues

Skin

Since modern radiation therapy is generally conducted with supervoltage equipment, severe late skin changes are infrequent. The use of bolus, radiation directed tangential to the skin surface, or the use of high-energy electrons will produce an increase in skin dose. Today, the only common indication for orthovoltage irradiation is skin cancer. Following orthovoltage treatment or supervoltage techniques that increase skin dose, there is usually epidermal atrophy and sometimes telangiectasis. The skin is hairless and dry because the function of sweat and sebaceous glands ceases. Some patients find it necessary to regularly apply petrolatum in order to keep the skin pliable and prevent fissuring. Acne does not occur in the irradiated field. Pigment changes may also occur; if the treatment was not well-fractionated, a thin, achromic, and telangiectatic scar develops. Achromia results from melanocyte destruction. Such areas readily sunburn. If the skin is severely damaged, it may ulcerate, especially after trauma; sometimes grafting is required.

Subcutaneous Fibrosis

Although skin injury is rarely a major problem in modern-day therapy, late effects on subcutaneous tissues are still important. Subcutaneous fibrosis usually appears within 6–12 months after treatment and is slowly progressive. There is decreased pliability of the subcutaneous tissues. In severe cases, the tissues may have a woody texture and become fixed into a single hard mass in which the subcutaneous tissue is not separable from overlying skin or underlying muscle or bone. The high-dose area is atrophic and indented. If the radiation entered the patient tangential to the skin, then skin and subcutaneous changes occur simultaneously. Patients with a great amount of adipose tissue in the subcutaneous layer (e.g., the groins) tend to develop the most severe changes. Fibrosis is rarely painful.

After high-dose treatment of vocal cord cancer with a single ipsilateral 4 × 4- to 5 × 5-cm field, the only change is an unsightly puckered area with subcutaneous plaque-like thickening in the center of the field and extending posteriorly into the leading edge of the sternocleidomastoid muscle. Lesser subcutaneous changes are noted in the anterior half of the field and in the anterior midline. The maximum dose (at 5 mm) is related to the incidence of subcutaneous fibrosis for ^{60}Co in table V [23]. There

Table V. Dose to produce subcutaneous fibrosis following irradiation of T_1 and T_2 vocal cord cancer with a single open field (^{60}Co, SSD 80 or 100 cm, 25–28 fractions) [from ref. 23, p. 185]

Maximum dose at 5 mm, cGy[a]	Subcutaneous fibrosis
6,350–6,850	0/6
6,900–7,100	3/12
7,150–7,540	4/4

University of Florida data; patients treated 10/64–12/74; analysis 3/77 (minimum 2-year follow-up); SSD = source-to-skin distance.
[a] Collimation with penumbra trimmers or 3-cm lead blocks on wire mesh tray.

were no detectable subcutaneous changes below 6,850 cGy, even after many years of follow-up. When parallel opposed ^{60}Co portals are used to treat vocal cord cancer, late changes in the skin and subcutaneous tissues are mininal.

Large areas of fibrosis may be accompanied by a 'tight' constrictive sensation. Obstructive lymphedema may be associated with fibrosis and produce intermittent episodes of erysipelas.

High dose irradiation of metastatic lymphadenopathy results in greater subcutaneous fibrosis in the neck than does a comparable dose to a neck that has no palpable adenopathy; apparently the fibrous stroma that replaces the tumor mass contributes to the reaction. Large daily fractions also increase the risk of subcutaneous fibrosis. Although fat necrosis is a potential risk following high-dose irradiation, this condition has rarely been observed at the University of Florida.

References

1 Baris, G.; Visser, A. G.; Andel, J. G. van: The treatment of squamous cell carcinoma of the nasal vestibule with interstitial iridium implantation. Radiother. Oncol. *4:* 121–125 (1985).

2 Chahbazian, C. M.; Regato, J. A. del: Cobalt-60 teletherapy of early carcinoma of the vocal cords. Am. J. Roentg. Rad. Ther. nucl. Med. *99:* 333–335 (1967).

3 Del Regato, J. A.: Dental lesions observed after roentgen therapy in cancer of the buccal cavity, pharynx, and larynx. Am. J. Roentg. Rad. Ther. *42:* 404–410 (1939).

4 Del Regato, J. A.; Vuksanovic, M.: Radiotherapy of carcinomas of the skin overlying the cartilages of the nose and ear. Radiology *79:* 203–208 (1962).

5 Harwood, A. R.; Beale, F. A.; Cummings, B. J.; Hawkins, N. V.; Keane, T. J.; Rider, W. D.: T3 glottic cancer: an analysis of dose-time-volume factors. Int. J. Radiat. Oncol. Biol. Phys. *6:* 675–680 (1980).

6 Harwood, A. R.; Beale, F. A.; Cummings, B. J.; Keane, T. J.; Payne, D. G.; Rider, W. D.; Rawlinson, E.; Elhakim, T.: Supraglottic laryngeal carcinoma: an analysis of dose-time-volume factors in 410 patients. Int. J. Radiat. Oncol. Biol. Phys. *9:* 311–319 (1983).

7 Harwood, A. R.; Hawkins, N. V.; Rider, W. D.; Bryce, D. P.: Radiotherapy of early glottic cancer. Int. J. Radiat. Oncol. Biol. Phys. *5:* 473–476 (1979).

8 Keene, M.; Harwood, A. R.; Bryce, D. P.; Nostrand, A. W. P. van: Histopathological study of radionecrosis in laryngeal carcinoma. Laryngoscope *92:* 173–180 (1982).

9 Kim, J. C.; Elkin, D.; Hendrickson, F. R.: Carcinoma of the vocal cord: results of treatment and time-dose relationships. Cancer *42:* 1114–1119 (1978).

10 Mancuso, A. A.; Hanafee, W. N.: *Computed tomography and magnetic resonance imaging of the head and neck*; 2nd ed., p. 244 (Williams & Wilkins, Baltimore 1985).

11 Martin, C. L.; Martin, J. A.: Long time studies of advanced cancer of the ear treated with electrosurgery plus radiation. Am. J. Roentg. Radium Ther. nucl. Med. *117:* 584–594 (1973).

12 Mendenhall, N. P.; Parsons, J. T.; Cassisi, N. J.; Million R. R.: Carcinoma of the nasal vestibule treated with radiation therapy. Laryngoscope *97:* 626–632 (1987).

13 Mendenhall, W. M.; Million, R. R.; Sharkey, D. E.; Cassisi, N. J.: Stage T3 squamous cell carcinoma of the glottic larynx treated with surgery and/or radiation therapy. Int. J. Radiat. Oncol. Biol. Phys. *10:* 357–363 (1984).

14 Mendenhall, W. M.; Parsons, J. T.; Cassisi, N. J.; Million, R. R.: Squamous cell carcinoma of the pyriform sinus treated with radical radiation therapy. Radiother. Oncol. *9:* 201–208 (1987).

15 Mendenhall, W. M.; Parsons, J. T.; Mendenhall, N. P.; Million, R. R.: T2–T4 carcinoma of the skin of the head and neck treated with radical irradiation. Int. J. Radiat. Oncol. Biol. Phys. *13:* 975–981 (1987).

16 Mendenhall, W. M.; Parsons, J. T.; Million, R. R.; Fletcher, G. H.: T1–T2 squamous cell carcinoma of the glottic larynx treated with radiation therapy: relationship of dose-fractionation factors to local control and complications. Int. J. Radiat. Oncol. Biol. Phys. (in press, 1988).

17 Million, R. R.; Cassisi, N. J.: Carcinoma of the skin; in Million, Cassisi, *Management of head and neck cancer: a multidisciplinary approach*, pp. 475–512 (Lippincott, Philadelphia 1984).

18 Morrish, R. B.; Chan, E.; Silverman, S., Jr.; Meyer, J.; Fu, K. K.; Greenspan, D.: Osteonecrosis in patients irradiated for head and neck carcinoma. Cancer *47:* 1980–1983 (1981).

19 Murray, C. G.; Herson, J.; Daly, T. E.; Zimmerman, S.: Radiation necrosis of the mandible: a 10-year study. I. Factors influencing the onset of necrosis. Int. J. Radiat. Oncol. Biol. Phys. *6:* 543–548 (1980).

20 Murray, C. G.; Herson, J.; Daly, T. E.; Zimmerman, S.: Radiation necrosis of the mandible: a 10-year study. II. Dental factors: onset, duration, and management of necrosis. Int. J. Radiat. Oncol. Biol. Phys. *6:* 549–553 (1980).

21 Parker, R. G.; Wildermuth, O.: Radiation therapy of lesions overlying cartilage. I. Carcinoma of the pinna. Cancer *15:* 57–65 (1965).

22 Parsons, J. T.: Time-dose-volume relationships in radiation therapy; in Million, Cassisi, *Management of head and neck cancer: a multidisciplinary appraoch*, pp. 137–172 (Lippincott, Philadelphia 1984).

23 Parsons, J. T.: The effect of radiation on normal tissues of the head and neck; in Million, Cassisi, *Management of head and neck cancer: a multidisciplinary approach*, pp. 173–207 (Lippincott, Philadelphia 1984).

24 Parsons, J. T.; Bova, F. J.; Million, R. R.: A reevaluation of split-course technique for squamous cell carcinoma of the head and neck. Int. J. Radiat. Oncol. Biol. Phys. *6:* 1645–1652 (1980).
25 Parsons, J. T.; Mendenhall, W. M; Cassisi, N. J.; Isaacs, J. H., Jr.; Million, R. R.: Hyperfractionation for head and neck cancer. Int. J. Radiat. Oncol. Biol. Phys. *14:* 649–658 (1988).
26 Shukovsky, L. J.: Dose, time, volume relationships in squamous cell carcinoma of the supraglottic larynx. Am. J. Reontg. Rad. Ther. nucl. Med. *108:* 27–29 (1970).
27 Spaulding, C. A.; Krochak, R. J.; Hahn, S. S.; Constable, W. C.: Radiotherapeutic management of cancer of the supraglottis. Cancer *57:* 1292–1298 (1986).
28 Wang, C. C.; Doppke, K.: Osteonecrosis of the temporal bone. Consideration of nominal standard dose. Int. J. Radiat. Oncol. Biol. Phys. *1:* 881–883 (1976).
29 Weems, D. H.; Mendenhall, W. M.; Parsons, J. T.; Cassisi, N. J.; Million, R. R.: Squamous cell carcinoma of the supraglottic larynx treated with surgery and/or radiation therapy. Int. J. Radiat. Oncol. Biol. Phys *13:* 1483–1487 (1987).
30 Wong, C. S.; Cummings, B. J.; Elhakim, T.; Briant, T. D.: External irradiation for squamous cell caricnoma of the nasal vestibule. Int. J. Radiat. Oncol. Biol. Phys. *12:* 1943–1946 (1986).

Dr. R. R. Million, Department of Radiation Oncology, Box J-385,
J. Hillis Miller Health Center, Gainesville, FL 32610–0385 (USA)

Vaeth JM, Meyer JL (eds): Radiation Tolerance of Normal Tissues.
Front Radiat Ther Oncol. Basel, Karger, 1989, vol 23, pp 238–250

Complications from Radiation Therapy to the Eye

Luther W. Brady[a], *Jerry Shields*[b], *James Augusburger*[b], *Arnold Markoe*[a], *Ulf L. Karlsson*[a]

[a]Department of Radiation Oncology, Hahnemann University, Philadelphia;
[b]Oncology Unit, Wills Eye Hospital, Philadelphia, Pa., USA

Chalupecky [1] in 1897 first described the effects of ionizing radiation on the eye. Subsequent studies by Birch-Hirschfeld [2] in 1908 identified the first case of radiation cataract. The definitive investigations relative to the effects of ionizing radiation on the eye began with those by Rohrschneider [3]. This author described a gradient in radiosensitivity of the ocular structures extending from the lens (the most sensitive tissue) through conjunctiva, cornea, uvea, and the retina to the least sensitive tissue, the optic nerve. Poppe [4] further elucidated the work of Rohrschneider.

The purposes of this paper are to summarize the currently available clinical and experimental data on the effects of radiation on eye and ocular adnexa and to suggest guidelines for radiation tolerance of normal ocular tissues.

Even though many clinicians have an almost morbid fear of the harmful effects of irradiating the eye and orbit, modern contemporary and innovative radiation therapy techniques have allowed for appropriate programs of treatment to be administered with minimum complications. Table I illustrates the magnitude of the potential problem. Table II demonstrates the techniques and dosages generally used in radiation therapy of eye lesions [2].

The presence of complications, whether functional or cosmetic, will vary, depending upon a number of factors: (1) the cellular composition of the injured tissue (in the eye there is a broad diversity of tissues with

Table I. Malignant tumors in or near the orbit

Site	Number of patients
Head and neck	29,800
Central nervous system	14,700
Eye	1,900
Skin	100,000
Other rhabdomyosarcoma, lymphoma, etc.	3,000
Metastases	80,000

Table II. Usual radiation dosages (Gy) in the treatment of eye diseases

Ocular lesion	^{90}Sr radionuclinde plaques, low-energy X-rays	Medium- and high-voltage X-rays	Megavoltage X-rays, ^{60}Co high-energy electrons
Nonneoplastic lesions	30–60 in 2–6 weeks (10/week)	25–40 in 2–4 weeks (10/week)	25–40 in 2–4 weeks (10/week)
Malignant tumors of the eye	20–160 in 5 days to 12 weeks	40–60 in 2–6 weeks	35–75 in 3–8 weeks
Malignant tumors of or involving the orbit	–	–	35–75 in 4–7 weeks

differing types of cellular composition); (2) that tissue's functional reserve to withstand evolution of a clinically apparent complication, and (3) other factors such as the vascular-nutritional integrity of the organ. These three factors underlie a general scheme that can be applied to the eye and orbital contents. *Acute lesions* represent primary functional cell necroses affecting rapidly proliferating cells. Acute radiation-induced lesions may be defined as effects which occur either during the course of fractionated radiation therapy or within several weeks following completion of that radiation therapy. Recovery from these mild forms occur generally with proper medical management within several weeks after completion of the treatment. Such lesions typically occur in the eyelid skin (blepharitis), in the conjunctiva (conjunctivitis), and in the corneal epithelium (keratitis). Subsequent cellular recovery may be followed by delayed lesions which are predominately stromal in pathogenesis. These lesions may consist of edema followed by interstitial fibrosis. Pathogenic mechanisms include endothelial damage in the microcirculation with passage of proteinaceous fluid into the interstitial spaces through the damaged vascular barrier. *Late effects* may also occur coincidentally with permanent changes in arterioles and small arteries. Late tissue complications, particularly where there is a lack of rapidly proliferating cells, are thought to be due to the nutritional consequences of ischemic vascular damage. Typical delayed radiation-induced effects on the eye include cataract formation and radiation retinopathy. Such lesions commonly develop after a latent interval of at least several months. However, the latent period can vary widely (from a few months to many years), depending upon individual biologic factors and on dose. In general, the higher the dose employed, the earlier the particular response will be observed.

Factors which influence the probability for radiation injury may be categorized as technical and nontechnical. Technical factors include human mistakes in the delivery of the radiation therapy and systematic errors such as those due to inaccurate initial adjustment of equipment, incorrect procedures, or unrecognized deviation of a particular parameter with time. Estimates of the incidence and significance of mistakes in the delivery of the radiation therapy program range from 1 to 40%. The incidence varies according to the type of treatment and the complexity of the treatment technique.

Strict attention to detail is mandatory in radiation therapy programs for tumors in or about the eye, since precise and proper control of the technical components of the treatment will have a significant impact upon reducing the potential for radiation complications.

The important technical factors are fraction size, protection or length of the course of treatment, hyperfractionation, type of radiation (beta, photon, electrons, neutrons, etc.), the radiosensitivity of the tissues being irradiated, and the patient's age.

Nontechnical factors which modify radiation tolerance include the presence of a concurrent disease state which either compromises the tissue's arterial supply (such as diabetes mellitus and systemic hypertension) or increases the sensitivity of normal tissues to radiation damage, such as ataxia and telangiectasia, and the simultaneous or sequential treatment with chemotherapeutic agents may also modify radiation tolerance.

Merriam [5], Merriam and Focht [6, 7], and Merriam et al. [8] have summarized the reported clinical complications according to the ocular tissue involved, the latent period, and the dose responsible for each effect.

In the following paragraphs, a few comments will be made regarding the various ocular tissues and their responses to ionizing radiation.

Table III. Effects of radiation on the lid skin

Effect	Latent period		Dose, Gy	
	early	late	single	divided
Erythema	2–4 weeks		6	$600t^{0.33}$ daily schedule
Pigmentation	2–4 weeks		4–6	
Depigmentation		6–12 months		40–50 in 4–5 weeks
Telangiectasia		2–5 years		30–60 in 3–6 weeks
Moist desquamation	2–8 weeks			50–60 in 5–6 weeks
Scarring		>6 months		80 in 3–8 weeks

Lid Skin (table III)

Erythema of the lids develops in a fashion similar to other areas of skin irradiated. It generally develops early, is transient, and disappears promptly after completion of the radiation therapy. It is seen most commonly in those circumstances where basal cell or squamous cell carcinomas of the lid are irradiated definitively. Moist desquamation may be seen when higher doses are delivered, but even that heals promptly with appropriate and proper local care. Time-dose relationships for skin effects are critical in terms of their severity as well as the rapidity with which they disappear after treatment.

Hyperpigmentation and depigmentation of the eyelid skin have both been described; most commonly these pigmentary changes occur as late complications of the treatment, usually becoming manifest 12 months or longer after completion of definitive irradiation of the lid. Telangiectasia generally does not appear until 4–5 years after completion of the radiation therapy, producing no symptoms and representing essentially a cosmetic change. Ulceration of the skin is a direct relationship to fraction size and total dose delivered as well as the time during which the treatment is delivered. This complication is rarely seen with contemporary techniques of radiation therapy. Lid lymphedema may be seen as a late effect.

Rounding of the lid margins is another frequent complication of the treatment of eyelid tumors. One sees in the treated area the loss of cilia, rounding of the margins, and some thinning. However, no functional loss is noted, and the appearance is seldom a cosmetic problem. Ectropion or entropion are seldom seen with current dosage schedules. These abnormalities are usually associated with extensive scarring of the lids and adjacent conjunctiva.

Tarsus (table IV)

This fibrous plate in the lids can undergo late atrophy and thinning when dosages for curative levels are administered. It is most commonly seen in patients treated for basal cell or squamous cell carcinomas of the lid, but produces no functional impairment and is essentially a clinical observation.

Table IV. Effects of radiation on the tarsus

Effect	Latent period		Dose, Gy	
	early	late	single	divided
Atrophy	–	>6 months	–	40–60 in 4–6 weeks

Table V. Effects of radiation on the lid margin

Effect	Latent period		Dose, Gy	
	early	late	single	divided
Epilation	1–5 weeks		10	20–30 in 2–3 weeks
Rounding of				40–60 in 4–6 weeks
Ectropion	–	6–12 months	–	
Entropion	–	>1 year	–	60–100 1 day to 10 weeks

Table VI. Effects of radiation on the lacrimal gland

Effect	Latent period		Dose, Gy	
	early	late	single	divided
Atrophy	–	>6 months	20	50–60 in 5–6 weeks

Table VII. Effects of radiation on the conjunctiva

Effect	Latent period		Dose, Gy	
	early	late	single	divided
Hyperemia	immediate	–	–	>5
Conjunctivitis	1–3 weeks	–	–	50 in 4–5 weeks
Telangiectasis	–	2–5 years	–	30–60 in 3–6 weeks
Keratinization	–	>1 year	–	50–100 in 5–10 weeks
Symblepharon	–	>1 year	–	80–100 in 1 day to 8 weeks

Lid Margin (table V)

Lash loss may occur following therapeutic radiation and is directly dependent upon the dose delivered to the hair follicles. It may be temporary or permanent, depending upon the total dose delivered to the volume being treated. Lash loss is generally not a significant cosmetic blemish, but regrowth on occasion can produce trichiasis requiring treatment. Effective surgical techniques of management for inturned lashes are presently available.

Lacrimal Ducts

Radiation dosages at the curative level will cause obliteration of the puncta and usually the canaliculi. Symptoms associated with this radiation effect are generally minor in character; however, some patients develop bothersome epiphora following punctal and canalicular radiation damage.

Lacrimal Gland (table VI)

When the lacrimal gland has been included within the volume of treatment, atrophy of this gland and consequent reduction in the tear volume may occur. These effects are seen only at the higher dose levels used for curative treatment. This, plus invasion or destruction of the gland by tumor, can lessen the secretory ability of the gland and produce a dry eye. In most patients, symptoms related to radiation-induced 'dry eye' can be managed adequately by the use of artificial tears.

Conjunctiva (table VII)

Conjunctival hyperemia commonly develops when shielding is not possible during the radiation therapy program, as well as when conjunctival shields are not adequately coated to absorb low-energy secondary X-rays. It is a dose-related phenomenon and, at higher doses, can be associated with corneal complications and iritis. Conjunctival hyperemia may be a direct effect of the radiation therapy, but also may be secondary to involvement of other ocular structures.

Conjunctivitis of varying severity may accompany the hyperemia and may on occasion be associated with secondary infection. In most patients, however, it responds well to topical corticosteroids and antibiotics. It occurs more frequently at higher dose levels and is a dose-related phenomenon. It usually gradually subsides with appropriate medical management some 2–4 weeks after completion of the treatment.

Conjunctival telangiectasia is a frequent late complication seen with higher dose levels and is a dose-related phenomenon. The incidence increases with dose and is most apt to develop when curative doses of radiation are being delivered. It represents essentially a cosmetic problem, producing no symptoms.

Keratinization of the conjunctival epithelium, particularly the palpebral conjunctiva, has been observed with radiation dosages in excess of 5,000 rad delivered during period >5 weeks. In some instances, it may be asymptomatic. If the palpebral conjunctiva becomes keratinized, however, the patient may develop keratitis. This complication can usually be avoided by appropriate attention to total dose delivered and by providing adequate shielding.

Symblepharon represents a very severe radiation injury to the conjunctiva in which both the palpebral and bulbar conjunctiva are denuded of their epithelium, and the opposing surfaces become adherent. This results in adhesions of the lids to the globe with deformity of the lids and limitation of ocular movement. Surgical correction may be necessary to deal with this particular complication. In contemporary radiation therapy practice, this complication is rarely seen.

Cornea (table VIII)

In many instances, it is impossible to adequately shield the cornea during ocular radiation therapy. Punctate keratitis is an acute radiation effect in which multiple small defects develop in the corneal epithelium within several weeks to months after treatment. Symptoms include irritation of the eye with varying amounts of tearing. The injury can be seen with low doses of radiation in the range of 30–50 Gy delivered within 4–5 weeks. In general, it will subside over a period of 4–6 weeks with appropriate management using topical corticosteroids and antibiotics. Proper attention to the radiation therapy technique including proper coating of conjunctival shields to protect the cornea is critically important.

Stromal edema of the cornea has been observed with radiation dosages in the range of 40–50 Gy in 4–5½ weeks. In general, this complication is transient, lasting only 2–4 weeks. In some patients, however, it may persist longer. Stromal edema is generally seen with doses that are

Table VIII. Effects of radiation on the cornea

Effect	Latent period		Dose, Gy	
	early	late	single	divided
Punctate	–	–	–	–
Keratitis	several weeks	–	10	30–50 in 3–5 weeks
Edema	1–3 weeks	–	–	–
Mild ulceration	several weeks	–	–	30–40 in 2–3 weeks
Chronic ulceration	–	several months	20	>60 in 5–6 weeks
Perforation	–	4–12 months	–	>60 in 5–6 weeks
Thinning	–	several	–	30–50 in 3–5 weeks
Scarring	–	1 year	–	>60 in 5–6 weeks
Keratinization	–	1 year	–	>50 in 4–5 weeks
Vascularization	–	>1 year	–	>50 in 2–3 weeks
Lipid infiltration	–	>1 year	–	>70 in 5–7 weeks
Poor wound healing	–	–	–	>180

greater than 50 Gy and most commonly when dosages are in the range of 70–80 Gy. Appropriate and proper medical management with topical corticosteroids and antibiotics is indicated.

Corneal ulceration is a rare radiation-induced ocular tissue effect. In severe cases, the full-thickness cornea may melt away, leaving the eye at risk for overwhelming infection (endophthalmitis or panophthalmitis). Corneal ulceration has been reported to occur most commonly with radiation dosages exceeding 60 Gy in 6 weeks. Thinning and perforation of the cornea has been described at varying dose levels, but in general occurs at higher dose levels. If perforation occurs, the eye is often lost. In some cases, however, the perforation and resulting tissue dehiscence is repaired by regeneration of the corneal epithelium. Unfortunately, considerable visual disturbance usually results from such a perforation. The likelihood of corneal ulceration can be diminished, if care is taken to prevent corneal epithelial trauma and secondary infection.

Keratinization is a late corneal complication of radiation therapy which can result in severe visual loss. In general, it is more likely to develop when radiation dosages exceed 50 Gy within 4–5 weeks. It is often associated with varying degrees of scarring, thinning, and vascularization.

Corneal vascularization can occur as a late result of radiation therapy. It typically does not become manifest until several years after the treatment. It can result from conventional clinical radiation dosages, but generally occurs with much larger than normal dosages.

Lipid infiltration of the cornea has been reported as a late complication of ocular irradiation. This tissue effect has usually been observed with corneal dosages that exceed 75 Gy. The effect on vision depends upon the location and density of the lipid deposits.

Sclera (table IX)

Thinning of the sclera has been reported with dosages ranging from 15 Gy to 20 Gy on the surface. Localized areas of scleral thinning following ocular irradiation usually do not require any treatment. Perforation of the sclera occurs rarely, even with high local radiation dosages used in the treatment of malignant melanomas of choroid and ciliary bodies. In some cases, a scleral perforation can be repaired successfully with a scleral patch graft.

Iris (table X)

Radiation therapy to the iris may produce iritis, an acute and usually transient dose-related inflammation. Radiation-induced iritis often occurs conjointly with keratitis or corneal ulceration. Affected patients are usually severely photophobic. The inflammation commonly leads to pigment deposition on the anterior capsule of the lens. Various degrees of iris atrophy can also occur. Atrophy of the iris is usually localized to a sector and has been seen most often when beta irradiation has been used. It is a late effect, typically becoming manifest several years after the radiation event, but is essentially asymptomatic and remains localized. Trabecular meshwork glaucoma develops in some eyes in response to radiation therapy. These forms of glaucoma are often quite resistant to medical or surgical therapy. It usually occurs as a consequence of intraocular inflammation, which acts by clogging the trabecular meshwork with inflammatory cells or debris or closing the filtration angle with posterior synechiae, or leads to development of iris neovascularization (rubeosis iridis).

Lens (table XI)

Radiation effects on the lens are those directly related to the production of cataract. Animal work, clinical observation, and experience have identified the dose of various qualities of radiation that will produce a lens opacity, the manner in which the cataract develops, the time of onset, and the metabolic and pathologic changes that develop [6]. The amount of

Table IX. Effects of radiation on the sclera

Effect	Latent period		Dose, Gy	
	early	late	single	divided
Atrophy	–	several years	–	200–300

Table X. Effects of radiation on the iris

Effect	Latent period		Dose, Gy	
	early	late	single	divided
Iritis	several days	–	20	>60 in 5–6 weeks
Rubeosis	–	several months to several years	–	70–80 in 6–8 weeks
Atrophy	–	>3 years	–	170–250

Table XI. Effects of radiation on the eye lens

Effect	Latent period		Dose, Gy	
	early	late	single	divided
Cataract	–	>year	>2	$CD_{50} \sim$ 4 Gy $t^{0.17}$ (daily schedule)

radiation given to the lens will have an impact upon the degree of opacity: the time of onset of the cataract is directly dose related. It is evident that the lens is the most radiosensitive structure in the eye. In the overall consideration of the radiation therapy program, the acceptance of a radiation-induced cataract of the lens may be a necessary component of the treatment program for treating tumors in this area. It should be appreciated that a progressive cataract, when it develops with loss of vision, may be extracted as easily as a senile one with restoration of vision, provided the rest of the eye is unaffected. However, the time interval between the radiation event and the extraction of the lens of the eye should be at least 1 year or more before the surgical procedure is initiated.

Table XII. Effects of radiation on the retina

Effect	Latent period		Dose, Gy	
	early	late	single	divided
Edema	several months	–	–	20–35 in 2–4 weeks
Vascular occlusion	–	–	–	–
Telangiectasia	–	–	–	–
Hemorrhages	–	6 months to many years	–	30–60 in 3–6 weeks
Exudates	–	–	–	–
Degeneration	–	–	–	–
Atrophy	–	–	–	50–80 in 4–8 weeks

Retina (table XII)

Radiation injury to the retina occurs as a clinical entity in spite of the fact that the retina is quite radioresistant. Most radiation-induced retinal changes appear to be on the basis of retinal vasular damage. Clinical changes in the retina can be observed with radiation dosages as low as 35 Gy delivered within 3 weeks. With increasing dosage, there is an increased incidence of retina changes from the radiation therapy. Radiation effects on the retina have been observed in patients treated by external beam radiation therapy as well as in individuals treated with various radionuclide plaques for a malignant tumor involving the eye. Initially, edema of the retina may be noted early during the course of radiation therapy. This acute retinal edema commonly subsides within several weeks. In some eyes, retinal edema recurs as a late complication of treatment, often in association with intraretinal or preretinal hemorrhages and exudates. These effects appear to be secondary to progressive radiation-induced obliteration of the retinal vessels. Optic papillitis, retinal microaneurysms, and macular exudates may simulate the picture of severe arteriosclerotic-hypertensive retinopathy. New vessel formation (neovascularization) may occur in an aberrant attempt to improve the local circulation. The fragile new blood vessels commonly bleed into the vitreous, however, resultin in further visual impairment. The vitreous hemorrhage may become organized with retinitis proliferans, resulting in detachment of the retina. The entire retina occasionally becomes severely ischemic. This ischemia in turn leads to an ischemic ocular inflammation and neovascular glaucoma in some eyes.

Optic Nerve

The optic nerve can develop radiation-induced papillitis. This condition is characterized by hyperemic disc swelling, usually accompanied by circumpapillary exudates and profound visual loss. Optic nerve atrophy has also been observed in patients with severe retinal changes. This condition is characterized by disc pallor and severe visual loss. It is felt that this feature is generally secondary to retinal degeneration. However, the circulation to the nerve itself may be impaired and may result in optic atrophy.

Orbit (table XIII)

Radiation effects on the orbit are directly related to inhibition of the growth of bone. When the radiation therapy is delivered in childhood, such treatment can result in marked facial deformities. The typical deformity is a hollowed-out appearance in the temporal region due to failure of growth of the lateral wall of the orbit.

If the nasal bones are included within the fields of treatment, growth in the nasal bones may also be impaired, resulting in a saddle nose deformity. In general, these changes occur at radiation dosages that exceed 35 Gy delivered within 3–4 weeks in childhood.

The potential for the development of malignant tumors in the irradiated area is well known and has been reported by multiple investigators. Here again, the critical factors are the long survival of the patient with the tumor controlled and the total dose delivered to the areas of normal tissue. There is a direct relationship between the dose and the incidence of second radiation-induced tumors. In general, the criteria set forth by Cahan [10] must be met for diagnosis of a radiation-induced tumor: (1) the tumor develops within the irradiated field; (2) the tumor is of different histologic type than the original primary lesion; (3) the total radiation dose delivered to the normal tissues within the volume is in excess of 60 Gy within 6–7 weeks, and (4) the interval between the initial radiation

Table XIII. Effects of radiation on the orbit

Effect	Latent period		Dose, Gy	
	early	late	single	divided
Growth failure	–	several years	–	40–70 in 3–7 weeks

event and the development of the second tumor is in excess of 6–7 years. The latent period has been reported to range from 4 to 30 years with a mean of 11 years. When treating a malignant tumor, the possibility of a late radiation-induced cancer must be accepted, as well as other radiation complications, as a calculated risk.

In conclusion, the frequency of radiation complications to the eye and orbital structures can be diminished to minimal levels with appropriate and proper attention to carefully designed treatment programs and precise attention to detail in its delivery. This includes specific attention to the type of radiation instrument to be employed, whether electron beam, photon beam, or radioactive plaques. In general, the critical factors influencing radiation complications from treatment to the eye and orbital structures relate to the age of the patient, the number of fractions, the total dose and time during which the radiation dose is delivered to the normal structures within the volume being treated, and other coexisting medical conditions.

References

1 Chalupecky, H.: Über die Wirkung der Röntgenstrahlen auf das Auge and die Haut. Zentbl. Augenheilk. *21:* 234–368 (1897).

2 Birch-Hirschfeld, G. V. A.: Zur Wirkung der Röntgenstrahlen auf das menschliche Auge. Klin. Mbl. Augenheilk. *46:* 129 (1908).

3 Rohrschneider, W.: Experimentelle Untersuchungen über die Veränderungen normaler Augengewebe nach Röntgenbestrahlung. III. Mitteilung. Veränderungen der Linse der Netzhaut und des Sehnerven nach Röntgenbestrahlung. Graefes Arch. Ophthal. *122:* 282 (1929).

4 Poppe, E.: Experimental investigation of the effects of roentgen rays on the eye. Oslo (1942).

5 Merriam, G. R., Jr.: Late effects of beta radiation on the eye. AMA Archs Ophthal. *53:* 708 (1955).

6 Merriam, G. R., Jr.; Focht, E. F.: A clinical study of radiation cataracts and the relationship to dose. Am. J. Roentg. *77:* 759 (1957).

7 Merriam, G. R., Jr.; Focht, E. F.: A clinical and experimental study of the effect of single and divided doses of radiation on cataract production. Trans. Am. ophthal. Soc. *60:* 35 (1962).

8 Merriam, G. R., Jr.; Biavati, B. J.; Bateman, J. L.; Rossi, H. H.; Boud, V. P.; Goodman, L.; Focht, E. F.: The dependence of RBE on the energy of fast neutrons. IV. Indication of lens opacities in mice. Radiat. Res. *25:* 123 (1965).

9 Sagerman, R. H.; Cassady, J. R.; Tretter, P.; Elsworth, R. M.: Radiation induced neoplasia following external beam therapy for children with retinoblastoma. Am. J. Roentg. *105*: 529 (1969).

10 Cahan,

Luther W. Brady, MD, Department of Radiation Oncology,
Hahnemann University Hospital, Philadelphia, PA 19102 (USA)

Vaeth JM, Meyer JL (eds): Radiation Tolerance of Normal Tissues.
Front Radiat Ther Oncol. Basel, Karger, 1989, vol 23, pp 251–254

Discussion

Dr. Padulski: Dr. Brady, when one's treating children with acute lymphoblastic leukemia or medulloblastoma, one's treating the brain down to the cribriform plate. Even when the port sets up beautifully, one's got a very small margin between the field and the lens. I don't know how to accurately estimate the lens dose. We can't be putting the total lens dose right in the lens, and I wonder if anybody has done good determination of lens doses in these typical lateral field setups. What types of rates of cataract formation are people seeing years later in medulloblastoma and acute lymphoblastic leukemia patients?

Dr. Brady: From the standpoint of measuring the lens dose in the child, obviously it's very complicated to do. One can't put the TLD there to do that. On the other hand, one can set up phantoms to do those kinds of measurements. There is a large body of information having to do with scatter dose into adjacent structures relative to small field, large field, and intermediate-size field which would indicate that the lens in that kind of circumstance would be receiving a significant dose, 15–20%, depending upon the field setup and whether or not you have altered the beam so that you're dealing with divergence that isn't from the opposite field going through the lens.

In some of the early work, and I refer you to a very nice paper that was written by Betty Falk, who was a physicist at Memorial Hospital, working with George Marion. They looked at the dose to the lens to produce cataract. It occurred somewhere in the range of 1,100–1,200 rads, under the circumstances of their particular experiments and the animals with which they were working. Generally, speaking, the incidence of cataract developing of a punctate character or confluent character does not have to be the entire lens that's involved. Cataract production is in the range of about 1,100–1,200 rad by conventional fractionation schemes. Again I don't know the incidence in children. I think the more critically important point in that situation is to irradiate under the most ideal kinds of careful circumstance in the treatment program, recognizing that there is a certain amount of radiation dose to the lens. If indeed a cataract does develop, it won't develop in every child, and it can be managed at some point in the future by extraction. The ophthalmologists in the past were rather reluctant to deal with that kind of situation, but now we find that they are somewhat more sanguine. I can't really answer the two points you're asking: (1) what the dose is and (2) what the incidence of cataract is. In our observation, cataract production has been essentially nonexistent in the patients whom we've treated, and the data from the clinical observations and from the research efforts in that animal models show that somewhere in the range of 1,100–1,300 rad would be the dose at which one would begin to get cataract.

Dr. Wong: Dr. Brady, you mentioned the use of cataract extraction in the treated eye. Do you have any personal experience in the role for lens implant and/or the use of a contact lens after treatment to the eye? And is there a dose effect?

Dr. Brady: We found very quickly in the patients with whom we were dealing with plaques that to do the extraction within a short period after the radiation event nor during the time of an acute inflammatory reaction was a disaster in every instance. It resulted in enucleation of the eye. If one waits until the cataract matures, a year, a year and a half, or longer, then one deals with them exactly the way one would in any cataract that occurs in an aging individual. I don't think that they necessitate any particular kinds of special treatment in that circumstance.

Dr. Wong: Including the use of a lens implant?

Dr. Brady: Yes.

Dr. Parker: We've had some trouble in a couple of patients in placing lens implants after a fairly high dose of irradiation for treatment of sinus tumors. I advise not to do it. One can wear a contact lens if one still has moisture. If one doesn't have moisture left, or tears, one can't use it. That's really what it comes down to.

Dr. Keil: Dr. Parker, we're treating a lot of joints in soft-tissue sarcomas. Are there any data on degenerative arthritis or changes in the joint with partial joint irradiation or whole-joint irradiation?

Dr. Parker: I don't have any data. We, of course like you, attempt to avoid the joint. Our treatment pattern is different, so one can't extrapolate our data to anybody else's. Our doses are 3,500 in ten fractions. In that group we've had no joint problems. I would think if you went to higher doses, you certainly would.

Dr. Doggett: Dr. Brady, in the ^{90}Sr treatment for postoperative pterygia, is there any new information on dose-fractionation schedules? Some of our ophthalmologists want us to treat these people with a single fraction of 2,000 rad immediately after operation.

Dr. Brady: I don't think that's necessarily the problem, but it depends upon where the surgical procedure has been carried out and where the eversion of the base has occurred. If it's just off of the cornea, then I would be a little bit more reluctant to use a single fraction. I might even in that instance be a little more reluctant to treat the patient. On the other hand if it's far posterior, and the pteryqium has been dissected off and then turned on itself (everted), then giving a single fraction I think is alright. We prefer to do multiple fractions. It's just a personal feeling. We have less in the way of complications from the treatment program using strontium. There's some argument whether you would need to do it at all. It's a very critical question to me right now because I have a major pterygium which has to be removed, and whether I will or will not have the strontium treatment afterwards I haven't decided.

Dr. Doggett: What fractionation schedule would you use?

Dr. Brady: We have been using 1,000 rad/fraction once a week for four or five fractions over a 4- or 5-week period.

Dr. Parker: Do you need that much?

Dr. Brady: No, I don't know that you necessarily need that much, but that's what we have been doing by tradition for 35 years, so it's hard to change when it works. It may be that the surgical resection, if well done, works too.

Dr. Froud: I've noticed over the years, using electron therapy, that there's a persistence of skin tanning and pigmentation for much longer than I would see with photon therapy. I wonder if Dr. Parker or anybody else would care to comment on that. Could you give us some guidance as to the tolerance of and precautions to be used when you're irradiating tear ducts and lacrimal ducts in and around the eye? That's a constant problem for many of us.

Dr. Parker: I guess I've never noticed. If I had noticed, I assumed it was due to differences in dosimetry or in control. We haven't seen many tear duct problems with conventional treatment, but Mary Katterall described obliteration of the tear duct in previously normal tear ducts with neutron treatment around the eye.

Dr. Million: We tried to put some little polyethylene catheters down through the tear duct, particularly in patients who had basal cell cancers. It didn't work. We stopped doing it.

Dr. Brady: I think the more critical question really is the extent of the tumor you're treating. And if indeed you can, by virtue of the extent of the tumor exclude the lacrimal gland and duct. I think you should make shielding devices in order to do that. On the other hand, I think it's a triumph of hope over reason to try to spare the lacrimal duct which then carries with it a high risk of missing the tumor you're treating. Failure to control the tumor by inadequate and inappropriate radiation therapy is as bad a complication as anything else we've been talking about. Therefore, the critical question is, can you exclude it safely, and often times in eyelid cancer, one can very nicely make shielding devices for the lacrimal duct. On the other hand I would absolutely be against any kind of compromise in the treatment which has a high risk of missing the tumor in the treatment program. I haven't seen obliteration of the lacrimal duct. On the other hand the secretion of the lubricating fluids in the eye come not only from the lacrimal gland, but also from the myobia glands along the eyelids. Even with obliteration of the duct or obliteration of the gland, or atrophy of the gland, you may not necessarily have a clinical problem relative to dryness of the eye.

Dr. Million: If you get obstruction of the duct and you do sometimes, there were attempts made to correct that with a device called a Jones cannula. That doesn't work either.

Dr. Parker: I think it's pretty simple. If it's open, it rarely closes, and if it's closed, it rarely opens.

Dr. Rubin: I wish to address the issue of fractures. I don't think we should close before we talk about that, because that is a problem both in the mandible and in the femoral neck area. How does one manage those fractures, and what doses do you associate with non-healing? Rod, in a lot of the CT changes you're showing, e.g., calcified areas changing, the changes are really in the calcified cartilage which is more akin to bone. Cartilage is surprisingly resistant. We put isotopes into joints, into both articulate cartilage and regular cartilage and found that unless they're traumatized in some ways as you indicated, it is a very resistant tissue. I don't regard it as dose limiting as I do the ossified tissues. The problem of heterotopic bone formation can be blocked with a dose as low as 1,000 rad. One part of that process is really the conversion of the periosteal cell into a chondroblast. That outside of callous is really cartilage. That takes very small doses. One can block that, but the part inside the intramembranous bone, which is where one has to pin, is a much more difficult thing to block. What we have found, using a model that one of our residents will be reporting on, a dose of 5,000 rad seems to stop all bone healing. We get into this with grafts and fractures. Have you ever seen a bone that is fractured heal, and how do you handle that problem? You might want to mention a quick word about tooth extraction, too, from your experience, with regard to fracturing of mandibles.

Dr. Parker: Didn't you just answer your own question? That's such a complicated question, because we usually break bones that have been irradiated, and we don't have any control over the dose. If they break through a metastatic lesion, it's nothing to do with radiation dose symmetry. We put mechanical supports in bones that are threatened, and we haven't had any clinical disasters at all in 10 years.

Vaeth JM, Meyer JL (eds): Radiation Tolerance of Normal Tissues.
Front Radiat Ther Oncol. Basel, Karger, 1989, vol 23, pp 255–276

Response of Normal Lung to Irradiation

Tolerance Doses/Tolerance Volumes in Pulmonary Radiation Syndromes

Sandra McDonald[a], *Philip Rubin*[a], *Paula Maasilta*[b]

[a]Department of Radiation Oncology, University of Rochester Cancer Center, Strong Memorial Hospital, Rochester, N.Y., USA;
[b]Department of Pulmonary Medicine, Helsinki University Central Hospital, Helsinki, Finland

Introduction

Pulmonary radiation syndromes, with clinical manifestations ranging from pneumonitis to fibrosis, are recognized as a spectrum of histopathologic abnormalities that represent the expression of radiation injury to different target cells in the lung [1]. There are 40 different cell types present in the lung which produce an impressive sequence of events with adequate doses of irradiation, detected by both light microscopy and electron microscopy using transmission and scanning techniques [2]. Dramatic ultrastructural changes can be detected within 24 h of a lethal dose of radiation [3, 4]. Clinically, lung damage is not apparent immediately; a long latent interval exists between the damaging event and the detection of physiologic and morphologic abnormalities associated with pneumonitis [5]. This delay between irradiation and tissue response is related to the turnover of the target cells. Adult lung target cells consist of type I and II pneumocytes, fibrocytes, endothelial cells, and macrophages [4]. The mechanisms for radiation pneumonitis and fibrosis probably relate to injury to these different target cells which often involves interaction of these various cells and should not be viewed as a single event [4]. The sequence of these histologic events and how they are thought to relate to the pneumonitis and fibrosis process will be discussed.

Pulmonary function abnormalities such as a fall in lung compliance, impaired gas exchange, arterial hypoxemia, and increased respiratory frequency may take 2–3 months to become apparent [5, 6]. However, with new techniques, biochemical assays are being obtained in animals, as early as 7 days after the radiation injury [7, 8]. The lung is unusual in its reaction because both the initial pneumonitis – which can be considered the more acute event – is actually a late effect, as is the subsequent development of fibrosis. The clinical presentation of these two well-characterized sequelae will be discussed. It has been suggested that they may be interrelated [2, 9, 10]; however, these events can be dissociated. Note that fibrosis can develop without the outset of pneumonitis, although once pneumonitis occurs, fibrosis is almost certain to take place [2].

Radiation concepts of safe tolerance doses are being altered by a variety of factors which not only include the traditional time/dose fractionation factors; particular emphasis needs to be placed on lung volumes in the treatment fields. Modern techniques, particularly using total-body or hemibody irradiation, place the lungs at an increased risk for radiation injury [11]. The wider use of chemotherapy, in combination with radiation therapy, has dramatically added to the toxicity of this organ. In fact, the lung may be the most dose-limiting organ in bone marrow transplantations [12].

There is excellent information and data for lung tolerance based upon a variety of experiences both in the laboratory and the clinic. The tolerance dose for the lung will be presented as a function of both dose and volume to provide a better understanding of lung radiosensitivity. Pulmonary late effects are often tolerated because fields are shaped to minimize lung tissue exposed to radiation, and, therefore, radiation injury remains within organ tolerance. This assumes that the remaining lung can expand and compensate for the volume lost through irradiation. Toxicity scoring of acute and late effects of the relatively acute pneumonitis and later fibrosis is being standardized in cooperative group studies. This sharpens the end points that will be measured which determine the concept of tolerance. There is a need for predictive assays, and these are being actively pursued and developed in our laboratory studies which will be briefly reviewed.

Clinical Presentation

The clinical pathologic course of lung injury after irradiation is biphasic and is dependent upon dose and volume of lung exposed. As illustrated in figure 1, with high doses exceeding clinical thresholds, pulmonary reactions clinically express themselves as a pneumonitic process 1–3 months after the completion of thoracic irradiation. Lethality can occur if both lungs are irradiated to high doses. Recovery is possible, and the

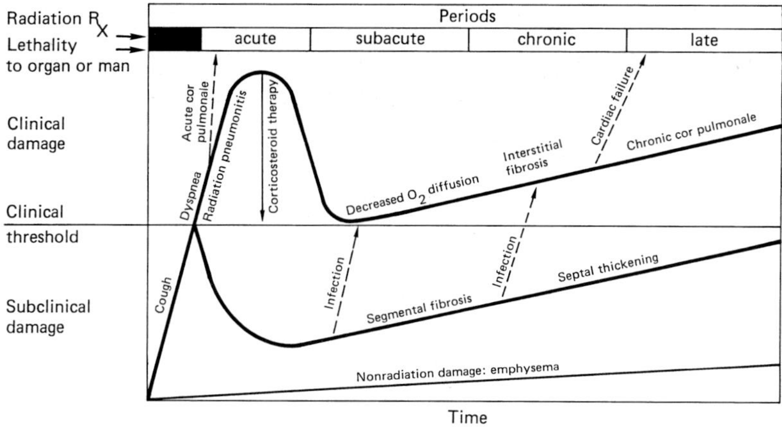

Fig. 1. Clinical pathologic course of the lung after high- and low-dose irradiation [from ref. 13, with permission].

second phase of fibrosis follows almost immediately and progresses in time. Lower doses of lung irradiation produce subclinical pathologic effects that can be expressed by added insult such as infection or drugs. A brief description of each clinical syndrome follows: radiation pneumonitis versus radiation fibrosis. The diagrams by Rubin and Casarett [13] of the clinical pathologic course have been confirmed by Travis [9] in her laboratory studies of postradiation histologic changes in mouse lungs. An acute, an intermediate, and a late effect are illustrated as a function of fractionation, dose, and intervals (fig. 2) producing similar 'roller coaster' curves.

Radiation Pneumonitis

The clinical syndrome of radiation pneumonitis usually occurs 3–6 months after the start of radiation in a large proportion (possibly 5–15%) of irradiated patients [5] (fig. 1). Acute radiation injury is more likely to be evident radiologically, particularly on computed tomographic (CT) studies [14], than symptomatically or on pulmonary function studies. During the period when clinical pneumonitis would occur, some radiologic abnormalities can be found in about 50% of all irradiated patients [5]. The severity of symptoms of the acute radiation pneumonitis syndrome is dependent on the degree of pulmonary involvement. There may be low-grade fever, nonspecific respiratory symptoms such as congestion, cough,

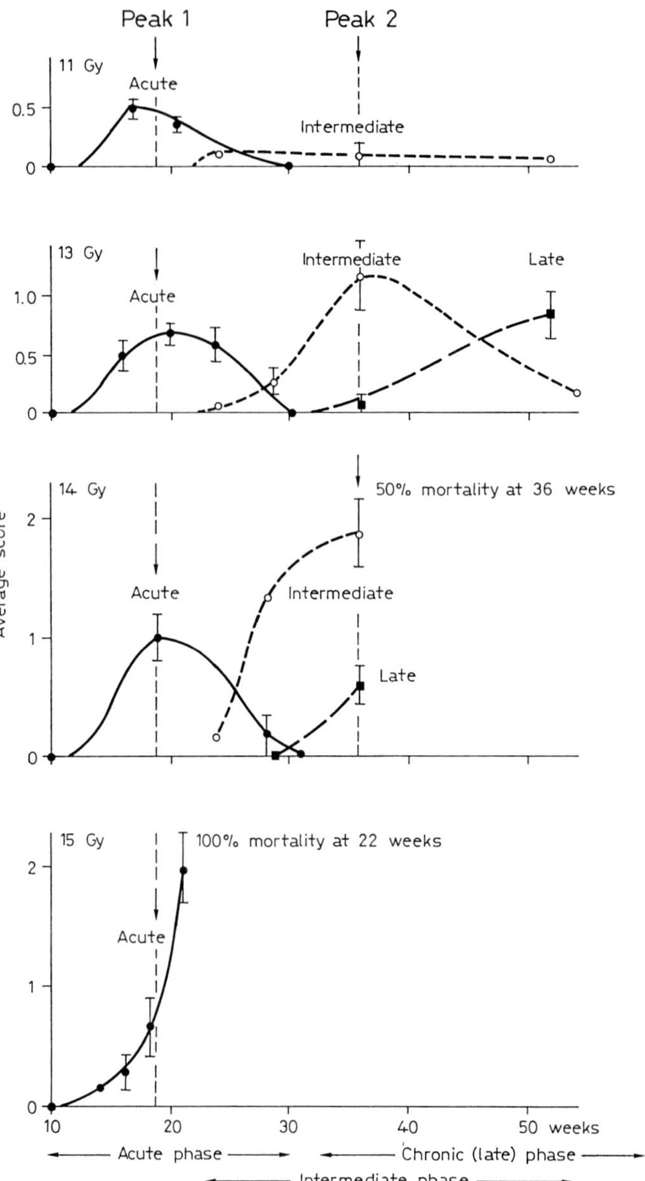

Fig. 2. Sequence of histologic changes in mouse lungs after irradiation utilizing four different single doses of 240-kV X-rays. Note the similarity of 'roller coaster' curves with clinical pathologic course. [From ref. 9, with permission].

and fullness in the chest. In more severe cases, dyspnea, pleuritic chest pain, and nonproductive cough may be present. Later, small amounts of sputum, that can be blood stained, may be produced. Physical signs in the chest are usually absent, but evidence of consolidation is sometimes found in the region corresponding to pneumonitis. Pleural friction rub or pleural fluid may be detected. If greater than 75% of the total lung parenchyma is irradiated in excess of 4,500 rad, the acute radiation pneumonitis can be very severe and produce acute respiratory distress with the patient experiencing spiking temperatures and acute cor pulmonale that can lead to death [13]. Patients who survive this phase experience a protracted period of pneumonitis – possibly for several months – that does not persist indefinitely [5]. This is the stage at which the mortality and most of the morbidity occurs.

No gross abnormalities in lung function occur before 4–8 weeks after completion of a course of radiotherapy. Restrictive changes gradually develop, with volume loss from each of several compartments being equivalent. This persists and progresses with time [15]. Gas exchange abnormalities occur approximately at the same time as the changes in lung volumes. These abnormalities consist of a fall in diffusion capacity and mild arterial hypoxemia that may be manifest only with exercise and with normal or low $PaCO_2$ levels. These changes appear to be consistent with a parenchymal lung defect and ventilation-perfusion inequality which results in a component of effective shunt [5]. Radionuclide evaluations have demonstrated underperfusion, rather than underventilation, to be the cause of these inequalities; this reflects radiation injury to the microvasculature [16–18]. However, most clinicians do not consider shunt of great practical importance, even in patients with massive radiation-induced pulmonary injury. At 1 month after radiotherapy for carcinoma of the lung, a decrease in diffusing capacity has been the single most significant pulmonary function abnormality, with a high statistical relationship to volume and dosage delivered to the thorax [19]. Larger doses of irradiation can lead to marked reductions in lung compliance which start at the time of acute pneumonitis and persist thereafter [20]. The compliance of the chest wall is usually much less affected. Sieman and Hill [21] found significant reductions in PaO_2 and elevations in $PaCO_2$ values 15 weeks after treatment in mice receiving radiation doses which would subsequently lead to lethality. In experiments with mice, at 10–15 weeks increased breathing rates, corresponding to pneumonitis and later fibrosis (on histology), are seen after lethal and sublethal doses of irradiation, with steep dose-response curves [22, 23].

The radiation injury seen on chest X-ray (1–3 months after the irradiation) is usually a diffuse infiltrate corresponding to the radiation field [6].

This appears as a result of an acute exudative edema, that is initially faint and progresses to homogenous or patchy air space consolidation. There is a frequently associated volume loss of the affected portion of the lung. These radiographic changes can occur even in an asymptomatic patient. Cases of radiographic changes outside treatment portals have been described [13], but this phenomenon is rare and has been attributed to opportunistic infections or other causes [24]. Computed tomographic (CT) studies of the lung used to evaluate for increased lung density have recently been correlated with radiation effects [25, 26]. Because of its sensitivity to slight changes in lung densities, CT is presently favored for diagnostic detection of pulmonary damage in humans [14, 25]. CT findings demonstrate a well-defined dose-response relationship [27]. Libshitz and Shuman [25] identified four patterns of radiation-induced changes in lung on CT: homogenous, slight increase in radiodensity; patchy consolidation; discrete consolidation; solid consolidation. These patterns appeared weeks to years after radiotherapy corresponding to both pneumonitis and fibrosis phases. In late-responding normal tissue such as lung, the latent time for expression of injury is dose dependent, occurring sooner after higher doses.

Radiation Fibrosis

In contrast to the acute reaction, the chronic effects of radiation are observed from months to years following treatment, even though histologic/biochemical changes are evident sooner. Pulmonary fibrosis develops insidiously in the previously irradiated field and stabilizes after 1 or 2 years [5] (fig. 1).

The clinical symptomatology related to radiographic changes is proportional to the extent of the lung parenchyma involved and the patients' preexisting pulmonary reserves. Most patients with radiation fibrosis are asymptomatic. In a few patients, particularly those with severe pneumonitis, chronic respiratory failure may be present: dyspnea on effort, reduced exercise tolerance, orthopnea, cyanosis, sometimes chronic cor pulmonale and finger clubbing. Symptoms are minimal if the fibrosis is limited to less than 50% of one lung [28]: if the volume increases above this limit, dyspnea may manifest clinically, and progressive chronic cor pulmonale leading to right-heart failure may occur.

A mild deterioration in pulmonary function may occur as fibrosis develops. There is a reduction in maximum breathing capacity which is particularly evident in patients with bilateral radiation fibrosis. The tidal volume usually decreases, and the frequency tends to increase, resulting in an overall moderate increase in minute ventilation [29]. Most studies have found these changes to persist indefinitely, with little recovery. Improvements in pulmonary function resulting from radiation response of lung tumors may compensate for losses due to radiation fibrosis [6, 30, 31]. Pulmonary function tests do not demonstrate significant changes when small volumes of lung are irradiated due to functional compensation of adjacent lung regions [17] and are, therefore, not an ideal end point for measurement of radiation-induced lung injury.

Radiologic changes consistent with fibrosis are seen in most patients who have received lung irradiation, even if they did not develop acute pneumonitis. Chest X-rays have the appearance of linear streaking, radiating from the area of previous pneumonitis which may extend outside the irradiated region, with concomitant regional contraction, pleural thickening, and tenting of the diaphragm. Hilum or mediastinum may be retracted with a densely contracted lung segment, resulting in compensatory hyperinflation of adjacent or contralateral lung tissue. This is usually seen 12 months to 2 years after irradiation [5]. CT is currently favored to image regions subjected to radiation therapy [14, 25, 26]. Magnetic resonance is being explored and may have promise in accurately distinguishing radiation fibrosis from recurrent tumor [32].

The late lung injury is characterized by progressive fibrosis of alveolar septa with the septa being thickened by bundles of elastic fibers. The alveoli collapse and are obliterated by connective tissue. These changes can lead to the radiographic appearance of lung scarring on chest radiography which corresponds to the shape of the radiation portal. Eventually, the previously irradiated lung can develop dense fibrotic nodules, especially in the area of previous tumor [33].

Late effects can occur without being preceded by acute effects [2, 34, 35]. Thus, the chronic phase of lung injury can occur without a prior history of an acute radiation pneumonitis. The radioprotector WR-2721 is more effective in protecting against the later phase than the pneumonitic phase, both with single and fractionated doses of irradiation [36, 37]; the reverse holds true for anesthetics [38].

Pneumonitis can be avoided by using low doses or fractionated schedules [39]; however, fibrosis is unavoidable. In rats, hyperfractionation protects against fibrosis, with no difference in acute toxicity when compared to conventional fractionation [40, 41]. The fact that these two phases of lung injury can be separated has been attributed to different target cell populations [1].

Although tolerance doses may be exceeded, not all patients will develop complications, since the likelihood of complications is a probability event. This probability is balanced against the probability of tumor control and leads to the discussion of lung tolerance as a function of both dose and volume.

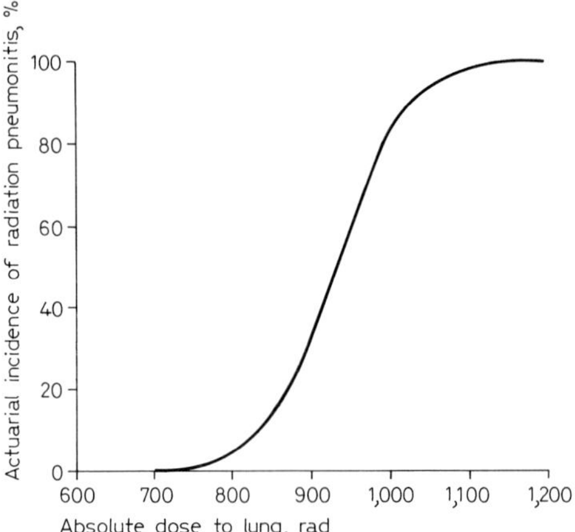

Fig. 3. Dose-response curve for radiation pneumonopathy in humans after upper hemibody irradiation [from ref. 11, with permission].

Tolerance Doses and Tolerance Volumes

Single Dose, Whole-Lung Volume

A considerable body of human data has accummulated since the introduction of total-body irradiation and half-body irradiation techniques. These techniques were applied often to doses of 8–10 Gy without lung correction factors. With total-body irradiation, bone marrow transplantation resulted in long-term survival for leukemia patients with death resulting from interstitial pneumonitis [12] which was often attributed to secondary opportunistic infection. With half-body irradiation for metastatic patients, the onset of pulmonary failure often 1–3 months later was mistaken for lymphangitic carcinomatosis. At autopsy, the presence of radiation pneumonopathy became evident, since no evidence of cancer spread to the lung was found. The studies of Keane et al. [11] and Fryer et al. [42] are an accurate portrayal of pulmonic lethality secondary to irradiation (fig. 3).

Precise dose-response curves were generated by these investigations with and without lung inhomogeneity correction. The threshold dose was 7 Gy, and the TD_5 was 8.2 Gy, and TD_{50} and TD_{90} are 9.3 and 11 Gy, respectively, corrected for pulmonary transmission. The dose response is so sharp that a difference of 2 Gy could change zero mortality to 50% lethality. Since the lung correction factor is 15–20% for telecobalt irradiation, failure to correct for lung transmission could be fatal for a 'safe'

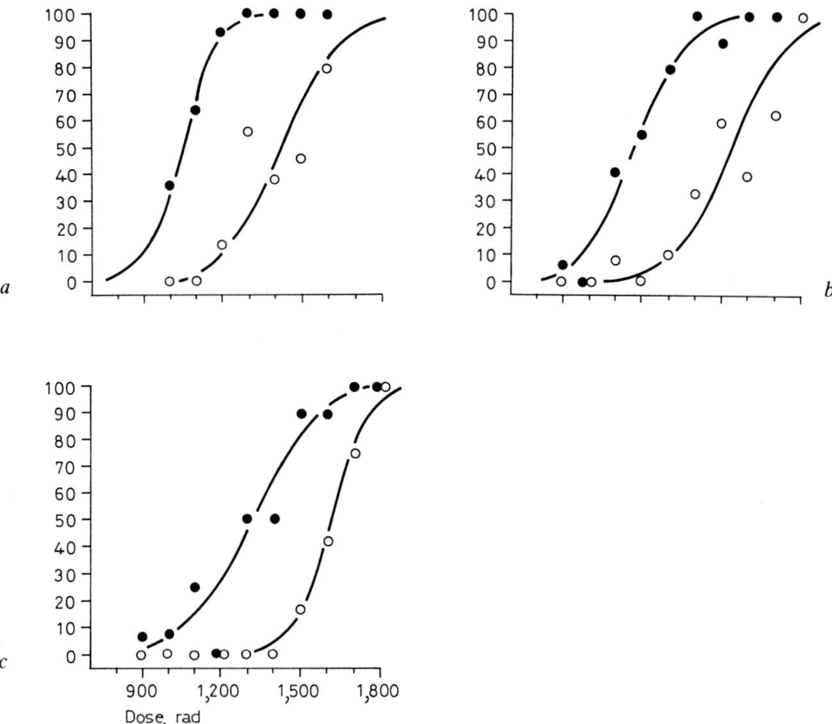

Fig. 4. Animal toxicity in LAFl mice *(a)* or C3H mice treated without *(b)* or with *(c)* a 1.0-mg/g dose of misonidazole at the time of irradiation. The percentage lethality as a function of radiation dose was assessed at either 180 (○) or 420 (●) days after treatment. [From ref. 43, with permission.]

threshold dose, if depth doses are chosen on routine charts. Low-dose rate irradiation is protective as used in total-body irradiation, but only shifts the lung dose response 2–3 Gy to the right [11]. There are numerous animal studies, particularly in mice, that produce similar steep dose-response curves, particularly in different murine strains [43] (fig. 4). The range for TD_5 is 9–12 Gy, and TD_{50} and TD_{90} are 10–15 and 12–18 Gy, respectively.

Fractionated Dose, Whole-Lung Volume

There are also well-documented fractionated dose-time data for lung in both animal models and in man that study a variety of pulmonary functions and lethality. Two excellent sources of human data are for whole-

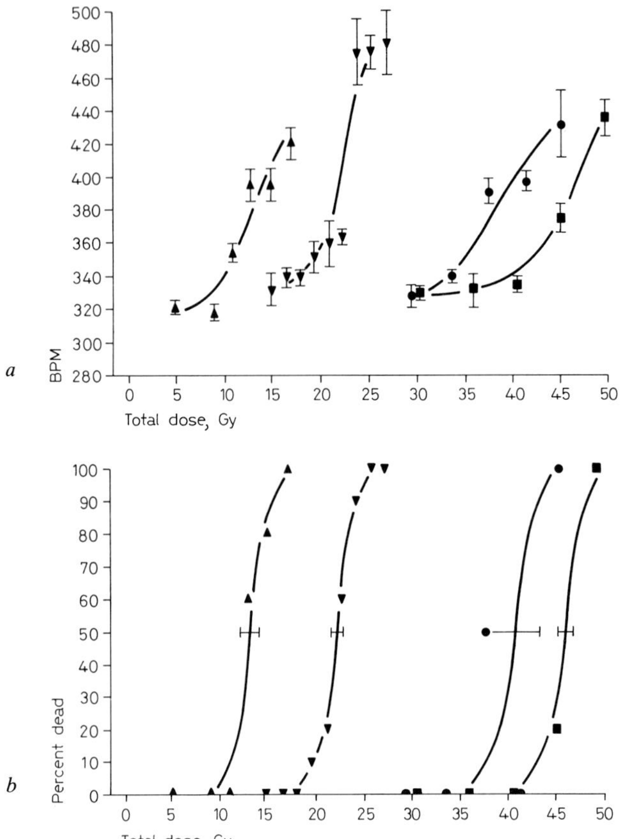

Fig. 5. Dose-response curves for fatal radiation pneumonopathy for different fractionation schedules, illustrating the sparing effects of decreasing fraction size, as determined after 16 *(a)* and 28 weeks *(b)*. That is, the fractional dose decreases, as the frequency of irradiation is increased from single dose (▲) to once a week (▼), to once a day (●), and to twice daily (■). [From ref. 39, with permission.] BPM in *a* = ■. BPM = breathing rate per minute.

lung irradiation in Wilms' tumor patients: the TD_5 is 25.6 Gy, and the TD_{50} is 30 Gy without dactinomycin. The LAF_1 mouse has been irradiated with a variety of schedules by Wara et al. [44], indicating a significant degree of recovery between fractions: with two fractions LD_{50} is 17 Gy, with 20 fx, LD_{50} is 47 Gy, indicating recovery of 30 Gy to achieve the same effect. This was further illustrated by Siemann et al. [39] with single-dose, 1 q week, 1 q day, and 2 q day schedules, simulating fractionation regimens used clinically, the LD_{50} was 13, 23, 41, and 46 Gy, respective-

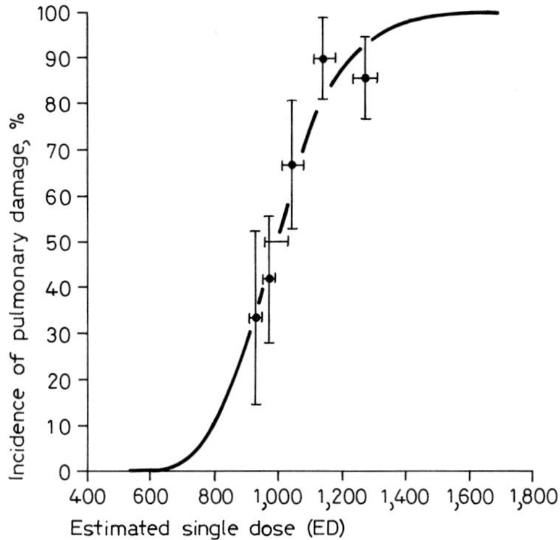

Fig. 6. Dose-response curve for radiation pneumonitis fibrosis. Partial lung volume irradation as a function of fractionated schedules. [From ref. 14, with permission.]

ly, in a similar mouse strain (fig. 5). This suggests slow repair and an α/β ratio in the range of 1.1–3.6 which has been confirmed by numerous radiation therapy investigators.

More interesting is the observation that fibrosis appears to be elicited at lower dose rates that those producing pneumonitis. As initially demonstrated by Travis [9] and Travis et al. [22], animals not dying of an early pulmonary pneumonitic death at 200 days developed increasingly rapid breathing rates, indicative of interstitial fibrosis (fig. 2). The deaths in our experiments that occurred at 400 days with the aforementioned schedules were with 11, 20, 38, 45 Gy, respectively. There was only a difference of 1.2–2.6 Gy between the absence of a recognizable clinical event and the lethal event. This was true for all daily or twice-a-day schedules. Thus, only a dose difference of 10–20% of the total dose depending upon the fractionation schemes can be the difference between life and death; the small dose percentage difference is accentuated with increasing fractionation.

Fractionated Dose, Partial Lung Volume

The most informative source of data regarding the clinical quanitification of dose and time for partial lung volume is the report by Mah et al. [14] (fig. 6). The end point utilized was an increase in lung density within the irradiated volume on CT during the posttreatment period. The estimated single dose (ED) model (ED = D $N^{0.058}$) best expressed the different fractionation schedules, and over the linear portion of the DIR curves a 5% ED increase predicts for a 12% increase in incidence of radiation-induced pneumonitis. Doses from 3,000 cGy in 10–15 days to 4,500–5,000 cGy in 25–30 days were yielding radiographic changes ranging from 30 to 90%. Dose-volume histograms correlated with CT findings could provide more accurate data for partial lung tolerance to irradiation.

Pathophysiology and Proposed Mechanisms

Histologically, lesions due to irradiation would most likely be found in all patients, even with very small doses. A great number of histologic changes have been documented in animals; however, data for humans are incomplete. The effects of irradiation on the lung parenchyma are evident within the first 24 h after exposure to radiation with resultant congestion and intra-alveolar edema. There is exudation of proteinaceous material into the alveoli, leading to impairment of gas exchange. An infiltration of inflammatory cells and desquamation of epithelial cells from the alveolar walls occurs [4]. The ultrastructural sequence of events is shown in table I. Within a few weeks the interstitial edema organizes into collagen fibrils which eventually leads to thickening of the alveolar septa. These changes may resolve within a few weeks to months. However, depending on the volume of lung parenchyma irradiated, the total dose, and the dose per fraction used, these pathologic exudative changes can result in an acute radiation pneumonitis. Although abnormalities are found in most elements, and no specific lesion is entirely characteristic of pneumonitis, current evidence [2, 45–47] suggests that damage to the type II pneumocyte and the endothelial cell is more closely linked to the pneumonitic process than the fibrotic.

The type II pneumocyte, which produces surfactant and maintains patent alveoli, has been widely studied. It is the most rapid in response to irradiation, as evidenced by a rapid decrease in the content of cytoplasmic surfactant containing lamellar bodies, occasional bizarre lamellar body development, and ultimate sloughing of some of the cells into the alveolar lumen [3, 48]. Changes in the surfactant system, leading to alterations in alveolar surface tension and low compliance, are most likely a direct result of the radiation [2, 7, 8], although it has been postulated to be a response to radiation-induced exudation of plasma proteins [5]. The latter mechanism seems unlikely; changes in surfactant appear sooner than vascular leakage. An increased level of alveolar surfactant is one of the earliest detectable changes following lung irradiation, starting within

Table I. Ultrastructural changes in lung postradiation in fatal radiation pneumonitis and fibrosis [from ref. 4, with permission]

Event	Time	Dose, Gy			
		0	5	9	13
Type II cell degranulation, surfactant release	1 h to 7 days	–	–	–	+
Loss of basal laminar proteoglycans	1 h to 7 days	–	±	+	++
Loss of alveolar macrophages	7 days	–	–	±	+
Surfactant recovery	4 weeks	–	–	–	+
Replacement of laminar proteoglycans	4–12 weeks	–	±	±	+
Radiation pneumonitis	12–30 weeks	–	–	–	+
Peak in soluble fibronectin	12–30 weeks	–	±	±	++
Fibrosis	30–60 weeks	–	±	+	+
Peak in insoluble fibronectin	30–60 weeks	–	+	+	++
Increased laminin	12–60 weeks	–	±	+	++

hours of irradiation and persisting a maximum of 2–6 weeks [7] (depending on the species studied). Subsequently, surfactant levels return to and remain at normal levels during the pneumonitis phase. During this phase, the exudation of plasma protein into the alveolar spaces is maximal; this may indicate that changes in surfactant are due to the direct effect of radiation on the type II cell rather than a response to increased alveolar fluid. The replicative activity of the type II cells in mouse lungs is elevated after irradiation during a time period that coincides with increased breathing frequency and histologic evidence of the presence of radiation pneumonitis [49]. Type II cell pleomorphism, degeneration, and hyperplasia persist for at least 1 year after irradiation of a single dose of 25 Gy [50].

Endothelial cell damage results in changes in perfusion and changes in permeability of vessel wall. In the first few days to weeks after irradiation, changes in the capillary endothelial lining become evident. The cells become pleomorphic, vacuolated, and may slough, producing areas of denuded basement membranes and occlusion of the capillary lumen by debris and thrombi [15, 51–53]. It must be noted that these phenomena are dose dependent and occur at lethal doses of irradiation. These effects are present well before the time of pneumonitis, but evidence of persistent damage and repair probably continues up to and beyond the phase of pneumonitis. Ward et al. [45, 54, 56], Gross et al. [49], and T'sao et al.

[55] have studied endothelial function, histopathology, ultrastructure, arterial perfusion, hydroxyproline accumulation, and several potential modifiers of radiation injury in the rat lung. Four markers of endothelial function (angiotensin-converting enzyme activity, plasminogen activator activity, and prostacyclin and tromboxane production) were routinely monitored. The first studies evaluated the effect of penicillamine, a collagen antagonist, showing that penicillamine delayed the onset, reduced peak severity, and/or accelerated recovery from radiation-induced events. This drug was slow acting, requiring administration over months, and did not seem to spare all four endothelial markers equally [57, 58]. The study has been repeated with angiotensin-converting enzyme inhibitors (captopril, CL 242817) which showed more effective and more uniform sparing of radiation lung damage [59]. These drugs might offer a new possibility to modify radiation-induced lung damage clinically in the future, although their mechanism of therapeutic action remain unclear today.

The late lung injury is characterized by progressive fibrosis of alveolar septa with the septa thickened by bundles of elastic fibers. The alveoli collapse and are obliterated by connective tissue. Although it has been suggested that the later fibrosis is a secondary consequence of the pneumonitis phase, it has been shown that the two phases can be dissociated. This probably relates to injury of different target cells – the lung consists of more than 40 cell types – and often times involves many different cells interacting and should not be viewed as a single event. The fibrosis process can be triggered by small doses of 5–10 Gy, and injury to the basement membrane of both endothelial cells and alveolar type I cells occurs [60]. Recently it has become increasingly clear, that the process leading to lung fibrosis is essentially a dynamic imbalance of collagen metabolism [61]. The surprising observation is that thickening of the interstitial membrane and increasing collagen deposition is occurring with small doses, i.e., <10 Gy as a dynamic process of deposition and absorption, rather than the view that the fibrosis is an end process or a scar. Experimental fibrosis might resolve spontaneously, if dense scars are not formed [62].

The mechanisms of chronic complications may be related to the effects of radiation on the vascular (endothelial cells) and/or the effects on somatic cells of the organ at risk. Each organ has a unique radiation tolerance, and thus a combination of vascular damage and somatic cell damage may be important in the development of late radiation injury. The nature of the triggering event in the pathogenesis of radiation fibrosis is unknown. Several hypotheses have been suggested: fibrosis is considered to follow parenchymal cell death, occurring when irradiated cells attempt to divide, the delay between irradiation and onset of fibrosis being ascribed to the long turnover times of parenchymal cells [63]. The dead parenchymal cells are then replaced by connective tissue. In another hypothesis, damage to the vasculature is considered to be the primary lesion [13, 64, 65]. The blood vessel damage leads to exudation of plasma proteins into the extravascular spaces, where this exudate initiates fibrosis. Damage to other cells that are involved in the synthesis and degradation of collagen, e.g., fibroblasts, might also be the triggering event. Law et al. [66] found no support for a causal relationship between exudation of vascular protein into tissue spaces and increases in collagen biosynthesis in the irradiated mouse lung. Alluding to the model of Rennard et al. [67], the alveolar macrophage and neutrophil is seen as crucial cells mediating fibrotic initiation through fibronectin and alveolar macrophage-derived growth factor. In radiation-induced fibrosis, the loss of macrophages as a very early consequence may be the pivotal event.

Chemotherapy Interactions with Radiation

In this era of combined modality cancer therapy, it is important to recognize that many antineoplastic agents induce lung damage or potentiate the damaging effects of radiations on the lung. Phillips and Margolis [51] and Wara et al. [44] showed that dactinomycin administration increased the incidence of radiation pneumonitis in humans receiving lung irradiation. The dose-response curve was shifted to the left (fig. 7). Testing effects of commonly used chemotherapeutic agents, Phillips et al. [24] reported that dactinomycin, cyclophosphamide, and, to a lesser extent, vincristine enhanced the lethality of thoracic irradiation. The effect of dactinomycin was seen if given as long as 30 days before, but not when given 30 days after the irradiation. Lung damage is a significant and often dose-limiting side effect of bleomycin. Up to 10% of patients treated with bleomycin develop pulmonary toxicity, and in 1% this is fatal [68]. Bleomycin, given with lung irradiation, produces lung toxicity greater than when either agent is given alone. Catane et al. [69] found 19% pulmonary toxicity, in 10% it was fatal. This effect might be maximal when bleomycin is given concurrently with the irradiation [70]. Collis et al. [71] assessed bleomycin- and radiation-induced lung damage in mice and found enhanced damage from combined treatment, with the extent of the lung damage dependent on schedule, mode of administration, and dose of the drug, but no time-dependent interaction was found. Cyclophosphamide also enhances radiation lung damage, but, in contrast to bleomycin, the enhancement has been found to be time dependent [72].

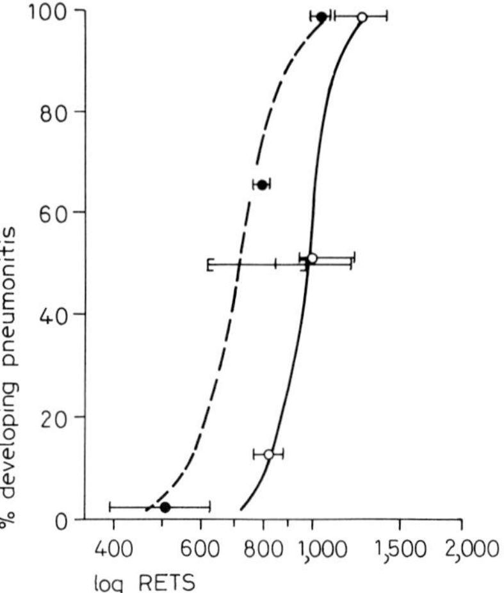

Fig. 7. Dose-response curve illustrating increased incidence of radiation pneumonitis with dactinomycin [from ref. 44, with permission].

The effects of irradiation are potentiated by doxorubicin. In addition to being observed in skin, intestines, and heart, the lung appears to be very sensitive to this combination [73, 74]. Of 24 patients treated with low-dose doxorubicin and irradiation, 13 developed pneumonitis [75]. Von der Maase et al. [76] assessed various antineoplastic drugs in combination with irradiation and found dose-enhancing effects of adriamycin, bleomycin, cyclophosphamide and mitomycin C at various time points. 5-Fluorouracil, methotrexate, and cisplatinum appeared to have no effect on the radiation response at the intervals investigated. Interferons have been shown to increase radiation cytotoxicity *in vitro* in a number of studies. Natural human leukocyte interferon [HuIFN-a (Le)] was the first interferon to be combined with radiation therapy in the treatment of small-cell lung cancer [77]. A potentiation of both antitumor effect and normal-tissue toxicity of radiations was observed in this treatment. In laboratory modeling at the University of Rochester Cancer Center, betaseron (recombinant human interferon betaser; fHuIFN-B_{ser}) appeared less toxic and beter tolerated than HuIFN-a (Le) and produced approximately the same potentiation effect *in vitro*. A clinical trial, combining thoracic irradiation with escalating betaseron doses, is presently being conducted. The mechanisms of these various drug radiation interactions in the lung are not clear, but the therapeutic implications are critical.

Predictive Assays for Late Effects in the Lung

There is a need for early biochemical markers of normal-tissue damage which would predict for late effects and which would allow the radiation oncologist and medical oncologist to determine if their treatment is exceeding the normal-tissue tolerance [78]. If biochemical markers of tissue damage could be detected during the subclinical phase, prior to the accumulation of significant injury, one could terminate therapy or institute treatment to prevent or attenuate later lesions. An ideal marker should be a simple and reproducible positive/negative biochemical test. As a consequence of early ultrastructural changes detected in irradiated lungs [3, 79] surfactant release has been studied as a measure of predicting later fatal radiation pneumonitis. Early release of surfactant during the 1st week following irradiation is quantifiable in bronchoalveolar lavage and correlates with later radiation pneumonitis. Surfactant is the first consistent early biochemical marker for later lethal radiation events in three murine strains and a rabbit model [7, 8]. Although these measurements are useful and sensitive, lung lavage profiles are dependent on relative increases which vary with alveolar surface area lavaged, and a constant baseline value is difficult to establish. Bronchoalveolar lavage is also a time-consuming invasive procedure and as such not suitable for clinical situations, when repeated measurements are needed. Detection of serum antigens released as byproducts of radiation-induced cell injury would allow for a positive-negative answer.

The protein components of surfactant, called 'apoproteins', have a high degree of specificity; the presence of this apoprotein in blood can be detected by sensitive immunoassays. The presence of surfactant apoprotein in blood would indicate damage to the capillary-alveolar membrane and leakage into serum. In the rabbit model, the first series of experiments indicated a correlation between surfactant released in bronchoalveolar fluid and surfactant detected in serum as a function of dose and time (fig. 8).

This is the first demonstration of unique cellular antigens in the serum detected by antibodies, supporting the concept that there may be an antigen-antibody reaction, occurring as part of the explanation for the progressive nature of both these processes as later effects. It may also account for the variations in expression of these injuries on different animal species and strains.

The ability to predict for potential severe late effects early after fractionated treatment or toward the end of a course of irradiation allows for intervention. The work of Shen et al. [80], utilizing Chinese herbal medicine, is impressive and is undergoing further assessment in our own

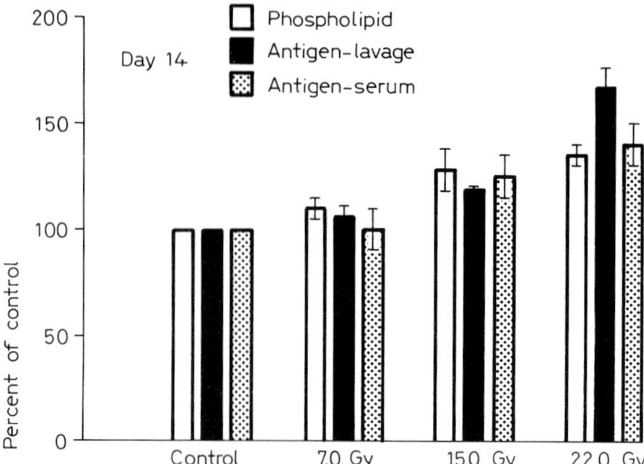

Fig. 8. Predictive assay. Correlation between alveolar surfactant increase and serum surfactant apoprotein levels.

laboratory models. This product was administered daily after high-dose unilateral lung irradiation in rats, well beyond tolerance, i.e., 30 Gy in a single dose. High alveolar surfactant levels never occurred, and late fibrosis was prevented months later. The major implications of their studies is that through intervention, a late effect did not occur, and the histopathologic events failed to appear.

Conclusions

(1) Radiation pneumonitis and radiation fibrosis are two distinct syndromes with probably different target cells; (2) dramatic ultrastructural changes occur rapidly: type II cell, endothelial basement membranes, and proteoglycans; (3) dose, time, and volume data for tolerance dose TD_{5-50} and tolerance volumes are well documented; (4) lung function measurements, radiologic imaging, and biochemical testing both in serum and BAL should be routine baseline studies; (5) volume-modifying factors need better definition and data similar to tolerance doses TD_{5-50}; (6) chemotherapy has altered the concept of 'early and late' effects and can produce adverse effects with and without radiation therapy; (7) predictive assays utilizing *serum* biochemical markers are possible and should make corrective actions feasible, and (8) corrective and preventive measures are possible, and late radiation effects should not be viewed as permanent and irreversible effects.

References

1 Travis, E. L.; Tucker, S. L.: The relationship between functional assays of radiation response in the lung and taret cell depletion. Br. J. Cancer *53:* suppl VII, pp. 304–319 (1986).
2 Penney, D. P.; Siemann, D. W.; Rubin, P.; Shapiro, D. L.; Finkelstein, J.; Cooper, R. A.: Morphologic changes reflecting early and late effects of irradiation on the distal lung of the mouse. Scanning Electron Microsc. *1:* 413–425 (1982).
3 Penney, D. P.; Rubin, R.: Specific early fine structural changes in the lung following irradiation. Int. J. Radiat. Oncol. Biol. Phys. *2:* 1123–1132 (1977).
4 Penney, D. P.: Ultrastructural organization of the distal lung and potential target cells of ionizing radiation. Int. Conf. on New Biology of Lung and Lung Injury and Their Implications for Oncology, Porvoo 1987.
5 Gross, N. J.: The pathogenesis of radiation-induced lung damage. Lung *159:* 115–125 (1981).
6 Gross, N. J.: Plumonary effects of radiation therapy. Ann. intern. Med. *86:* 81–92 (1977).
7 Rubin, P.; Shapiro, D. L.; Finklestein, J. N.; Penney, D. P.: The early release of surfactant following lung irradiation of alveolar type II cells. Int. J. Radiat. Oncol. Biol. Phys. *6:* 75–77 (1980).
8 Rubin, P.; Siemann, D. W.; Shapiro, D. L.; Finkelstein, J. N.; Penney, D. P.: Surfactant release as an early measure of radiation pneumonitis. Int. J. Radiat. Oncol. Biol. Phys. *9:* 1669–1673 (1983).
9 Travis, E. L.: The sequence of histological change in mouse lungs after single doses of X-rays. Int. J. Radiat. Oncol. Biol. Phys. *6:* 345–347 (1980).
10 Field, S. B.; Hornsey, S.: Slow repair after X-rays and fast neutrons. Br. J. Radiol. *50:* 600–601 (1977).
11 Keane, T. J.; Van Dyk, J.; Rider, W. D.: Idiopathic interstitial pneumonia following bone marrow transplantation: the relationship with total body irradiation. Int. J. Radiat. Oncol. Biol. Phys. *7:* 1365–1370 (1981).
12 Bortin, M. M.; Kay, H. E. M.; Gale, R. P.; Rimm, A. A.: Factors associated with interstitial pneumonitis after bone-marrow transplantation for acute leukaemia. Lancet *II:* 437–439 (1982).
13 Rubin, P. and Casarett, G. W.: Clinical radiation pathology (Saunders, Philadelphia 1968).
14 Mah, K.; Van Dyk, J.; Keane, T.; Poon, P. Y.: Acute radiation-induced pulmonary damage: a clinical study on the response to fractionated radiation therapy. Int. J. Radiat. Oncol. Biol. Phys. *13:* 179–188 (1987).
15 Gross, N. J.: Experimental radiation pneumonitis, IV. Leakage of circulatory proteins onto the alveolar surface. J. Lab. clin. Med. *95:* 19–31 (1980).
16 Prato, F. S.; Kurdyak, R.; Saibil, E. A.; Rider, W. D.; Aspin, N.: Regional and total lung function in patients following pulmonary irradiation. Investive Radiol. *12:* 224–237 (1977).
17 Prato, F. S.; Kurdyak, R.; Saibil, E. A.; Rider, W. D.; Aspin, N.: Physiological and radiographic assessment during the development of pulmonary radiation fibrosis. Radiology *122:* 389–397 (1977).
18 Vieras, F.; Bradley, E. W.; Alderson, P. O.; Jacobus, J. P.; Grissom, M. P.: Regional pulmonary function after irradiation of the canine lung: radionuclide evaluation. Radiology *147:* 839–844 (1983).
19 Brady, L. W.; Germon, P. A.; Cander, L.: The effects of radiation therapy on pulmonary function in carcinoma of the lung. Radiology *85:* 130–134 (1965).
20 Phillips, T. L.; Wyatt, J. P.: Radiation fibrosis; in *Fishman, Pulmonary diseases and disorders*, vol. I, pp. 658–675 (McGraw-Hill, New York, 1980).

21 Sieman, D.W.; Hill, R.P.: Quantitative changes in the arterial blood gases of mice following localized irradiation of the lungs. Radiat. Res. *93:* 560–566 (1983).
22 Travis, E.L.; Down, J.D.; Holmes, S.J.; Hobson, B.: Radiation pneumonitis and fibrosis in mouse lung assayed by respiratory frequency and histology. Radiat. Res. *84:* 133 (1980).
23 Travis, E.L.; Tucker, S.L.: The relationship between functional assays of radiation response in the lung and target cell depletion. Br. J. Cancer *53:* 304–319 (1986).
24 Phillips, T.L.; Wharam, M.D.; Margolis, L.W.: Modification of radiation injury to normal tissues by chemotherapeutic agents. Cancer *35:* 1678–1684 (1975).
25 Libshitz, H.I.; Shuman, L.S.: Radiation induced pulmonary change: CT findings, J. Comput. assist. Tomogr. *8:* 15–19 (1984).
26 Van Dyk, J.; Hill, R.P.: Postirradiation lung density changes measured by computerized tomography. Int. J. Radiat. Oncol. Biol. Phys. *9:* 847–852 (1983).
27 Mah, K.; Poon, P.Y.; Van Dyk, J.; Keane, T.J.; Majesky, L.F.; Rideout, D.F.: Assessment of acute radiation-induced pulmonary changes using computed tomography. J. Comput. assist. Tomogr. *10:* 736–743 (1986).
28 Weichselbaum, R.R.; Awan, A.M.: Principles of radiation oncology; in Bitran, Golomb, Little, Weishelbaum, *Lung cancer – a comprehensive treatise*, pp. 61–70 (Grune and Stratton: Orlando, 1987).
29 Shrivastava, P.N.; Hans, L.; Concannon, J.P.: Changes in pulmonary compliance and production of fibrosis in X-irradiated lungs of rats. Radiology *112:* 439–440 (1974).
30 Germon, P.A.; Brady, L.W.: Physiologic changes before and after radiation treatment for carcinoma of the lung. J. Am. med. Ass. *206:* 808 (1968).
31 Evans, R.F.; Sagerman, R.H.; Ringrose, T.L.: Pulmonary function following mantle field irradiation for Hodgkin's disease. Radiology *111:* 729 (1974).
32 Glazer, H.S.; Lee, J.K.T.; Levitt, R.G.; Heiken, J.P.; Ling, D.; Totty, W.G.; Balfe, D.M.; Emani, B.; Wasserman, T.H.; Murphy, W.A.: Radiation fibrosis: differentiation from recurrent tumor by MR imaging. Radiology *156:* 721–726 (1985).
33 Rubin, P.: The Franz Busche Lecture. Late effects of chemotherapy and radiation therapy: a new hypothesis. Int. J. Radiat. Oncol. Biol. Phys. *10:* 5–34 (1984).
34 Rubin, P.: Radiation toxicity: quantitative radiation pathology for predicting effects. Cancer *39:* suppl. 2, pp. 729–736 (1977).
35 Siemann, D.W.; Hill, R.P.; Penney, D.P.: Early and late pulmonary toxicity in mice evaluated 180 and 420 days following localized lung irradiation. Radiat. Res. *89:* 396–407 (1982).
36 Travis, E.L.; Parkins, C.S.; Holmes, S.J.; Down, J.D.; Fowler, J.F.: WR-2721 protection of pneumonitis and fibrosis in mouse lung after single dose of X-rays. Int. J. Radiat. Oncol. Biol. Phys. *10:* 243 (1984).
37 Travis, E.L.; Meistrich, M.L.; Finch-Neimeyer, M.V.; Watkins, T.L.; Kiss, I.: Late functional and biochemical changes in mouse lung after irradiation: differential effects of WR-2721. Radiat. Res. *103:* 219 (1985).
38 Down, J.D.; Collis, C.H.; Jeffery, P.K.; Steel, G.G.: The effects of anesthetics and misonidazole on the development of radiation-induced lung damage in mice. Int. J. Radiat. Oncol. Biol. Phys. *9:* 221 (1983).
39 Siemann, D.W.; Rubin, P.; Penney, D.P.: Pulmonary toxicity following multifraction radiotherapy. Br. J. Cancer *53:* 365–367 (1986).
40 Giri, P.G.S.; Kimler, B.F.; Giri, U.P.; Cox, G.G.: Hyperfractionation protects against long-term fibrosis in rat lung. Br. J. Cancer *53:* 324–326 (1986).
41 Rongen, E. van; Tan, C.H.T.; Durham, S.K.: Late functional biochemical and histo-

logical changes in the rat lung after fractionated irradiation to the whole thorax. Radiol. Oncol. *10:* 231–246 (1987).

42 Fryer, C. J. H.; Fitzpatrick, P. J.; Rider, W. D.; Poon, P.: Radiation pneumonitis: experience following a large single dose of radiation. Int. J. Radiat. Oncol. Biol. Phys. *4:* 931–936 (1978).

43 Siemann, D. W.; Hill, R. P.; Penney, D. P.: Early and late pulmonary toxicity in mice evaluated 180 and 420 days following localized lung irradiation. Radiat. Res. *89:* 396–407 (1982).

44 Wara, W. M.; Phillips, T. L.; Margolis, L. W., Smith, V.: Radiation pneumonitis: a new approach to the derivation of time-dose factors. Cancer *32:* 547–552 (1973).

45 Ward, W. F.; Molteni, A.; Solliday, S. H.; Jones, G. R.: The relationship between endothelial dysfunction and collagen accumulation in irradiated rat lung. Int. J. Radiat. Oncol. Biol. Phys. *11:* 1985–1990 (1985).

46 Travis, E. L.; Hanley, R. A.; Fenn, J. O.; Klobukowski, C. J.; Hargrove, H. B.: Pathologic changes in the lung following single and multifraction irradiation. Int. J. Radiat. Oncol. Biol. Phys. *2:* 475–490 (1977).

47 Travis, E. L.: Early indicators of radiation injury on the lung: are they useful predictors for late changes? Int. J. Radiat. Oncol. Biol. Phys. *6:* 1267–1269 (1980).

48 Penney, D. P.; Shapiro, D. L.; Rubin, P.; Finkelstein, J.; Siemann, D. W.: Effects of radiation on the mouse lung and potential induction of radiation pneumonitis. Virchows Arch. Abt. B Zellpath. *37:* 327–336 (1981).

49 Gross, N. J.; Narine, K. R.; Colletti-Squinto, L.: Replicative activity of lung type 2 cells following lung X-irradiation. Radiat. Res. *111:* 143–150 (1987).

50 Port, C. D.; Ward, W. F.: The ultrastructure of radiation injury in rat lung: modification by *D*-penicillamine. Radiat. Res. *92:* 61–82 (1982).

51 Phillips, T. L.; Margolis, L.: Radiation pathology and the clinical response of lung and esophagus. Front. Radiat. Ther. Onc., vol. 6, pp. 254–273 (Karger, Basel 1972).

52 Leroy, E. P.; Liebner, E. J.; Jensick, R. J.: The ultrastructure of canine alveoli after supervoltage irradiation of the thorax. Lab. Invest. *15:* 1544–1558 (1966).

53 Maisin, J. R.: The influence of radiation on blood vessels and circulation. III. Ultrastructure of the vessel wall. Curr. Top. Radiat. Res. Q. *10:* 29–57 (1974).

54 Ward, W. F.; Solliday, N. H.; Molteni, A.; Port, C. D.: Radiation injury in rat lung. II. Angiotensin-converting enzyme activity. Radiat. Res. *96:* 294–300 (1983).

55 T'sao, C. H.; Ward, W. F.; Port, C. D.: Radiation injury in rat lung. III. Plasminogen activator and fibrinolytic inhibitor activities. Radiat. Res. *96:* 284–293 (1983).

56 Ward, W. F.; Molteni, A.; T'sao, C.; Solliday, N. H.: Pulmonary endothelial dysfunction induced by unilateral as compared to bilateral thoracic irradiation in rats. Radiat. Res. *111:* 101–106 (1987).

57 Ward, W. F.; Shih-Hoellwarth, A.; Tuttle, R. D.: Collagen accumulation in irradiated rat lung: modification by *D*-penicillamine. Radiat. Biol. *146:* 533–537 (1983).

58 Ward, W. F.: Radiation-induced pulmonary arterial perfusion defects: modification by *D*-penicillamine. Radiology, *139:* 201–204 (1981).

59 Ward, W. F.; Kim, Y. T.; Molteni, A.; T'sao, C. H.; Solliday, N. H.: Modification of radiation pneumonitis and pulmonary fibrosis in rats. Int. Conf. on New Biology of Lung and Lung Injury and Their Implications for Oncology, Porvoo 1987.

60 Rosenkrans, W. A.; Penney, D. P.: Cell-cell matrix interactions in induced lung injury. III. Long-term effects of X-irradiation on basal laminar proteoglycans. Anat. Rec. *215:* 127–133 (1986).

61 Murray, J. C.: What is pulmonary fibrosis (Editorial). Thorax *43:* 9–11 (1986).

62 Pickrell, J. A.; Diel, J. H.; Slauson, D. O.; Halliwell, W. H.; Mauderly; J. L.:

Radiation-induced pulmonary fibrosis resolves spontaneously if dense scars are not formed. Exp. molec. Path. *38:* 22–32 (1983).
63 Withers, H. R.; Peters, L. J.; Kogelnik, H. D.: The pathology of late effects of irradiation; Meyn, Withers, *Radiation biology in cancer research*, pp. 439–448 (Raven Press, New York 1980).
64 Jennings, F. L.; Arden, A.: Development of radiation pneumonitis: time and dose factors. Archs Path. *74:* 351–360 (1961).
65 Law, M. P.; Thomlinson, R. H.: Vascular permeability in the ears of rats after X-irradiation. Br. J. Radiol. *51:* 895–904 (1978).
66 Law, M. P.; Ahier, R. G.; Coultas, P. G.: The role of vascular injury in the radiation response of mouse lung. Br. J. Cancer *53:* suppl. VII, pp. 327–329 (1986).
67 Rennard, S. I.; Bitterman, P. B.; Crystal, R. G.: Current concepts of the pathogenesis of fibrosis: lessons from pulmonary fibrosis; in Prog. Clin. Biol. Res. *154:* 359–377, 1984.
68 Blum, R. H.; Carter, S. K.; Agre, K.: A clinical review of bleomycin. A new antineoplastic agent. Cancer *31:* 903–914 (1973).
69 Catane, R.; Schwade, J. G.; Turrisi, A. T.; Webber, B. L.; Muggia, F. M.: Pulmonary toxicity after radiation and bleomycin: a review. Int. J. Radiat. Oncol. Biol. Phys. *5:* 1513–1518 (1979).
70 Einhorn, L.; Krause, M.; Hornback, N.; Furnas, B.: Enhanced pulmonary toxicity with bleomycin and radiotherapy in oat cell lung cancer. Cancer *37:* 2414–2416 (1976).
71 Collis, C. H.; Down, J. D.; Pearson, A. E.; Steel, G. G.: Bleomycin and radiation-induced lung damage in mice. Br. J. Radiol. *56:* 21–26 (1983).
72 Collis, C. H.: The response of the lung to ionizing radiation and cytotoxic drugs; thesis Cambridge 1981.
73 Cassady, J. R.; Richter, M. P.; Piro, A. J.; Jaffe, N.: Radiation-adriamycin interactions: preliminary clinical observations. Cancer *36:* 946–949 (1975).
74 Chan, P. Y. M.; Kagan, A. R.; Byfield, J. E.; Rao, A. A.; Gilbert, H. A.; Nussbaum, H.: Pulmonary complications of combined chemotherapy and radiotherapy in lung cancer. Front. Radiat. Ther. Onc., vol. 13, pp. 136–144 (Karger, Basel 1979).
75 Verschoore, J.; Lagrange, J. L.; Boublil, J. L.; Aubanel, J. M.; Blaive, B.; Pinto, J.; Namer, M.: Pulmonary toxicity of a combination of low-dose doxorubicin and irradiation for inoperable lung cancer. Radiother. Oncol. *9:* 281–288 (1987).
76 Von der Maase, H.; Overgaard, J.; Vaeth, M.: Effect of cancer chemotherapeutic drugs on radiation-induced lung damage in mice. Radiother. Oncol. *5:* 245–257 (1986).
77 Mattson, K.; Holsti, L. R.; Niiranen, A.; Kiuisaari, L.; Ivanainen, M.; Sorijärvi, A.; Cantell, K.: Human leukocyte interferon as part of a combined treatment for previously untreated small cell lung cancer. J. Biol. Response Mod. *4:* 8–17 (1985).
78 Rubin, P.; Finkelstein, J. N.; Siemann, D. W.; Shapiro, D. L.; Van Houtte, P.; Penney, D. P.: Predictive biochemical assays for late radiation effects. Int. J. Radiat. Oncol. Biol. Phys. *12:* 469–476 (1986).
79 Moosavi, H.; McDonald, S.; Rubin, P.; Cooper, R.; Stuard, D.; Penney, D.: Early radiation dose-response in lung: an ultrastructural study. Int. J. Radiat. Oncol. Biol. Phys. *2:* 921–931 (1977).
80 Shen, Y.; Yang, X.; Zhan, Q.; Guo, R.; Liu, J.; Yang, C.: The use of Chinese herb medicine in experimental radiotherapy. Int. J. Radiat. Oncol. Biol. Phys. *16:* To be published (1988).

Sandra McDonald, MD, Department of Radiation Oncology,
University of Rochester Cancer Center, PO Box 647, 601 Elmwood Avenue,
Rochester, NY 14642 (USA)

Vaeth JM, Meyer JL (eds): Radiation Tolerance of Normal Tissues.
Front Radiat Ther Oncol. Basel, Karger, 1989, vol 23, pp 277–298

Gastrointestinal Tract Radiation Tolerance

Leonard L. Gunderson, James A. Martenson, Jr.
Division of Radiation Oncology, Mayo Clinic, Rochester, Minn., USA

Gastrointestinal (GI) radiation tolerance was summarized by Rubin and Casarett (table I) [1], Roswit et al. [2], and Phillips and Margolis [3] at the 1971 symposium on normal-tissue tolerance. The recommended tolerance doses of Rubin and Casarett [1] were based on 1,000 cGy/week – 200 cGy/fraction for 5 days.

The intent of this chapter is to reevaluate acute and chronic GI radiation tolerance as a function of treatment with radiation alone versus combined with other modalities and to determine the influence of organ status with regard to uninvolved versus involved by tumor. Since 1971, the use of aggressive combinations of radiation and chemotherapy has increased for both thoracic and abdominal malignancies. For many abdominal malignancies, stomach and small intestine are the dose-limiting structures in such treatment combinations. When an organ is involved by malignancy, tolerance may be more difficult to define, as recurrent tumor can cause the same signs and symptoms as treatment-related complications.

Table I. Radiation tolerance doses – GI [modified from ref. 1]

Organ	Injury at 5 years	1–5% $TD_{5/5}$	25–50% $TD_{50/5}$	Volume or length
Esophagus	ulcer, stricture	6,000	7,500	75 cm^3
Stomach	ulcer, perforation	4,500	5,000	100 cm^3
Intestine	ulcer, stricture	4,500	6,500	100 cm^3
Colon	ulcer, stricture	4,500	6,500	100 cm^3
Rectum	ulcer, stricture	5,500	8,000	100 cm^3
Pancreas	secretory functions	—	—	—
Liver	liver failure, ascites	3,500	4,500	whole
Biliary ducts	stricture, obstruction	—	—	—

Data based on supervoltage (1–6 MV), 1,000 cGy/week (5 × 200)

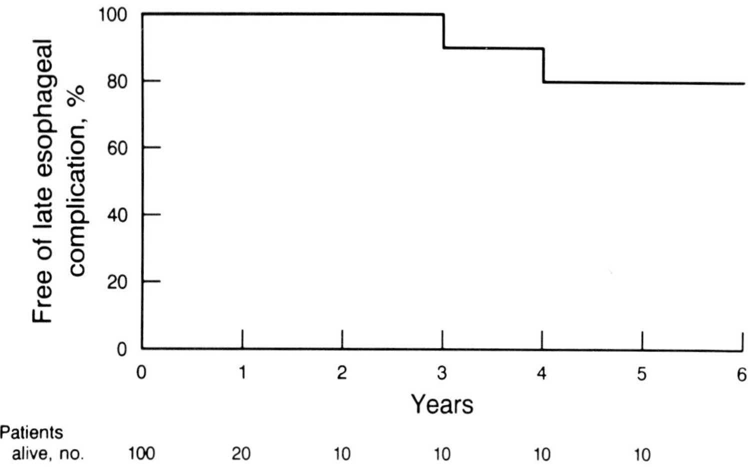

Fig. 1. A theoretical Kaplan-Meier curve showing the risk of late esophageal complications in a lung cancer population of 100 patients with a high mortality rate resulting in a survival curve of 10% between 2 and 5 years. Two late complications occur in this population, 1 at 3 and 1 at 4 years. The crude late complication rate is 2%, but the risk of a late esophageal complication at 5 years is 20%. The use of crude complication rates underestimates the actual risk of a complication in a long-term survivor by a factor of ten.

In addition, a higher incidence of complications may be acceptable with an involved versus uninvolved organ and with unresectable versus resected disease.

Esophagus

Available human and animal data regarding the tolerance of the esophagus to irradiation are often difficult to interpret [3]. Most information is derived from groups of patients treated by radiation therapy for lung cancer (organ uninvolved) or esophageal cancer (organ involved). Both of these patient populations have a short survival, and, therefore, few patients are generally at risk for late complications. Moreover, reported complication rates virtually always use the original patient population as the denominator and, therefore, underestimate the rate of serious toxicity relative to the actual number of patients at risk at any given point in time (fig. 1). Finally, in esophageal cancer patients, radiation toxicity is difficult to distinguish from effects of the primary tumor [4, 5]. For example, in a Princess Margaret Hospital series, 67% of the patients developed a stricture following radiation therapy for esophageal cancer [5]. By clin-

Table II. Incidence of severe acute and chronic esophageal complications in lung cancer patients treated on RTOG Protocol 73–01 [7]

Dose-Fractionation	Esophageal Dose, Gy[a]	Number of Patients	Incidence of Severe Acute Esophagitis	Incidence of Esophageal Stricture
40 Gy split	25 Gy	93	1	0
40 Gy continuous	40–45 Gy	97	3	1
50 Gy continuous	40–45 Gy	91	1	0
60 Gy continuous	40–45 Gy	84	1	1

[a]Estimate, based on upper limit of dose to spinal cord.

ical criteria, 27% of the strictures were felt to be due to benign causes, while 73% were felt to be caused by recurrent tumor. However, 5 patients who were felt before death to have benign stricture by clinical criteria (including negative endoscopic biopsy) came to autopsy. Recurrent tumor was found at the site of the stricture in 4 of these 5 patients. Overall, it was estimated that postradiation esophageal stricture represents recurrent tumor 95% of the time.

Organ Uninvolved

Normal esophagus is usually included in the radiation field of patients undergoing treatment for lung cancer. When conventional fraction sizes are used, acute symptoms of substernal burning or dysphagia are almost always observed after 20–40 Gy [6]. When total doses do not exceed 45 Gy, severe acute esophagitis is rare [6, 7] (table II).

The lung cancer literature also serves as the principle source of human data regarding late complications following irradiation of the normal esophagus. Esophageal stricture following doses ≤ 45 Gy in this clinical setting is very rare [7] (table II). Results from a small group of patients treated at the Mallinkrodt Institute of Radiology for lung cancer suggest that above doses of approximately 60 Gy, the risk of clinically significant long-term damage to the esophagus is appreciably increased (fig. 2) [6]. The only chronic problem that occurred at < 60 Gy was due to a short time-dose fractionation scheme.

Chemotherapeutic agents can markedly influence the incidence of significant toxicity in patients who receive irradiation to the normal esophagus [8–10]. In a group of lung cancer patients treated at the Mayo Clinic with a combination of radiation therapy, cyclophosphamide, adriamycin, cisplatin, and bleomycin, the incidence of severe esophagitis was 20–50% and was directly related to the dose of bleomycin [10] (table

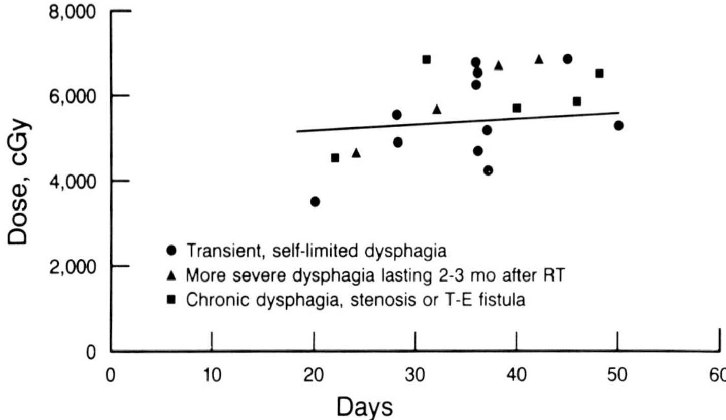

Fig. 2. The relationship between total dose, duration of treatment, and esophageal complications in a group of 20 lung cancer patients treated at the Mallinkrodt Institute of Radiology. Doses in the region above the exclusion line were associated with a 58% rate of moderate or severe complications, while doses below the exclusion line were associated with a 25% rate of moderate or severe complications. [From ref 6: The ordinate was modified to account for a conversion from roentgens, in the original figure, to cGy in the above figure. The exclusion line was not present in the original figure.]

III). Other agents which appear to increase acute radiation esophagitis include actinomycin D and vinblastine [8, 9] (table III).

Organ Involved

In patients with esophageal cancer, treatment with radiation therapy alone generally results in an incidence of severe acute esophagitis of less than 10% [11–13] (table IV). The addition of a variety of chemotherapeutic agents has not resulted in an obvious increase in severe acute or late complications (13–17), with the possible exception of the Harvard–New England Deaconess experience with continuous infusion of 5-fluorouracil [17] (table IV). As previously noted, however, the rate of esophageal complication rates reported in esophageal cancer literature must be interpreted with caution, since it is not always possible to distinguish between tumor and treatment-related toxicity.

Summary

In summary, doses from 45 to 60 Gy in standard fractionation, alone or in combination with chemotherapy, usually result in acceptable chronic tolerance of the normal esophagus. When certain types of chemotherapy are combined with irradiation, there is an increase in the incidence of acute esophagitis: bleomycin, actinomycin D, vinblastine, ? infusion

Table III. Incidence of radiation esophagitis in lung cancer patients treated with and without chemotherpy

Authors	Institution	Number of patients	Radiation dose	Fraction size	Chemotherapy	Esophagitis		Comments
						n	%	
Hall et al. [8]	Eastern Solid Tumor Group	115	5,000 R	200 R	None	17	15	randomized prospective study
		113	5,000R	200R	5-fluorouracil	15	13	
		114	5,000 R	200 R	actinomycin D	24	21	
Coy [9]	British Columbia Cancer Institute	93	40 Gy	5 Gy	none	13	14	choice of treatment made by date of birth
		101	40 Gy	5 Gy	vinblastine	30	30	
Eagan et al. [10]	Mayo Clinic	12	40 Gy	4 Gy	CAP-BLEO	8[a]	67	bleomycin dose 10 U twice weekly
		10	40 Gy	4 Gy	CAP-BLEO	6[a]	60	bleomycin dose 5 U twice weekly

R = Roentgen; CAP-BLEO = cyclophosphamide, adriamycin, platinum, bleomycin.

[a]Severe or life-threatening toxicity was observed in 6 of 12 (50%) patients with a bleomycin dose of 10 U twice weekly and in only 2 of 10 (20%) patients with a bleomycin dose of 5 U twice weekly.

Table IV. Acute and late toxicity in esophageal cancer patients treated by radiation therapy and/or chemotherapy

Authors	Institution	Number of patients	Radiation dose, Gy	Fraction size, Gy	Chemotherapy	Acute esophagitis[a]		Late esophageal complications[b]	
						n	%	n	%
Elkon et al. [11]	Rush Presbyterian St. Luke's Hospital	55c	variable	not stated	none	none noted		3	5
Langer et al. [12]	Massachusetts General Hospital	46	50–69	1.8	none	4	9	9	20
Richmond et al. [13]	Henry Ford Hospital	17	40–60	2–2.5	none	none noted		2	12
		25	56–60	2–2.5	5-FU, CDDP	none noted		1	4
Keane et al. [14]	Princess Margaret Hospital	35	25–50	2.5	5-FU, Mito-C	none noted		8	23
Marcial et al. [15]	Radiation Therapy Oncology Group	25d	50	2.5	VCR, BLEO, MTX, 5-FU, FA	2	8	none noted	
Byfield et al. [16]	University of California, Davis	6	50–60	2.5	5-FU	0	0[e]	none noted	
Lokich et al. [17]	Harvard New England Deaconess	12	44–69	1.8–2.0	5-FU	2	17	4	57[f]

5-FU = 5-Fluorouracil; CDDP = cisplatin; Mito-C = mitomycin-C;
VCR = vincristine; BLEO = bleomycin; MTX = methotrexate; FA = folinic acid.

[a] Includes esophagitis described as 'severe' or of suffiicient intensity to require treatment interruption.

[b] Includes stenosis, fistula, perforation, bleeding.

[c] Number of patients treated for cure.

[d] Number of patients evaluable for toxicity.

[e] One patient complained of esophageal pain.

[f] Only 7 patients at risk for late esophageal complications.

5-fluorouracil. When the esophagus is involved by malignancy, we must either establish the diagnosis when the lesion is smaller or develop better combined treatment modalities. Until either or both occurs, the most common cause of esophageal stricture will continue to be uncontrolled or recurrent disease.

Anus

In most clinical situations, including lower pelvic irradiation, if multiple-field techniques are used, the full circumference of the anus is quite often spared. Therefore, most information regarding anal tolerance is derived from series in which the anus is involved with malignancy. Tolerance will be evaluated with different treatment modalities including external beam irradiation alone or in combination with chemotherapy, or brachytherapy with or without external irradiation.

External Radiation and/or Chemotherapy

Nearly all patients who receive irradiation to the anus will experience an acute, self-limited perineal skin reaction which can range from mild, nearly asymptomatic tanning of the skin to intense erythema and moist desquamation. The frequency and severity of reported significant acute toxicity varies widely in the medical literature [18–20]. Cantril et al. [18], for example, described acute toxicity among 39 patients treated with radiation therapy for anal cancer (92% by external beam radiation therapy alone) with daily fraction sizes of 1.8–2.25 Gy to total doses of 44–80.5 Gy [18]. Eighteen percent experienced a 'moderate' acute perineal skin reaction, 20% experienced a 'severe' acute perineal skin reaction, and 62% experienced a 'mild' or no reaction. In contrast, in a Princess Margaret Hospital series using a larger fraction size of 25 Gy, 'virtually all' patients developed moist desquamation, even after doses as low as 25 Gy in ten fractions [20].

The use of combined chemotherapy and radiation therapy does not appear to result in a large increase in acute perineal toxicity when compared to radiation therapy alone [20–22]. In the Princess Margaret experience, for example, moist desquamation was common, regardless of whether the patients were treated by radiation therapy alone or radiation therapy combined with infusion 5-fluorouracil and mitomycin C [20]. In the series of these authors, a treatment break had to be introduced in order to achieve acceptable acute tolerance. Byfield et al. [21] reported moist desquamation in 6 of 11 patients treated by 3–5 cycles of 5-fluorouracil 25 mg/kg/24 h over 5 days in combination with 10 Gy of radiation therapy per week, given in 2.5-Gy fractions, with a minimum of 9 days rest between cycles.

Significant late complications following radiation therapy for anal cancer include anal necrosis, ulceration, stricture, and chronic bleeding. In patients with large, extensively infiltrating, or circumferential tumors, late complications may occur in a setting where the neoplasitc process itself has significantly damaged normal anatomy. Even when tumors totally regress as a function of treatment, late anal complications may occur because the normal tissues are unable to totally repair themselves because of preexistent neoplastic destruction. In the Institut Gustave-Roussy series, for example, severe grade 3 complications were 'often associated with rectovaginal fistulae and destruction of the anal canal by extensive tumors' [19]. The frequency of severe grade 3 complications was directly related to the size of the tumor. Among patients with T_1 and T_2 tumors, only 2 of 33 (6%) developed severe complications. In contrast, 3 of 25 (12%) with T_3 tumors and 4 of 6 (67%) with T_4 tumors developed severe complications.

The overall rate of serious anal complications following external radiation therapy for anal cancer ranges from 0 to 22%, with 0–13% requiring a colostomy as a result of anal complications [18–20, 22] (table V). No obvious differences exist in late severe complication rates for patients treated by irradiation alone versus combined irradiation and chemotherapy (table V).

Implant and/or External Beam Irradiation

Data regarding the tolerance of the anus to interstitial radiation therapy is somewhat limited [18, 23–26] (table VI). Interstitial doses of 55–60 Gy in a single implant are associated with significant acute and long-term toxicity. Dalby and Pointon [23] found that 23 of 98 patients (24%) treated by such an approach developed necrosis. The overall rate of colostomy due to complications was 6%. A 2- to 4-week hospitalization was required for most patients following implant removal to allow for recovery from the acute perineal radiation reaction. A small study of 6 patients with anal cancer by Ramming et al. [25] suggests that interstitial implantation of the anus may be better tolerated when combined with external beam treatment. Following combined external interstitial doses of 65–70 Gy, none of the 6 patients experienced severe complications. Alternatively, fractionation of implants when doses exceed 40 Gy also appears to result in a lower rate of complications that lead to colostomy [24].

Summary

Significant self-limited acute toxicity is seen in the vast majority of patients treated for anal cancer. Long-term complications of anal necrosis, stricture, and/or bleeding are seen in up to 25% of the patients (range 0–25%) treated by external and/or interstitial irradiation

Table V. Severe late anal complications following external radiation therapy (RT)

Authors	Total tumor dose, Gy	Daily fraction size, Gy	Duration of RT[a]	Chemo-therapy	Number of patients	Patients with severe late complications		Patients with colostomy resulting from complications	
						n	%	n	%
Cantril et al. [18]	44.1–80.5	1.8–2.25	not noted	none	32[b]	7	22	2[c]	6
Eschwege et al. [19]	60–65	usually 2.0	6–6½ weeks	none	64	9	14	not noted	
Cummings et al. [20]	45–60	usually 2.5	4–6 weeks	none	25	3	12	1	4
	50	2.5	4 weeks	5-FU, Mito-C	30	4	13	4	13
Flam et al. [22]	30.9–48.6	none noted	3–6½ weeks	5-FU, Mito-C	11	0	0	0	0

5-FU = 5-Fluorouracil; Mito-C = mitomycin C.

[a]The duration of RT is given exclusive of treatment breaks.

[b]Includes 1 patient treated preoperatively who subsequently refused surgery and excludes patients who underwent radioactive implantation.

[c]One case treated via an external ^{137}Cs source to 110 Gy (maximum dose); the other case was a patient with an 8-cm tumor treated to a total of 69 Gy.

Table VI. Severe anal complications following interstitial implantation with or without external irradiation for anal cancer

Authors	Interstitial total dose, Gy	External beam tumor dose, Gy	Total dose Gy	Number of patients	Patients with severe complications		Patients with colostomy resulting from severe complications	
					n	%	n	%
Dalby and Pointon [23]	55–60	0	55–60	98	23	24	6	6
Papillon [24]								
Implant only	30–90[a]	0	30–90	98	24[b]	24	≤4[b]	≤4
External RT plus implant	NS	30	NS					
Ramming et al. [25]	20–50	25–46	65–70	6	0	0	0	0
Hintz et al. [26]	37–38	43–56	81–94	2	1			1
Cantril et al. [18]	not noted	not noted	approximately 59–80.5	3	2			2

RT = Radiation therapy.
[a] When doses exceeded 40 Gy, 2–3 implants were used.
[b] Four patients had severe radionecrosis and required ‘radical surgery’; the remaining 20 had ‘milder ulceronecrotic reactions’, and all healed within <4 months with sphincter function preservation.

with or without chemotherapy. The incidence of colostomy for complications is 4–5% in most series. In many cases, these complications result from destruction of the normal anatomy by the neoplastic process itself rather than by radiation-induced damage. Although the precise tolerance of the anus remains unknown, doses in the range typically used for treating anal cancer leave the majority of patients with functional anal anatomy.

The incidence of both acute and chronic complications due to the nonsurgical treatment approaches discussed in this section must be kept in perspective by considering alternative treatment. A decade ago, the treatment of choice for most anal cancers was abdominoperineal resection. In the current irradiation and/or chemotherapy series, the colostomy-free survival ranges from 70 to >90% (including colostomies performed for disease persistence as well as for complication).

Large Bowel

With large-bowel cancers, irradiation is rarely used as the solitary method of treatment, except for select early lesions for which endocavitary irradiation may be an acceptable alternative. Most information regarding large-bowel radiation tolerance has, therefore, been obtained in the setting of an uninvolved organ being included in the radiation field of another malignancy (i.e., rectum and/or sigmoid included in anteroposterior/posteroanterior and lateral fields for prostate, bladder, and gynecologic malignancies). In such a situation, severe chronic complication rates greater than 5% would usually be unacceptable for primary irradiation of early-stage disease or for adjuvant irradiation combined with resection. (The circumference of the rectum can be irradiated to a dose of 5,500–6,000 cGy in 180-cGy fractions with a chronic severe risk ≤ 5%.) For more locally advanced lesions, a toxicity risk of 10–25% may be accepted by patient and physician. The mid and lower rectum are often carried to higher radiation doses than other sites in the large bowel, as dose limiting small bowel and stomach can be excluded.

In this section, large-bowel tolerance will be evaluated with external irradiation alone or in combination with intraoperative electrons. Comments regarding external irradiation will be limited to rectal tolerance generated in prostate cancer series. Although rectal tolerance information exists in the gynecological literature, external irradiation is usually combined with brachytherapy (data discussed in the chapter by Rotman). Some animal data will also be presented that discuss the influence of diet and medications on rectal healing after radiation injury.

External Irradiation and/or Implant

The majority of prostate radiation series use multiple-field techniques, with boost field doses to 65–70 Gy, that spare the posterior wall of the rectum. A number of analyses have shown that the incidence of bowel

Table VII. Rectal tolerance in the irradiation of prostate cancer

Institution	Stage	Dose to prostate, Gy	Number of patients	Colostomy incidence, %	Radiation ulcer, %
External					
M.D. Anderson [31]	C	65–70 (10/week, 4-field)	165	6	—
Mallinkrodt [30]	B and C	65–70 (10/week AP-PA)	267	0.37	—
External plus implant					
Memorial Medical Center [32]	A_2–C	40/4–4½ weeks (external)	100	5	6
	A_2–B_1	30 (implant)			
	B_2–C	35 (implant)			
Mayo Clinic/William Beaumont Hospital [34][a]	bulky C	35.6 (external)[b] 35 (implant)	30	16.7	37
Mayo Clinic/William Beaumont Hospital [35][a]	bulky C and B	35.6 (external)[b] 35 (implant)	18	0	5.5

AP = Anteroposterior; PA = posteroanterior.
[a] Technical modification of implant was implemented in 1985 and used in 18 additional patients – 4 had bulky stage B disease.
[b] 5 Gy × 1 prior to implant, 17 × 1.8 Gy after implant – 4-field.

complications increases with doses in excess of 70 Gy [27–30]. While the colostomy incidence is at or below 1% in most series (table VII), an exception to this was a 6% incidence in an M. D. Anderson Hospital series [31]. Table VIII evaluates local control and complications in the M. D. Anderson Hospital series as a function of stage and dose. The only severe complication seen at the 65-Gy level at this institution was in a patient treated with large-field rotation ^{60}Co. Most of the severe problems were at the 70-Gy dose level. Prior to 1976, although four-field techniques were utilized, most patients had only one field per day treated. Since 1976, there have been no colostomies in the M. D. Anderson prostate series with the dose limited to 65 Gy in most patients [Hussey, personal commun.].

When interstitial implants with a perineal template were combined with external irradiation in an attempt to improve local control and survival, the incidence of rectal complications was initially excessive [32–35] (table VII). Techniques have been modified to reduce both the rectal dose and associated complications.

Intraoperative Radiation Therapy (IORT)

While tolerance with IORT will not be discussed in detail, 4 of 51 patients in a Mayo analysis of complications with pelvic IORT had large bowel in the IORT field [36, 37]. Severe chronic sequelae have not been noted in any of those patients. One had proctitis for 3 months and 1 patient an inflammatory ulcer for 1 month. In 2 of the 4 patients, large bowel had not been bypassed; the other 2 had a previously constructed Hartman pouch rectal stump that was within the IORT field.

Table VIII. Local control and complication rates (%) for prostate cancer by tumor dose (M.D. Anderson Hospital) [modified from ref. 31]

	Local control		Complications[a]	
Stage	~65 Gy	~70 Gy	~65 Gy	~70 Gy
C_1	94 (16/17)	92 (68/74)	6 (1/17)	11 (8/74)
C2	62 (8/13)	79 (27/34)	0 (0/13)	12 (4/34)
Total	80 (24/30)	88 (95/108)	3 (1/30)	11 (12/108)

[a]The only complication in the group receiving ~65 Gy was in patient treated with large fields using a rotation technique with ^{60}Co.

Animal Data

As noted in an animal model by Trott et al. [38], a number of factors can alter the severity of chronic large-bowel damage. In that trial a 24-mm segment of Wistar rat large bowel was irradiated with 23 Gy in a single fraction, and 90% developed a chronic radiation ulcer. The modification of the ulcer-healing process in control animals which were irradiated and did not receive any special treatment was compared with that found in animals treated with cortisone, neomycin, Metamucil (laxative), or combinations thereof. Some animals were fed a standard rodent diet, others a residue-free synthetic diet, and some received both in sequence. Survival was increased in animals that received daily cortisone enemas plus neomycin in the drinking water after irradiation or in those who had Metamucil added to their diet. Animals that received the synthetic diet after irradiation survived as long as the diet was continued, but over 90% developed progressive large-bowel obstruction when the synthetic diet was stopped and the subject placed on normal diet. (Hard pellet-like stools were produced which abraded the surface of the bowel and did not allow the radiation-induced ulcer to heal.)

Summary

The animal model reflects what can be seen in the clinical setting in which radiation damage can be modified by sterodis, stool softener or Metamucil, and diet. When radiation ulcers will not heal with conservative management, diversion with a temporary colostomy can be successful. Biopsies of heavily irradiated rectal wall could cause ulceration if performed repetitively. In summary, the damage caused by irradiation can be modified for better or worse by later diagnostic and treatment choices.

Stomach

With respect to gastric injury, the classic data generated by Friedman and others in the Walter Reed testicular experience was summarized by Roswit et al. [2] in 1972 (table IX). The treatment technique was usually one field per day with doses delivered over 3–4 weeks with a 1-MV supervoltage machine. In view of the low-kilovoltage, short-time dose fractionation schemas, etc., tolerance data generated from that series are not very applicable.

With higher energy supervoltage machines and standard fractionation of 180–200 cGy/fraction 5 days/week, most data suggest that the $TD_{5/5}$ for stomach is probably 45–50 Gy. In data from the M.D. Anderson Hospital [39], the stomach was within a para-aortic field for both cervix and testicular cancers. The chronic risk varied from 2 to 8%, with total doses varying from 4,000 to 5,000 cGy at 180–200 cGy/fraction.

Table IX. Gastric injury (Walter Reed data) [modified from ref. 2]

	Dose, R			
	2,500–3,400	3,500–4,400	4,500–5,400	5,500–6,400
Total number of cases	15	32	61	22
Percent with problems	20	25	50	63
Dyspepsia	13	3	2	—
Gastritis	—	21	21	32
Ulcer	7	—	15	14
Ulcer and perforation or obstruction	—	—	11	18

[a] Radiation usually given over 3–4 weeks (short-fractionation schemes) with low kV (≤1 MeV); treatment of 1 field/day.

In a Massachusetts General Hospital series, a group of 46 patients with gastric cancer were irradiated [40]. In most patients, the irradiated stomach was uninvolved by malignancy, since the gastric lesion had been resected, but in 13 patients the lesion was not resected. The entire stomach or remaining stomach was usually included to a minimum dose of 4,500 cGy in 25 fractions over 5 weeks, and protions of the stomach were sometimes included within a reduced field to 50.4–52.2 Gy. Most patients were treated with 10-MV photons with parallel opposed fields. Forty of 46 patients received chemotherapy in conjunction with their irradiation. From a chronic toxicity standpoint, 34 patients were at risk ≥ 12 months and 25 at risk ≥ 18 months. There was no evidence of chronic injury to either stomach or liver in this series of patients.

In a Mayo Clinic phase I/II tolerance study of multiple daily fractions and/or 5-fluorouracil, we attempted to combine two fractions of irradiation per day with 5-fluorouracil [41]. Both 165 as well as 150 cGy/fraction were intolerable from an acute GI end point. Patients had prolongatioin of acute symptoms persisting for as long as 2–4 weeks after completion of combined modality treatment. Normally, with 1 fraction of 180 cGy/day plus 5-fluorouracil, most acute GI symptoms ameliorate within several days to 1 week of completion of treatment. When two fractions of 150 cGy/day were given without 5-fluorouracil, the tolerance was improved and was more comparable to one fraction of 180 cGy plus 5-fluorouracil.

A good analysis of gastric and duodenal tolerance exists in biliary duct data from Buskirt et al. [42, 43] at our institution. For locally unresectable or residual biliary cancer, the following aggressive treatment regimens were utilized: external irradiation alone or combined with 5-

fluorouracil, 4,500 cGy/25 fractions in 5 weeks to a tumor/nodal field with a reduced field boost for 1,000–2,000 cGy in 200-cGy fractions, and similar external beam irradiation to a tumor nodal field combined with a boost with intraoperative electrons or brachytherapy. Distal stomach and duodenal C loop are usually included to 4,500 cGy [42]. With brachytherapy, the patients received a dose of 1,500–2,500 cGy which was usually calculated at a 1-cm radius from the transcatheter iridium. A dose versus complication analysis was performed in patients who received external alone or external combined with IORT electrons (with IORT, one could exclude duodenum and stomach). With external doses ≤ 5,500 cGy to duodenum and/or stomach, the risk of severe GI complications varied from 5 to 10%, depending on which parameter was evaluated. At doses >5,500 cGy, 180-cGy fractions/5 days a week, 33% of patients developed severe problems. In patients who received external irradiation plus iridium, the dose to the external field was limited to 50.4 Gy, but most received additional radiation dose to duodenum and/or stomach from the iridium boost (higher doses with distal lesions). There was a 30- to 40% incidence of severe complications in the duodenum or stomach in this group of patients.

Summary

With 180-Cgy fractions and 6–10 + MeV photons, one can safely treat all or the majority of the stomach to a dose of 45–50 Gy with a 5- to 10% risk of severe radiation damage. If doses exceed 55 Gy, the incidence of severe complications rises sharply to 30–40%, suggesting a steep dose-response tolerance curve for stomach and/or duodenum.

Small Intestine

Irradiation Alone

When parallel opposed fields are used for postoperative irradiation of rectal cancer instead of four-field techniques, the incidence of small-bowel obstruction requiring reoperation nearly doubles when compared with surgery alone [44] (table X). With multiple-field techniques, the risk of small-bowel obstruction is equivalent to surgery alone, although reoperation in the irradiated group is going to be more difficult. When small-bowel series are obtained with cross-table lateral views, a moderate amount of anteriorly located small intestine will be noted, much of which can be excluded if lateral fields are used for a component of treatment [44, 45]. Since complications from radiation have a volume-dose relationship for most tissues and organs, multiple-field treatment techniques to decrease the volume of irradiated small bowel should be used whenever feasible.

Table X. Incidence of small-bowel obstruction versus field design – adjuvant rectal [from ref. 44]

	M.D. Anderson Hospital %[a]	LDSH %[a]	Massachusetts General Hospital %[b]
Operation along	5	—	5
Operation plus post-operative irradiation	10–12[c]	10	4

X-ray technique: [a]anteroposterior/posteroanterior; [b]anteroposterior/posteroanterior plus laterals. [c]The original incidence of 17.5% was reduced to 10–12% by reduction of superior field extent.

If postoperative irradiation is used in an adjuvant setting for colon cancer, multiple-field techniques can rarely be used to decrease the volume of irradiated small bowel. The preoperative diagnostic studies commonly obtained do not allow adequate reconstruction of the target volume which could result in a more limited treatment field. (Barium enema plus pathologic findings reconstruct only cephalocaudad tumor extent; routine use of preoperative computerized tomography would not be cost-effective.) In the publication by Duttenhaver et al. [46], 80 patients with colon cancer were treated in an adjuvant setting at the Massachusetts General Hospital with the same dose criteria that were used as in their rectal series (4,500 cGy, 25 fractions/5 weeks to a tumor and/or nodal field, 5,000 cGy within boost). By using the specialized technique of decubitus position for a portion of treatments, one can often get shift of small bowel and decreased volume within irradiation fields when compared with a more standard supine treatment position. In that series, morbidity was analyzed as a function of the degree of shift of small bowel. Five of 80 patients developed severe morbidity, but only 2 (2.5%) required operative intervention.

An excellent analysis of the dose-volume relationship regarding small-bowel complications was performed by Gallagher et al. [45]. The volume of small bowel within radiation fields was reconstructed for a variety of irradiated sites. The patients that had no prior surgery or a pelvic operation other than abdominoperineal resection had substantially less volume of small bowel within irradiated field than those patients who had abdominoperineal resection. Moderate to marked differences occurred with anteroposterior/postenoanterior versus four-field techniques, and some advantage was found for the prone position with external compression and bladder distension. Dose and volume had a relationship to both acute and chronic effects. Five patients subsequently developed small-bowel obstruction (0 of 75 with no previous pelvic surgery, 3 of 25 or 12% with abdominoperineal resection, and 2 of 50 or 4% with other pelvic operations).

Radiation and Chemotherapy

Since standard treatment for rectal cancer has evolved to irradiation plus chemotherapy in many centers on the basis of randomized GI Tumor Study Group [47] and Mayo/NCCTG trials [48], the tolerance of small bowel with combined modality regimens needs to be reviewed. In the earlier GI Tumor Study Group trial which used parallel opposed fields, severe small-bowel complications appeared excessive with irradiation plus chemotherapy (bolus 5-fluorouracil weeks 1 and 5; maintenance 5-fluorouracil + MeCCNU). The Mayo/NCCTG trial was the first combined modality rectal trial that mandated multiple-field irradiation techniques. In the last analysis in March of 1988 with minimum 2-year follow-up, there was no difference in severe small-bowel complications with an incidence <5% with irradiation +/− chemotherapy. Further follow-up is necessary to be certain that chronic tolerance is acceptable with combined modality approaches.

Summary

A 1988 interpretation of radiation tolerance doses for GI organs is shown in table XI. At the 1971 symposium, tolerance data presented by Rubin and Casarett [1] were based on daily fractions of 200 cGy and lower energy supervoltage equipment. The upper estimates of tolerance in the $TD_{5/5}$ column in the current table are based on the availability of higher energy supervoltage machines in most institutions and the use of 180-cGy fractions 5 days/week. For those who deliver 1,000 cGy/week in five fractions, the lower estimates of tolerance are recommended. The main differences in the 1988 update relate to clarification of gastric and colon tolerance and inclusion of tolerance information on anus and bile duct. As was the case in the original tolerance estimates by Rubin and Casarett [1], the current recommendations are based on our interpretation of the literature combined with our personal experience.

Since the mid 1970s, the use of combined modality treament has markedly increased in an attempt to achieve radiation sensitization with chemotherapy or radiation dose modifiers and to decrease the high incidence of systemic metastases. For most GI malignancies, combinations of radiation and chemotherapy have become increasingly common, if not the accepted standard, as either primary treatment (anus and/or esophageal; unresectable pancreas, large bowel, and/or gastric) or adjuvant treatment after resection (rectum, pancreas and/or other). Since optimal treatment regimens do not yet exist for most locally advanced malignancies, an ongoing evaluation of normal-tissue tolerance by modality will be necessary.

Table XI. Radiation tolerance doses – GI[a]

Organ	Injury at 5 years	1–5% TD5/5	25–50% TD50/5	Volume or length
Esophagus	ulcer, stricture	6,000–6,500	7,500	75 cm³
Stomach	ulcer, perforation	4,500–5,000	5,500	100 cm³
Intestine (small)	ulcer, stricture	4,500–5,000	5,500	100 cm³
Colon	ulcer, stricture	5,500–6,000	7,500	100 cm³
Rectum	ulcer, stricture	5,500–6,000	7,500	100 cm³
Anus	ulcer, stricture	6,000–6,500	≥7,500	whole
Pancreas	secretory functions	—	—	—
Liver	liver failure, ascites	3,500	4,500	whole
Biliary ducts	stricture, obstruction	5,000	7,000[b]	—

[a]Compiled by Gunderson and Martenson, 1988 (literature interpretation, personal experience). Based on supervoltage 4–10 MV, 900 cGy/week (5 × 180).
[b]External to 5,000/28 × 180/5$\frac{1}{2}$ week + 2,000 cGy at 1 cm with ^{192}Ir.

Acknowledgements

The authors appreciate the efforts of Julie Chambers and Bonnie Espy for assistance in the preparation of the manuscript. We are indebted to our wives and families for the support received in personal and professional endeavors.

References

1 Rubin, P.; Casarett, G.: A direction for clinical radiation pathology – the tolerance dose; in Vaeth, Front. Radiat. Ther. Onc., vol. 6, pp. 1–16 (University Park Press, Baltimore 1972).

2 Roswit, B.; Malsky, S. J.; Reid, C. B.: Radiation tolerance of the gastrointestinal tract; in Vaeth, Front. Radiat. Ther. Onc., vol. 6, pp. 160–181 (University Park Press, Baltimore 1972).

3 Phillips, T. L.; Margolis, L.: Radiation pathology and the clinical response of lung and esophagus; in Vaeth, Front. Radiat. Ther. Onc., vol. 6, pp. 254–273 (University Park Press, Baltimore 1972).

4 Cederqvist, C.; Nielsen, J.; Bertelsen, A.; Hansen, H. S.: Cancer of the oesophagus. II. Therapy and outcome. Acta. chir. scand. *144:* 233–240 (1978).

5 Beatty, J. D.; DeBoer, G.; Ricer, W. D.: Carcinoma of the esophagus: pretreatment assessment, correlation of radiation treatment parameters with survival, and identification and management of radiation treatment failure. Cancer *43:* 2254–2267 (1979).

6 Seaman, W. B.; Ackerman, L. V.: The effect of radiation on the esophagus: a clinical and histologic study of the effects produced by the betatron. Radiology *68:* 534–541 (1957).

7 Perez, C. A.; Stanley, K.; Rubin, P.; Kramer, S.; Brady, L.; Perez-Tamayo, R.; Brown, G. S.; Concannon, J.; Rotman, M.; Seydel, H. G.: A prospective randomized study of various irradiation doses and fractionation schedules in the treatment of inoperable non-oat-cell carcinoma of the lung. Cancer *45:* 2744–2753 (1980).

8 Hall, T. C.; Dederick, M. M.; Chalmers, T. C.; Krant, M. J.; Shnider, B. I.; Lynch, J. J.; Holland, J. F.; Ross, C.; Koons, C. R.; Owens, A. H.; Frei, E.; Brindley, C.; Miller, S. P.; Brenner, S.; Hosley, H. F.; Olson, K. B.: A clinical pharmacologic study of chemotherapy and X-ray therapy in lung cancer. Am. J. Med. *43:* 186–193 (1967).

9 Coy, P.: A randomized study of irradiation and vinblastine in lung cancer. Cancer *26:* 803–807 (1970).

10 Eagan, R. T.; Fleming, T. R.; Lee, R. E.; Ingle, J. N.; Frytak, S.; Creagan, E. T.: Chemotherapy response as a prognosticator for survival in patients with limited squamous cell lung cancer treated with combined chemotherapy and radiotherapy. Int. J. Radiat. Oncol. Biol. Phys. *6:* 879–883 (1980).

11 Elkon, D.; Lee, M. S.; Hendrickson, F. R.: Carcinoma of the esophagus: sites of recurrence and palliative benefits after definitive radiotherapy. Int. J. Radiat. Oncol. Biol. Phys. *4:* 615–620 (1978).

12 Langer, M.; Choi, N. C.; Orlow, E.; Grillo, H.; Wilkins, E. W.: Radiation therapy alone or in combination with surgery in the treatment of carcinoma of the esophagus. Cancer *58:* 1208–1213 (1986).

13 Richmond, J.; Seydel, H. G.; Bae, Y.; Lewis, J.; Burdakin, J.; Jacobsen, G.: Comparison of three treatment strategies for esophageal cancer within a single institution. Int. J. Radiat. Oncol. Biol. Phys. *13:* 1617–1620 (1987).

14 Keane, T. J.; Harwood, A. R.; Elhakim, T.; Rider, W. D.; Cummings, B. J.; Ginsberg, R. J.; Cooper, J. C.: Radiation therapy with 5-fluorouracil infusion and mitomycin C for oesophageal squamous carcinoma. Radiother. Oncol. *4:* 205–210 (1985).

15 Marcial, V. A.; Valez-García, E.; Cintrón, J.; Ydrach, A. A.: Radiotherapy preceded by multidrug chemotherapy in carcinoma of the esophagus: a pilot study of the Radiation Therapy Oncology Group. Cancer clin. Trails *3:* 127–130 (1980).

16 Byfield, J. E.; Barone, R.; Mendelsohn, J.; Frankel, S.; Quinol, L.; Sharp, T.; Seagren, S.: Infusional 5-fluorouracil and X-ray therapy for non-resectable esophageal cancer. Cancer *45:* 703–708 (1980).

17 Lokich, J. J.; Shea, M.; Chaffey, J.: Sequential infusional 5-fluorouracil followed by concomitant radiation for tumors of the esophagus and gastroesophageal junction. Cancer *60:* 275–279 (1987).

18 Cantril, S. T.; Green, J. P.; Schall, G. L.; Schaupp, W. C.: Primary radiation therapy in the treatment of anal carcinoma. Int. J. Radiat. Oncol. Biol. Phys. *9:* 1271–1278 (1983).

19 Eschwege, F.; Lasser, P.; Chavy, A.; Wibault, P.; Kac, J.; Rougier, P.; Bognel, C.: Squamous cell carcinoma of the anal canal: treatment by external beam irradiation. Radiother. Oncol. *3:* 145–150 (1985).

20 Cummings, B.; Keane, T.; Thomas, G.; Harwood, A.; Rider, W.: Results and toxicity of the treatment of anal canal carcinoma by radiation therapy or radiation therapy and chemotherapy. Cancer *54:* 2062–2068 (1984).

21 Byfield, J. E.; Barone, R. M.; Sharp, T. R.; Frankel, S. S.: Conservative management without alkylating agents of squamous cell anal cancer using cyclical 5-FU alone and X-ray therapy. Cancer Treatment Rep. *67:* 709–712 (1983).

22 Flam, M. S.; John, M.; Lovalvo, L. J.; Mills, R. J.; Ramalho, L. D.; Prather, C.; Mowry, P. A.; Morgan, D. R.; Lau, B. P.: Definitive nonsurgical therapy of epithelial malignancies of the anal canal. Cancer *51:* 1378–1387 (1983).

23 Dalby, J. E.; Pointon, R. S.: The treatment of anal carcinoma by interstitial irradiation, Am. J. Roentg. Rad. Ther. nucl. Med. *85:* 515–520 (1961).
24 Papillon, J.: Radiation therapy in the management of epidermoid carcinoma of the region. Dis. Colon Rectum *17:* 181–187 (1974).
25 Ramming, K. P.; Juillard, G.; Parker, R.; Eilber, F.: Management of carcinoma of the rectum and anus without abdominoperineal resection. Am. J. Surg. *152:* 16–20 (1986).
26 Hintz, B. L.; Charyulu, K. N.; Sudarsanam, A.: Anal carcinoma: basic concepts and management. J. surg. Oncol. *10:* 141–150 (1978).
27 Leibel, S. A.; Hanks, G. A.; Kramer, S.: Patterns of care outcome studies: results of the national practice in adenocarcinoma of the prostate. Int. J. Radiat. Oncol. Biol. Phys. *10:* 401–409 (1984).
28 Pilepich, M. V.; Asbell, S. O.; Krall, J. M.; Baerwald, W. H.; Sause, W. T.; Rubin, P.; Emami, B. N.; Pidcock, G. M.: Correlation of radiotherapeutic parameters and treatment-related morbidity. Analysis of RTOG study 77–06. Int. J. Radiat. Oncol. Biol. Phys. *13:* 1007–1012 (1987).
29 Pilepich, M. V.; Krall, J. M.; Sause, W. T.; Johnson, R. J.; Russ, H. H.; Hanks, G. E.; Perez, C. A.; Zinninger, M.; Martz, K. L.; Gardner, P.: Correlation of radiotherapy parameters and treatment-related morbidity in carcinoma of the prostate. Analysis of RTOG study 75–06. Int. J. Radiat. Oncol. Biol. Phys. *13:* 351–357 (1987).
30 Pilepich, M. V.; Perez, C. A.; Walz, B. J.; Zivnuska, F. R.: Complications of definitive radiotherapy for carcinoma of the prostate. Int. J. Radiat. Oncol. Biol. Phys. *7:* 1341–1348 (1981).
31 Hussey, D. H.; Chan, R. C.: Patterns of failure in patients treated by radiotherapy for genitourinary tumors. Cancer Treatment Symp. *2:* 51–57 (1983).
32 Puthawala, A. A.; Nisar Syed, A. M.; Tansley, A. A.; Shanberg, A.; Austin, P. A.; McNamara, C. S.: Temporary iridium-192 implant in the management of carcinoma of the prostate. Endocurie Hypertherm. Oncol. *1:* 25–34 (1985).
33 Brindle, J. S.; Benson, R. C.; Martinez, A.; Edmundson, G. K.; Zincke, H.; Utz, D. C.: Acute toxicity and preliminary therapeutic results of pelvic lymphadenectomy combined with transperineal interstitial implantation of ^{192}Ir and external beam radiotherapy for locally advanced prostate cancer. Urology *25:* 233–238 (1985).
34 Martinez, A.; Benson, R. C.; Brindle, J. S.; Schray, M. F.; Zincke, H.; Edmundson, G. K.; Diokno, A.: Pelvic lymphadenectomy and transperineal interstitial implantation of iridium-192 combined with external beam radiotherapy for patients with bulky prostatic carcinoma (Abstract). Endocurie Hypertherm. Oncol. *4:* (1988).
35 Brindle, J. S.; Martinez, A.; Benson, R. C.; Schray, M. F.; Zincke, H.; Dionko, A.; Edmondson, G. K.; Gonzalez, J.: Pelvic lymphadenopathy and transperineal interstitial implantation of iridium-192 combined with external beam radiotherapy for patients with bulky prostatic carcinoma. ASTRO Proc. Int. J. Radiat. Oncol. Biol. Phys. *15:* 133 (1988).
36 Shaw, E. G.; Gunderson, L. L.; Martin, J. K.; Beart, R. W.; Nagorney, D. M.; Podratz, K. C.: Toxicity and results of intraoperative radiation therapy for primary unresectable and recurrent pelvic malignancies. ARS Proc. Am. J. clin. Oncol. *10:* 105 (1987).
37 Gunderson, L. L.; Martin, J. K.; Beart, R. W.; Nagorney, D. M.; Fieck, J.; Wieand, H. S.; Martinez, A.; O'Connell, M. J.; Martenson, J. A.; McIlrath, D. C.: Intraoperative and external beam irradiation for locally advanced colorectal cancer. Annls Surg. *27:* 52–60 (1988).
38 Trott, S. R.; Breiter, N.; Spiethoff, A.: Experimental studies on the pathogenesis of the chronic radiation ulcer of the large bowel in rats. Int. J. Radiat. Oncol. Biol. Phys. *12:* 1637–1643 (1986).

39 Goldstein, H. M.; Rogers, L. F.; Fletcher, G. H.; Dodd, G. D.: Radiological manifestations of radiation induced injury to the normal upper gastrointestinal tract. Radiology *117:* 135–140 (1975).

40 Gunderson, L. L.; Hoskins, B.; Cohen, A. M.; Kaufman, S.; Wood, W.; Carey, R.: Combined modality treatment of gastric cancer. Int. J. Radiat. Oncol. Biol. Phys. *9:* 965–975 (1983).

41 O'Connell, M. J.; Gunderson, L. L.; Moertel, C. G.; Kvols, L. K.: A pilot study to determine clinical tolerability of intensive combined modality therapy for locally unresectable gastric cancer. Int. J. Radiat. Oncol. Biol. Phys. *11:* 1827–1831 (1985).

42 Buskirk, S. J.; Gunderson, L. L.; Adson, M. A.: Martinez, A.; May, G. R.; McIlrath, D. C.; Nagorney, D. M.; Edmundson, G. K.; Bender, C. E.; Martin, J. K.: Analysis of failure following curative irradiation of gallbladder and extrahepatic bile duct carcinoma. Int. J. Radiat. Oncol. Biol. Phys. *10:* 2013–2023 (1984).

43 Buskirk, S. J.; Gunderson, L. L.; Nagorney, D. M.; Martenson, J.; Bender, C.; May, G. R.; Williams, H. J.; Adson, M. A.; McIlrath, D. C.; Martin, J. K.; Themaine, W. J.: Analysis of failure following curative irradiation of extrahepatic bile duct carcinoma. ASTRO Proc. Int. J. Radiat. Oncol. Biol. Phys. *12:* Suppl. 1, p. 120 (1986).

44 Gunderson, L. L.; Russell, A. H.; Llewellyn, H. J.; Doppke, K. P.; Tepper, J. E.: Treatment planning for colorectal cancer: radiation and surgical techniques and value of small bowel films. Int. J. Radiat. Oncol. Biol. Phys. *11:* 1379–1393 (1985).

45 Gallagher, M. J.; Brereton, H. D.; Rostock, R. A.; Zero, J. M.; Zekoski, D. A.; Poyss, L. F.; Richter, M. P.; Kligermann, M. M.: A prospective study of treatment techniques to minimize the volume of pelvic small bowel with reduction of acute and late effects associated with pelvic irradiation. Int. J. Radiat. Oncol. Biol. Phys. *12:* 1565–1573 (1986).

46 Duttenhaver, J. D.; Hoskins, R. B.; Gunderson, L. L.; Tepper, J.; Willett, C.: Adjuvant postoperative radiation therapy in cancer of the colon. Cancer *57:* 955–963 (1986).

47 Gastrointestinal Tumor Study Group: Prolongation of the disease-free interval in surgically resected rectal cancer. New Engl. J. Med. *312:* 1465–1472 (1985).

48 Gunderson, L. L.; Collins, R.; Earle, J. D.; Wieand, H. S.; Moertel, C.; Krook, J.; Martenson, J. A.; Beart, R. W.; Kubista, T.: Adjuvant treatment of rectal cancer. Randomized prospective study of irradiation + chemotherapy. A NCCTG Mayo Clinic Study. ASTRO Proc. 1986. Int. J. Radiat. Oncol. Biol. Phys. *12:* suppl. 1, p. 169 (1986).

Leonard L. Gunderson, MD, Division of Radiation Oncology, Mayo Clinic, Rochester, MN 55905 (USA)

Vaeth JM, Meyer JL (eds): Radiation Tolerance of Normal Tissues.
Front Radiat Ther Oncol. Basel, Karger, 1989, vol 23, pp 299–301

Discussion

Dr. Kelman: This is a question concerning the biliary duct tumor that is 2½ cm in size involving the left and right ducts for which we have now done a drainage procedure. Given that one expects to use 5-fluorouracil probably and it's a small tumor, and one might have a possibility of being able to treat it with some control with irradiation, what's the most imaginative procedure that you can come up with?

Would you include twice-daily fractions, a field within a field, how would you treat his otherwise very healthy lady most aggresively?

Dr. Gunderson: This conference is on tolerance as opposed to treatment. but I will use it as an opportunity to make some statements about tolerance to bile duct itself because I didn't earlier due to time.

We use three approaches: either (1) radiation therapy plus chemotherapy with boosts of up to 7,000 rad; (2) irradiation plus transcatheter, or (3) irradiation plus interoperative electron boost.

What we have noted is that with both the transcatheter boost with iridium as well as with interoperative electrons, one has major problems with stenosis of bile ducts. Most of these patients have circumferential tumors. Even if we find ways of controlling the lesions, we're left with a total circumferential tumor problem which the body has to heal. It's not really surprising that even if we end up with better methods of control, we are going to end up with stenosis. We are going to have to find ways to overcome that, e.g., with laser.

There is a major problem with interoperative electrons. We get a fibrous problem in the hilum of the liver when we use IORT electrons. With transcatheter iridium, we get stenosis of the ducts that come into the main duct. It's not surprising, since some of those areas are going to be receiving up to 10,000 cGy with the combined external beam and transcatheter iridium.

Dr. Kelman: Do you think that the problem can be reduced by twice-daily treatment; maybe 100 twice a day, 110 twice a day?

Dr. Gunderson: I'm not convinced that a change in dose fractionation is going to alter the bile duct problems that we see when the entire circumference of the duct is involved. It may be a combined factor of the length of duct and the involvement circumferentially. But I'm convinced that we will overcome the stenosis problem in a small lumen structure that is totally involved with tumor. Take the ureter, for example, with a circumferential lesion. If you control the tumor with irradiation, you have a total lumen that has been replaced by fibrosis.

Dr. Boutin: Unfortunately, normal tissue does not always mean healthy tissue. I was wondering, Dr. Gunderson, if you had any recommendations for what we should consider normal liver tolerance in patients who may have some sclerosis or some normal tissue replaced by metastatic disease. What is a safe dose for those patients?

Dr. Gunderson: The safest dose is to not treat the total liver. I have treated patients with bile duct cancer, and I try to treat tumor plus 2-cm margins instread of tumor plus 5-cm margins. I would hesitate to treat the whole liver of a patient with underlying sclerosis because I would anticipate that the tolerance would be markedly reduced.

Dr. Travis: Just a comment about the incidence of late complications after combined drug therapy and radiation therapy. Clearly, experimental data are very few, and clinical data are also just as scarce, but it is possible that if you have two different target cells for an acute effect and a late effect in a tissue and the drug that you use may be specific for only those target cells for the acute effects. If you have equal toxic acute effects, one would not expect to have an increased incidence of late effects, so the problem of late effects after drugs and irradiation may not be as great if we titrate our doses of one or the other. Any comments?

Dr. Rubin: It's a very interesting idea, but, as you pointed out, we need so much more information about how these drugs are acting. This is one of the major points that I have been trying to make. We really need to know the radiation pathology, the chemopathology/physiology just as we have to know the radiation effects to be able to optimally combine modalities and avoid toxicities. But I don't know how good the chemotherapy literature is. I think outside of Cytoxan, the Ditman study, it's very difficult to come up with programs that are completely safe.

Dr. Gunderson: With the liver, for example, the feelings are changing on what the pathology is. It was just back in 1982 that Phil was saying that most of the chemotherapy problems with liver were hepatocellular, but now we have the chemotherapist saying that we are seeing classic veno-occlusive phenomena with certain drugs.

As patients undergoing aggresive chemotherapy live longer, our whole understanding of some of the pathology and some of the problems that occur long-termwise are going to change.

Dr. Rubin: That's a good point. With methotrexate, there was a lot of hepatocellular damage. With the use of BCNU, one runs into the nonocclusive disease. One has to know which compartment you're acting on in order to be able to figure out how to optimally combine therapies.

Dr. Travis: But it may be possible that we won't see the increase in late effects because drugs are far more selective in their injury than are radiations.

Dr. Rubin: I agree.

Dr. Gunderson: It's true that with gastric tissue and large-bowel tissue, for example, we are primarily seeing drugs that have a mucoserosal effect. Therefore, we see a marked increased in the acute sort of problems. But you're right, we may not see an increase in chronic changes.

Dr. Rubin: We didn't show the bleomycin story. If you give the bleomycin first and then the radiation therapy and one then brings separating them, what one sees with a simultaneous program is completely different from that with a separation. We have clearly shown that if one gives the bleomycin first and separate it by weeks to a month, you won't even recognize that it was given. But if you give radiation therapy first and then follow with bleomycin, weeks to a month later, you will recognize that, and you will increase the damaging effect. I think that one has to do timing studies and then see what the pathophysiology is.

Dr. Travis: We have done the Cytotoxan in lung followed by irradiation similar to the studies that I presented. It is a very different pattern. It seems that the damage is done very quickly with drugs, but then nothing changes unlike with irradiation where things change over at least a 6-month period.

Dr. Rubin: I think, as a practical rule, if you have to give drugs and irradiation, one's better off giving the drugs first because the odds are that one will clear that out. One may not have any injury occurring there; where as if one does it the other way around (and liver is a good example), one can have a lot of effects not only there, but agents that are not metabolized. Metothrexate, e.g., can create havoc with bone marrow. One has to be careful, not only with the organ that one's dealing with, but if it doesn't really handle the drug properly, it will dump it somewhere else, and very severe toxicity results.

Dr. Gunderson: The one caution that I would make with the liver is that the changes that are occurring are those where the patient received chemotherapy. One ends up with a sensitized liver. Coming back with radiation treatment later gives many changes. If using drugs that can produce chemical hepatitis, one better be aware that tolerance is reduced.

Vaeth JM, Meyer JL (eds): Radiation Tolerance of Normal Tissues.
Front Radiat Ther Oncol. Basel, Karger, 1989, vol 23, pp 302–309

Normal Tissue Tolerance to Irradiation of the Cardiovascular System

J. Robert Stewart

Division of Radiation Oncology, Department of Radiology, Utah Regional Cancer Center, University of Utah Health Sciences Center, Salt Lake City, Utah, USA

Introduction

In the interval since the publication in 1972 of the San Francisco Cancer Symposium on tolerance of normal tissue to irradiation [1], it has become well recognized that the heart frequently is the dose-limiting organ to consider when planning radiation therapy to neoplasms in the thorax. A number of papers have appeared in recent years which comment on various aspects of radiation-induced heart disease [2–8], and extensive reviews have been published to which the interested reader is directed for more detailed information [9, 10]. The purpose of this brief review of clinical and experimental material is not to provide comprehensive coverage of the subject, but rather to concentrate on certain aspects of clinical relevance and review some data newly acquired since the previous symposium.

Clinical Description

Radiation-induced heart disease most commonly presents clinically with pericardial disease several months following radiation therapy either as a pericardial effusion or as acute pericarditis. Either of these syndromes may be accompanied by tamponade which may require treatment. A number of other manifestations have been described, and the spectrum of syndromes is shown in table I. Pericarditis is in quotes in the second entry to call attention to the fact that that syndrome may be due to effects in the tumor contiguous with the heart rather than the heart itself. The most serious complication, pancarditis, shows involvement of all layers of the heart and presents clinically as relentless myocardial failure in addition to a clinical course characterized by dominant pericardial dis-

Table I. Clinical syndromes associated with cardiac irradiation

Temporally closely related to the irradiation
Transient physiological changes (rhythm, blood pressure, pulse rate, ECG changes, etc.)
Acute 'pericarditis' during treatment of mass contiguous to the heart
Delayed months to years following irradiation
Acute pericarditis
Pericardial effusion
Pancarditis (severe pericardial and myocardial disease)
Functional valvular defects
Cardiac conduction abnormalities
Coronary artery disease

ease. Pathologically, the hallmark of pericardial disease is fibrous thickening of the organ accompanied by fibrinous exudate and in the myocardium a diffuse interstitial fibrosis. The pathology of the disease has been described in detail by Fajardo et al. [11]. The findings, as in radiation damage to other organs, are characteristic of radiation-induced heart disease but nonspecific. This review will discuss (1) evidence supporting a radiation dose-response in the heart; (2) reiteration of the concept of tolerance dose; (3) supporting evidence for an effect of fractionation on incidence; (4) pathogenesis of myocardial damage and tolerance of capillaries, and (5) the effect of radiations on coronary artery disease. Little new information is available to review that bears on radiation sensitivity of the remaining elements of the cardiovascular system such as the larger arteries and veins. For a more detailed description of the clinical syndromes listed in Table I, the reader is referred to the review by Stewart and Fajardo [10].

Dose Response

We reported in the previous symposium [12] evidence from clinical data which suggested clearly that there was a dose response and that the dose response varied with the volume of heart irradiated. For instance, when greater or equal to 60% of the cardiac volume was included as in mantle irradiation for Hodgkin's disease, the dose to produce pericarditis was less than when a smaller volume of the cardiac silhouette was included as in adjuvant treatment for breast carcinoma [9, 10, 13]. The dose response for Hodgkin's disease shown in figure 1 was plotted by probit analysis of our previously published data [13]. A dose response was confirmed by us in experimental radiation-induced heart disease in rabbits [13], and subsequently there have been confirmatory reports based on analysis of clinical material [5] and in experimental models utilizing rats [14] and dogs [15] as subjects.

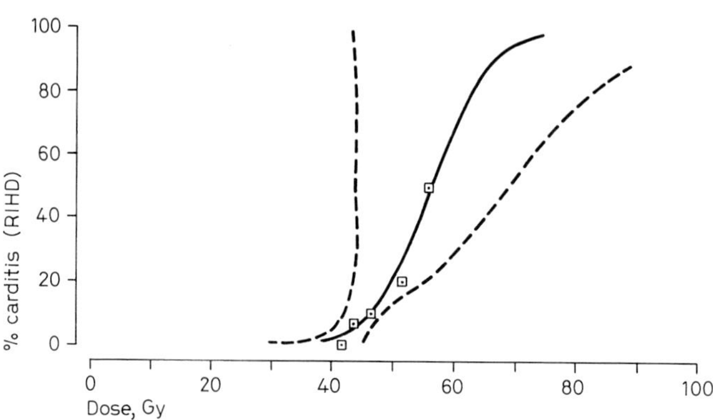

Fig. 1. Probit analysis of dose response for radiation-induced heart Disease (RIHD). The curve is derived by replotting by probit of the analysis of 318 determinant cases of Hodgkin's disease previously reported by Stewart and Fajardo [13]. □ = Data by Stewart and Fajardo [13]; ——— = fitted probit curve; ----- = 95% confidence limits. LD_5 = 43.3 Gy (40.3–46.4 95% confidence limits).

Tolerance Dose

Based on the dose-response analysis of clinical material, we previously defined tolerance dose as the dose to produce an incidence of no greater than 5% of mild pericarditis [13]. For large heart volumes, this figure was approximately 40 Gy in 4–5 weeks, 4–5 fractions/week. When small volumes of the heart were irradiated as in adjuvant irradiation postmastectomy for breast cancer, the tolerance dose appeared to be closer to 60 Gy in standard 1.8- to 2-Gy fractions.

Importance of Dose per Fraction

Comparison of cases of Hodgkin's disease treated at the Stanford University with a similar analysis from the University of California, San Francisco, revealed that the incidence of pericarditis was higher in the Stanford series [9, 10, 13]. The total dose was slightly higher in the Stanford cases, but even more striking was the difference in fractionation with consistently higher dose per fraction. This suggested the possibility of a fractionation effect. When Hodgkin's disease was treated with predominantly anterior field weighting for mediastinal disease, there resulted a higher total dose to the cardiac structures as well as a larger dose per fraction. In those cases a high incidence of cardiac damage was noted [2], again suggesting the possibility of a dose per fraction effect. Based on this information, changes were made in the approach to treatment of the mantle at Stanford as reported by Carmel and Kaplan [16]. These

Table II. Alpha/beta ratio 6 months after irradiation

	α/β Gy
Connective tissue	
Low dose	2.9
High dose	2.6
Vascular component	1.8
Ventricular wall thickness	3.5

Based on Gillette et al. [15]

changes consisted of a maintenance of the total dose at 44 Gy, while decreasing the dose per fraction, and, when possible, shielding the cardiac apex and much of the ventricular volume by subcarinal blocking for at least part of the dose. This resulted in a dramatic drop in incidence of cardiac disease. In my own practice since the early 1970s I have consistently attempted to confine the cardiac dose to 40 Gy or less in 1.8 Gy-fractions and frequently have used apical and subcarinal blocking when feasible, often with partial transmission blocks which reduce the dose per fraction to portions of the heart. Integral with this technique was consistently treating both the anterior and posterior fields on each treatment day with equal weighting to avoid inhomogeneities that result in a large dose/per fraction. With this approach cardiac complications have all but disappeared. These data are complicated to interpret because they involve changes in dose per fraction, volume of heart irradiated and, in some cases, of total dose; however, they do suggest the possibility of an important dose per fraction effect. This question has recently been addressed specifically in beagle dogs, and the importance of dose per fraction in a number of cardiac end points has been shown by a low α/β ratio consistent with many other late-responding tissues [15]. These findings are summarized in table II.

Pathogenesis of the Myocardial Lesion

Clinical and pathological analysis of our extensive clinical material [9–13, 17, 18] provided few clues as to the pathogenesis of pericardial fibrosis or the pronounced diffuse myocardial fibrosis characteristic of late-stage pancarditis. We, therefore, turned to an animal model and selected the rabbit. We found in this animal that the histological lesions produced by single doses or fractionated radiation were identical to those in humans [19–21] and that there was a pronounced and steep dose response similar to the patient material [13]. Acutely after a single dose of irradiation, there was a transient acute reaction with inflammatory cells present throughout all layers of the heart. This cleared in a few days, after which there was a long latent period with no evident histological change. After about 70 days the late phase began with progressive focal myocardial fibrosis, invariably accompanied by pericardial disease similar to the situation in humans with pancarditis. This progressive histological change was often accompanied by signs of cardiac failure and spontaneous deaths of the animals.

A closer look at the events occurring during the latent stage by electron microscopy showed that there were dramatic changes in the endothelial cells of myocardial capillaries, and the damage was accompanied by evidence of capillary regeneration as reflected by tritiated thymidine studies showing increased DNA synthesis [21]. As time progressed and the diffuse fibrosis increased, there was an approximately 50% decrease in the number of capillaries present. More recently, early capillary damage has been shown by Gillette et al. [15] in dogs and by Lauk et al. [14] in rats. Since in the rabbit the histological changes following fractionated and single-dose irradiation were identical to those seen in humans after fractionated radiation therapy, we proposed that the primary lesion in myocardial fibrosis was injury to endothelial cells in the microvasculature. Replacement of these cells was attempted, as reflected by an increase in the number of cells undergoing DNA synthesis. This attempt was not totally successful, leading to a quantitative decrease in the number of capillaries and, therefore the circulatory capacity of the myocardium which in turn led to the fibrosis. If this hypothesis is correct and the capillary injury model translates to fractionated irradiation, it would appear that capillary tolerance in myocardium might be somewhat lower than that estimated by Rubin and Cassarett [22] at the previous symposium. The work of Gillette et al. [15] documents the steep dose response for capillary loss (table II), and their data suggest a lower than 60-Gy threshold, at least for 4-Gy fractions. Our studies and those of others have not provided direct evidence for explanation of the pathogenesis of radiation pericarditis.

Coronary Artery Disease

Anecdotal reports of precocious coronary artery disease in survivors of cancer who have been irradiated to the heart have raised the concern that irradiation may cause or aggravate a susceptibility to coronary artery disease. This has been based mainly on reports summarized by Fajardo [23] and by Kopelson and Herwig [24]. The latter authors could find only 10 cases under the age 30 years. The concern, however, is especially relevant in view of the large number of long-term survivors with Hodgkin's disease previously irradiated. As this population ages and is subject to other risk factors of coronary artery disease such as smoking and dietary factors, we might expect an increasing morbidity and mortality from coronary artery disease. This has been looked for specifically by Boivan and Hutchison [25] in follow-up of over 900 patients previously irradiated for Hodgkin's disease, but no statistically significant increase in coronary artery disease mortality could be measured, and, therefore, the study would be interpreted as negative evidence, albeit based on a limited number of patients and somewhat limited follow-up. More recently Host et al. [26] have reported follow-up of a large series of patients with breast cancer who had been randomized to receive or not receive radiation therapy following mastectomy. In the irradiated group there were 10 coronary artery deaths versus 1 in the nonirradiated population. This difference was statistically highly significant, therefore, suggesting positive correlation between irradiation and subsequent coronary artery disease. At this time I would consider the issue unsettled as to the role of irradiation in this potentially important complication. Further long-term population studies of previously treated Hodgkin's disease should add relevant information concerning the risk of coronary artery disease.

Conclusions

Radiation-induced heart disease is now a well-established complication of thoracic irradiation, and the heart is often the dose-limiting organ in the region. There are well-established risk factors for development of radiation-induced heart disease including the total dose administered, the dose per fraction (low alpha/beta ratio), and the volume of heart irradiated. The myocardial component of radiation-induced heart disease is preceded by capillary damage and by a decrease in the microcirculation, suggesting that myocardial fibrosis has an ischemic cause. Evidence for damage to the capillaries in myocardium suggests that the tolerance dose of radiation may be lower than suggested by Rubin and Cassarett [22] in 1972 for skin capillaries. Finally, the risk of coronary artery disease following cardiac irradiation remains controversial and incompletely assessed at this point.

Acknowledgments

I wish to acknowledge the help and stimulus resulting from collaboration over the years with J. Martin Brown, Keith F. Cohn, James R. Eltringham, E. W. Hancock, Henry

S. Kaplan, Melvin R. Klauber, and Vera Page. A special acknowledgment is due to my good friend and colleague, Luis J. Fajardo, whose interest in this project and the field of radiation pathology has contributed so greatly to radiation oncology. My thanks to Edward L. Gillette and Huib S. Reinholt for helpful suggestions and to Marie Grossi for preparation of the manuscript.

References

1 Vaeth, Front. Radiat. Ther. Oncol., vol. 6, (Karger, Basel 1972).
2 Byhardt, R.; Brace, K.; Ruckdeschel, J.: Dose and treatment factors in radiation-related pericardial effusion associated with the mantle technique for Hodgkin's disease. Cancer *35:* 795–802 (1975).
3 Westerhof, P. W.; Putte, C. J. van der: Radiation pericarditis and myocardial fibrosis. Eur. J. Cardiol. *4:* 213–218 (1976).
4 Brosius, F. C.; Waller, B. F.; Roberts, W. G.: Radiation heart disease: analysis of 16 young (aged 15 to 33 years) necropsy patients who received over 3,500 rads to the heart. Am. J. Med. *70:* 519–530 (1981).
5 Mill, W. B.; Baglan, R. J.; Kurichety, P., et al.: Symptomatic radiation-induced pericarditis in Hodgkin's disease. Int. J. Radiat. Oncol. Biol. Phys. *10:* 2061–2065 (1984).
6 Morgan, G. W.; Freeman, A. P.; McLean, R. G., et al.: Late cardiac, thyroid, and pulmonary sequelae of mantle radiotherapy for Hodgkin's disease. Int. J. Radiat. Oncol. Biol. Phys. *11:* 1925–1931 (1985).
7 Green, D. M.; Gingell, R. L.; Pearce, J., et al.: The effect of mediastinal irradiation on cardiac function of patients treated during childhood and adolescence for Hodgkin's disease. J. clin. Oncol. *5:* 239–245 (1987).
8 Pohjola-Sintonen, S.; Toterman, K.; Salmo, M., et al.: Late cardiac effects of mediastinal radiotherapy in patients with Hodgkin's disease. Cancer *60:* 31–37 (1987).
9 Fajardo, L. F.; Stewart, J. R.: Radiation-induced heart disease. Human and experimental observations; in Bristow, Drug-induced heart disease, pp. 241–261 (Elsevier, Amsterdam 1980).
10 Stewart, J. R.; Fajardo, L.: Radiation-induced heart disease: an update. Prog. in cardiovasc. Dis. *27:* 173–194 (1984).
11 Fajardo, L. F.; Stewart, J. R.; Cohn, K. E.: Morphology of radiation-induced heart disease. Archs Path. *86:* 512–519 (1968).
12 Stewart, J. R.; Fajardo, L. F.: Radiation-induced heart disease; in Vaeth, Front. Radiat. Ther. Onco., vol. 6., pp. 274–288 (Karger, Basel 1972).
13 Stewart, J. R.; Fajardo, L. F.; Dose response in humans and experimental radiation-induced heart disease. Application of the nominal standard dose (NSD) concept. Radiology *99:* 403–408 (1971).
14 Lauk, S.; Kiszel, Z.; Buschmann, J., et al.: Radiation-induced heart disease in rats. Int. J. Radiat. Oncol. Biol. Phys. *11:* 801–808 (1985).
15 Gillette, E. L.; McChesney, S. L.; Hoopes, P. J.: Isoeffect curves for radiation-induced cardiomyopathy in the dog. Int. J. Radiat. Oncol. Phys. *11:* 2091–2097 (1985).
16 Carmel, R. J.; Kaplan, H. S.: Mantle irradiation in Hodgkin's disease. Cancer *37:* 2813–2815 (1976).
17 Cohn, K. E.; Stewart, J. R.; Fajardo, L. F., et al.: Heart disease following radiation. Medicine *46:* 281–298 (1967).
18 Stewart, J. R., et al.: Radiation-induced heart disease. A study of twenty-five patients. Radiology *89:* 302–310 (1967).

19 Stewart, J. R.; Fajardo, L. F.; Cohn, K. E., et al.: Experimental radiation-induced heart disease in rabbits. Radiology *91:* 814–817 (1968).
20 Fajardo, L. F.; Stewart, J. R.: Experimental radiation-induced heart disease. I. Light microscopic studies. Am. J. Path. *59:* 299–316 (1970).
21 Fajardo, L. F.; Stewart, J. R.: Pathogenesis of radiation-induced myocardial fibrosis. Lab. Invest. *29:* 244–257 (1973).
22 Rubin, P. R.; Casarett, G.: A direction for clinical radiation pathology: the tolerance dose; in Vaeth, Front. Radiat. Ther. Onc., vol. 6, pp. 1–16 (Karger, Basel 1972).
23 Fajardo, L. F.: Radiation-induced coronary artery disease. Chest *71:* 563–564 (1977).
24 Kopelson, G.; Herwig, K. J.: The etiologies of coronary artery disease in cancer patients. Int. J. Radiat. Oncol. Biol. Phys. *4:* 895–906 (1978).
25 Boivin, J. F.; Hutchison, G. B.: Coronary heart disease mortality after irradiation for Hodgkin's disease. Cancer *49:* 2470–2475 (1982).
26 Host, H.; Brennhovd, I.O.; Loeb, M.: Postoperative radiotherapy in breast cancer. Long-term results from the Oslo study. Int. J. Radiat. Oncol. Biol. Phys. *12:* 727–732 (1986).

J. Robert Stewart, MD, Division of Radiation Oncology,
University of Utah Health Sciences Center, 50 North Medical Drive,
Salt Lake City, UT 84132 (USA)

Vaeth JM, Meyer JL (eds): Radiation Tolerance of Normal Tissues.
Front Radiat Ther Oncol. Basel, Karger, 1989, vol 23, pp 310–322

Radiation Effects on Renal Function

Arnold M. Markoe[a], *Luther W. Brady*[a], *Charles Swartz*[b], *Odette Campbell*[a], *Kristina Antoniades*[c]

[a] Department of Radiation Oncology, Hahnemann University Hospital;
[b] Department of Internal Medicine, Division of Nephrology, Hahnemann University Hospital, Philadelphia, Pa.;
[c] Department of Pathology, Crozer-Chester Medical Center, Chester, Pa., USA

Introduction

The fact that irradiation can damage the kidney has long been established [17]. This damage can run the gamut from subclinical changes to clinically significant hypertension and renal failure [5]. Changes occur in renal morphology as well as in function [17]. The initial report of the possible renal effects of irradiation appeared between 1904 and 1907 [17], although radiation nephropathy as an entity may have been recognized by Gassman several years earlier [5]. Table I outlines the important clinical observations leading up to the classic presentation by Kunkler and Luxton [12] and Luxton and Kunkler [13] who attempted to define the total dose associated with a high risk for development of severe radiation nephritis in adults treated with fractionated radiation therapy. Table II gives the five clinical types of radiation nephropathy these authors defined. They suggested that 2,800 rad to both kidneys within 5 weeks was the limit of tolerance [13], revised upward from their earlier limit of 2,300 cGy within 5 weeks [12]. Subsequent studies have tended to support this tolerance dose level in adults [10, 11]. Unfortunately, the clinical data of Kunkler and Luxton [12] and Luxton and Kunkler [13] were derived from patients treated prior to the advent of high-energy radiation equipment and with fractionation schemes that are not the current practice.

Animal experimentation with respect to radiation effects on the kidney also has suffered, until recently, from experimental design that was inconsistent with clinical practice. Animals have been unilaterally nephrectomized and the remaining kidney irradiated at varying times thereafter, and kidneys have been exteriorized for irradiation. Most animal studies have utilized highly selected inbred strains, have anesthetized the animals for treatment, and have employed single large fractions

Table I. Historical overview

1907	Initial report of possible renal effects of radiation [20].
1920s	Experimental animal radiation nephritis.
1927	Azotemia, proteinuria, and hypertension in patients receiving renal irradiation [4].
1944	Nephrectomy can relieve radiation-induced hypertension [3].
1952	Initial detailed reports of human experience and radiation nephritis.
1964	Definition of clinical syndromes – suggestion of tolerance doses [12, 13].

Table II. Five syndromes of radiation nephritis in man

Acute radiation nephritis
Onset 6–13 months after radiotherapy in adults
Lesser latent period in children
Hypertension/anemia/proteinuria is major triad of symptoms
Chronic radiation nephritis
May succeed acute radiation nephritis or occur without prior acute radiation nephritis
Hypertension/anemia/proteinuria/azotemia
Benign hypertension
Hypertension and variable proteinuria
Late malignant hypertension
>1–1½ years after radiotherapy in adults, may rapidly progress
Responds to antihypertensive medication
Responds to nephrectomy of atrophic kidney if 1 of 2 kidneys is contracted
Asymptomatic proteinuria

of radiation. Even more recent studies, utilizing varying fractionation schemes and daily doses, more in keeping with clinical reality, to treat unoperated animals to both kidneys have had to employ anesthesia or restraint of the animal.

We will report on a small series of random-bred dogs who were trained to stand in stanchion for irradiation and who were treated to both kidneys in an unanesthetized state. We will also present clinical data on a mixed series of patients irradiated to one or both kidneys as a consequence of receiving adequate radiation therapy for their malignant disease and will examine these patients for the incidence of radiation nephropathy.

Methods

For canine experiments, random-bred dogs (a majority of German Shepards) were acclimatized in our animal colony. Animals were allowed food and water as demanded.

During the acclimatization period, each dog was trained to stand in stanchion within a wooden box which provided only mild restraint to motion.

All animals were irradiated unanesthetized using an orthovoltage unit operating at 210 kVp energy and 15 mA and utilizing a Thoreus II filter. The half-value layer of the beam was described as HVL = 2.15 mm Cu. All animals were irradiated by a single posterior portal measuring 10 × 15 cm (length × width) with the central 3 cm blocked with lead to avoid any treatment over the spinal cord. All animals were treated to both kidneys simultaneously at 5 cm depth, and the adrenal glands were also included within the portal. We irradiated 3 animals each to 2,500, 3,000 or 3,500 cGy. Animals were irradiated daily, with no treatment on weekends, and the total treatment time was kept constant at 16–17 days. Therefore, the fraction size was allowed to vary somewhat. Animals irradiated to 2,500 cGy received 10 fractions at 200 cGy, followed by 2 fractions of 250 cGy. Dogs irradiated to 3,000 cGy received 12 fractions of 250 cGy each. Those animals treated to 3,500 cGy received 12 fractions of 292 cGy each.

The animals were anesthetized only for the purpose of obtaining experimental data. Data was obtained before irradiation during the acclimatization period and then at intervals after therapy. Pentobarbital anesthesia was used throughout experimentation (30 mg/kg induction dose). At each determination point, blood was obtained for blood urea nitrogen, creatinine, hematocrit, and white blood cell determinations. Arterial blood pressure was evaluated and the bladder catheterized for determination of creatinine clearance and for renal plasma and blood flow determinations. Urine was obtained for urinary sodium and potassium levels after 30 min of intravenous hydration. The bladder was then fully expressed of contents, lavaged with double distilled water and evacuated, and the catheter attached to a graduate for urine collection. Three separate 20-min urine samples were obtained for creatinine clearance and for excretion of *p*-aminohippurate. Animals had been previously primed with 24 mg/kg creatinine and 20 mg/kg *p*-aminohippurate. Quantitation of creatinine and *p*-aminohippurate was done by the nephrology laboratory at Hahnemann University Hospital. The glomerular filtration rate was calculated as were renal blood and plasma flow and the filtration fraction derived. Glomerular filtration rate and renal blood and plasma flow were corrected for animal body weight, since these parameters are known to be dependent upon animal weight [1, 8]. Data were accessioned periodically over at least 1 year following therapy.

We have also examined our clinical records for patients treated to the entire abdomen in whom the kidneys were in the treatment portal or under posterior 5% transmission blocks for all or a portion of their therapy. These patients fell into three primary disease categories. They were mostly patients treated for ovarian cancer or lymphoma, but a few patients treated to the whole abdomen for testicular tumors were also found. Unfortunately, the vast majority of the 103 patients identified had advanced or massively recurrent disease and were not expected to survive beyond 6 months prior to their irradiation. After exclusion of these patients as well as those lost to follow-up, we were able to collect 21 patients for analysis. Of these 21 patients, 12 died and are examined separately. Table III gives the pertinent characteristics of these patients. Table IV shows the same characteristics for the remaining 9 patients who are still alive at times ranging from 27 months to 14 years after treatment.

Results

The animal data are shown graphically in figures 1–7. Figure 1 indicates that there was meaningless change in the arterial blood pressure of

Table III. Patients failing to survive after abdominal radiotherapy

Number of patients = 12 (all female)
Average age = 49.6 years (range 31–69 years)
Ovarian carcinoma = 10 (stage I_C = 2, stage II_B = 1, stage III = 7)
Lymphoma = 2 (stage II_A DHL, stage III_B DPDLL)
Irradiation: All treatment using 6 MV photon beam
100–150 cGy/fraction
Posterior 5% transmission block over kidneys at variable times
Average renal dose = 2,377 cGy (range 1,650–3,025 cGy)
Average unblocked dose = 1,990 cGy (range 900–3,025 cGy)
Median survival = 12 months (only patients surviving > 6 months included in this series, range 6–28 months)
Renal symptoms = 0/12
Cause of death
Disease: 8/12
Sepsis: 1/12
PE: 1/12
Complications: 1/12 (bowel obstruction ? Due to radiotherapy)
Unknown: 1/12

Table IV. Patients surviving after abdominal radiotherapy

Number of patients = 9 (female = 5, male = 4)
Average age = 48.8 years (range 20–71)
Ovarian carcinoma = 5 (stage I_C = 2, stage II_B = 3)
Lymphoma = 2 (stage IV_A NPDLL and stage IV_A unclassified)
Testicular = 2 (stage II_B teratocarcinoma and stage III seminoma)
Irradiation shown in table III
Average renal dose = 2,766 cGy (range 1,845–4,950, highest dose to only 1 of 2 kidneys, the other kidney full shielded)
Average unblocked dose = 2,364 cGy
Median survival = 11 years (range 27 months to 14 years, all patients with last follow-up examination within 1987 or 1988)
Renal symptoms = 1/9

the dogs measured up to 2½ years after completion of therapy. Certainly, there is no increase in pressure of any significance, nor does there appear to be any time dependency exhibited. A similar situation appears to obtain for the hematocrit value which remains between 90 and 110% of pretreatment values over the duration of our monitoring of values (fig. 2). Blood urea nitrogen shows somewhat more variability (fig. 3), but again appears to hunt around the 100% of pretreatment value.

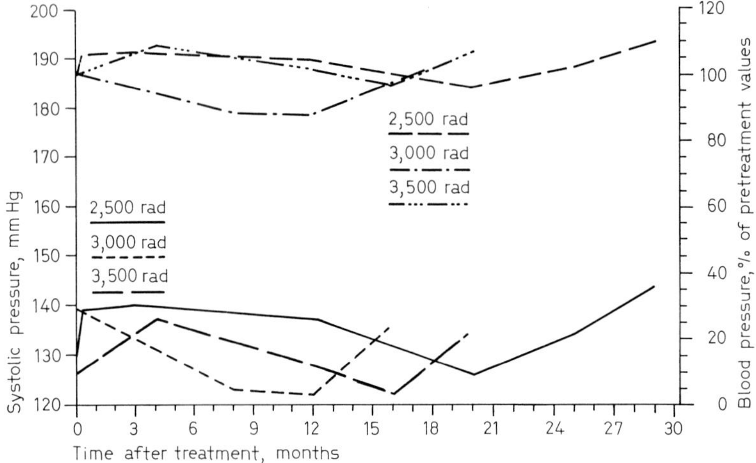

1

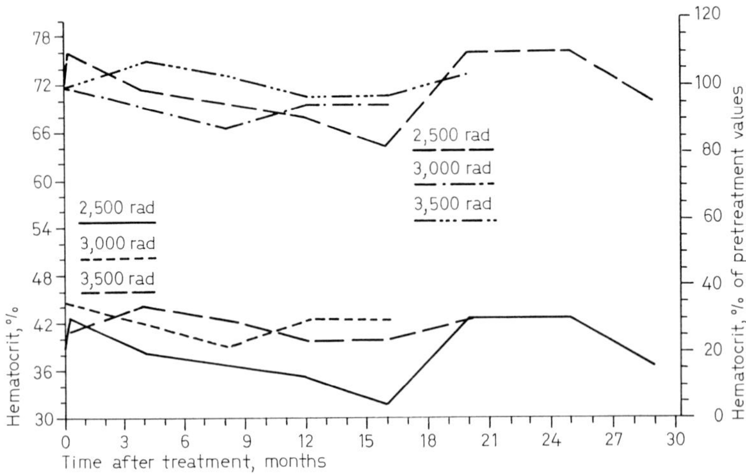

2

Fig. 1. Radiation effects on kidney: blood pressure. The lower curves give the measured systolic pressure and refer to the left axis, and the top set of curves gives the same data as percent of pretreatment values and refer to the right axis.

Fig. 2. Radiation effects on kidney: hematocrit. The lower curves give the measured value for hematocrit and refer to the left axis, and the upper set of curves gives the same data as percent of pretreatment values and refer to the right axis.

Fig. 3. Radiation effects on kidney: blood urea nitrogen. The lower curves give the absolute value measured for blood urea nitrogen and refer to the left axis, and the topmost set of curves give the same data as percent of petreatment values and refers to the right axis.

Fig. 4. Radiation effects on kidney: glomerular filtration rate. Data presented as percent of pretreatment values.

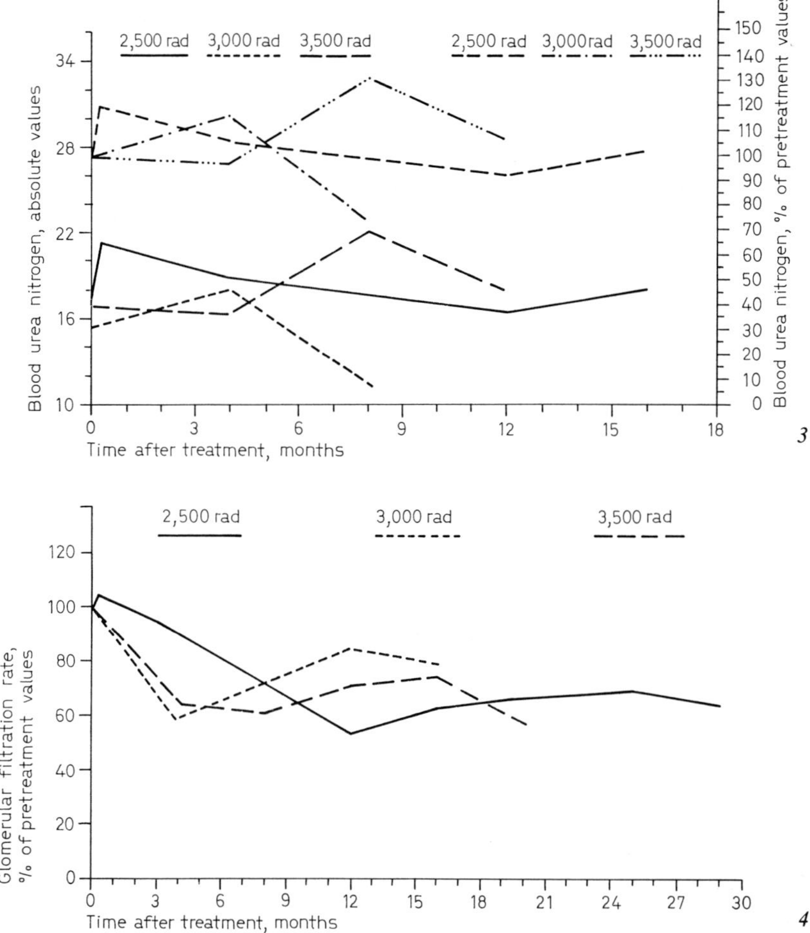

3

4

However, when we examine renal function parameters, a different picture emerges. Figure 4 clearly shows that irradiation produces depressions of the glomerular filtration rate that appear after 3 months following treatment and which appear to persist thereafter. We did not see any dose-response effect over the narrow range that we have studied, nor did we see any real time dependence of effect after 4–12 months. A similar situation is seen with respect to renal blood flow and renal plasma flow estimates shown in figures 5 and 6, respectively. The filtration fraction, defined as the ratio of glomerular filtration rate to renal plasma flow is shown in figure 7 not to vary significantly from pretreatment values.

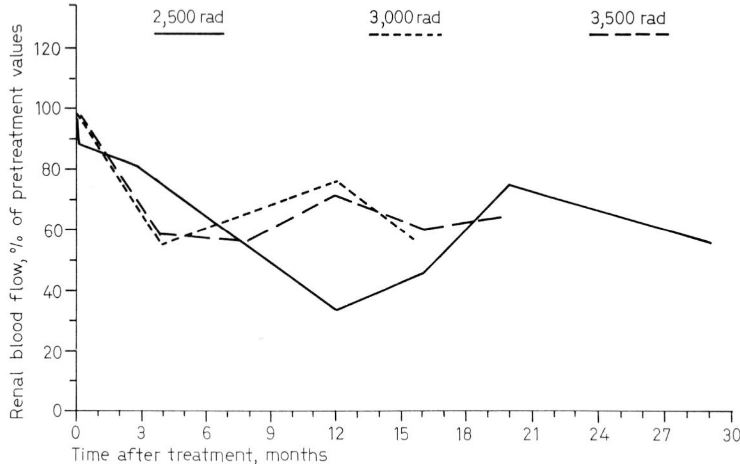

5

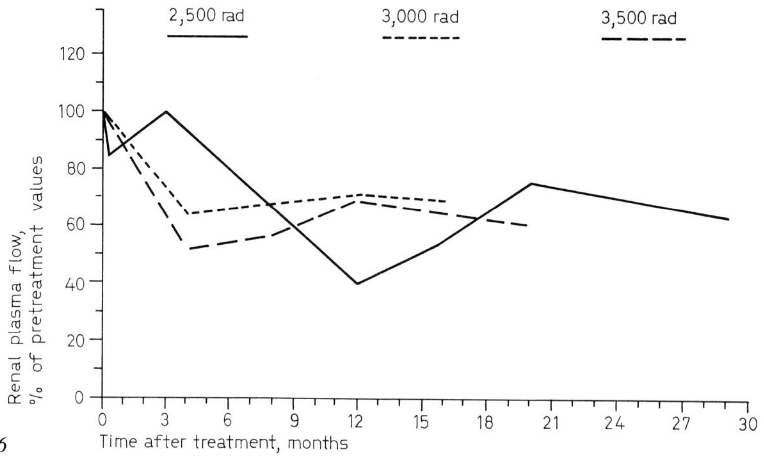

6

Fig. 5. Radiation effects on kidney: renal blood flow. Data presented as percent of pretreatment values.

Fig. 6. Radiation effects on kidney: renal plasma flow. Data presented as percent of pretreatment values.

Fig. 7. Radiation effects on kidney: filtration fraction. Data presented as percent of pretreatment values.

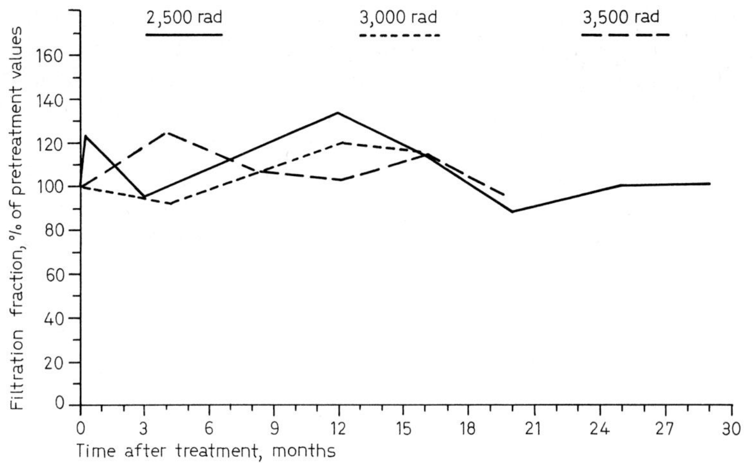

7

We were also able to subject 4 kidneys from 2 animals receiving 2,500 cGy renal irradiation to light microscopy 30 months after irradiation. One kidney from each animal was fixed in formalin without any other preparation, but the other was injected with latex to better delineate the vascular structure. All kidneys showed evidence for glomerulosclerosis with glomeruli smaller than expected and with a moderate increase of mesangial matrix. The capillaries were somewhat swollen. Edema of the intermediate arteries was an inconstant finding. The larger arteries appeared uninvolved. There was mild tubular dilatation, and the tubular lining cells were foamy and vacuolated. These findings of glomerular and tubular damage are well documented in the literature [5, 6, 9, 14, 15].

In our companion clinical series, none of the 12 patients who have died after their radiation therapy showed any signs of the acute phase of renal damage. Nine of the 12 patients died of their disease, 2 patients died of unrelated causes (pulmonary embolus in 1 and sepsis in the other) and 1 patient was considered to have succumbed to treatment-related toxicity of intestinal obstruction, but no postmortem examination was performed to rule out ovarian carcinoma involving the bowel. In these patients the kidneys received doses ranging from 1,650 to 3,025 cGy, usually 150 cGy/fraction or less. In the 9 patients alive after therapy, all but 2 patients have maintained normal blood pressures and blood urea nitrogen levels. One patient had essential hypertension prior to the radiation therapy, and there have not been any changes in her blood pressure over the 11 years following treatment. However, we found a single patient who developed hypertension 13 years after irradiation. Both kidneys had received 3,187 cGy. The initial 2,500 cGy was received through unblocked anterior and posterior portals with both fields being treated daily. An additional 1,375-cGy tumor dose was delivered with the kidneys blocked from the posterior portal only, and the estimated (conservative) dose received by each kidney was approximately 50% of the tumor dose at midline. The patient was treated at 125 cGy per fraction throughout her course of therapy. This patient was further studied 1 year after developing hypertension because she had, by then, developed azotemia and hyperkalemia, although her hypertension was controlled by Lopressor. A renal flow and function scan was performed and revealed a glomerular filtration rate of only 48 ml/min with the right kidney performing 61% of the total renal function. The calculated renal plasma flow was 261 ml/min with the right kidney having 67% of the total flow. A static renal scan indicated a normal right kidney and a left kidney with delayed perfusion but apparently normal excretion. The impression from the study was of bilateral renal vascular disease, worse in the left kidney than the right, and a question of left renal artery stenosis.

The other patients in this study segment all had bilateral renal doses ranging from 1,845 to 2,775 cGy at 125–150 cGy/fraction. However, 1 patient had unilateral kidney irradiation for bulky pararenal and nodal disease from testicular tumor. His right kidney only was treated to 4,950 cGy. He remains alive, free of disease, and free of renal problems 11 years after irradiation.

Discussion

The animal experimentation reported in this paper represents results obtained irradiating both kidneys in intact, unanesthetized dogs using daily doses and schedules within the realm of clinical application of radiation therapy. Thus, unlike experimentation where unilaterally nephrectomized animals are irradiated with large single fractions, in the anesthetized state, to the remaining kidney or to one exteriorized kidney, these experiments do not suffer from questions regarding potentially altered states. The data presented clearly show that there is a diminution of renal function, particularly with respect to glomerular filtration rate and renal blood and plasma flow of a magnitude quite consistent with that reported by Mendelsohn and Caceres [16] in the unilaterally nephrectomized dog whose remaining kidney was irradiated to 2,010, 2,750, or 3,780 cGy within 13 days. These authors reported that both glomerular filtration rate and renal plasma flow gradually fell to40% of control values and then rose somewhat. Mendelsohn and Caceres [16] reported that loss of function was proportional to the dose. In our study, we document loss of function to 50–80% of pretreatment glomerular filtration rate values and to 40–60% of pretreatment renal plasma and renal blood flow values. However, we are not able to define any true dose-reponse effect for these parameters. Additionally, we find no real change in filtration fraction, implying that glomerular filtration rate and renal plasma flow changes are proportionate. This is not in agreement with the human data reported by Avioli et al. [2] who found that the filtration fraction progressively rose as a consequence of a disproportionate decrease in renal plasma flow in 10 patients receiving 2,000–2,400 cGy within 3–4 weeks for treatment of intraabdominal or retroperitoneal malignancies. Our data are more in keeping with that obtained in rabbits by Hamada [7], indicating a slight, but transient, rise in filtration fraction followed by a gradual recovery.

Surprisingly, the changes observed in glomerular filtration rate and renal plasma and blood flow were unaccompanied by significant changes in blood urea nitrogen, hematocrit, or blood pressure. Nor were there any consistent patterns found in urinary sodium or potassium levels. The fact that hematocrit remains constant in the face of diminished renal function was unexpected, since Stewart et al. [18] have demonstrated that the degree of anemia as assessed by hematocrit measurements is an early indicator of the extent of renal damage after irradiation.

It has been shown in both animal experimentation and in clinical series that renal damage appears to be both dose- and time-dependent. We did not observe this in our study over the limited dose range and a narrow range of fraction size employed.

With respect to our patient population, none of the total of 21 patients were seen to develop any syndrome consistent with acute radiation nephropathy at renal doses ranging from 1,650 to 4,950 cGy (the latter to one kidney only). There were 10 patients evaluable (dead or alive) who lived >18 months after irradiation, and only 1 of these patients developed a chronic nephropathy, presumed secondary to prior irradiation. This patient developed hypertension 13 years after treatment, and renal function abnormality was documented approximately 1 year later. The elevated blood pressure has been controlled with antihypertensive medication, the renal function tests remain to be repeated.

It is interesting that the dogs showed no changes consistent with acute nephropathy up to 29 months after irradiation, although they certainly exhibited alterations in renal function. They were followed, therefore, for an equivalent maximum time of nearly 17 human years! The failure to observe any evidence of radiation nephropathy, either on an acute or chronic basis, suggests that the kidney may be able to tolerate somewhat higher doses than previously anticipated. Stewart et al. [18] have recently

Table V. Effect of fraction size on renal function [data approximated from ref 18]

Fraction size cGy	*Isoeffective dose* cGy
1,500	approximately 1,500
1,000	2,200
800	2,400
600	3,000
400	3,800
300	4,200
250	4,800
200	5,000
180	5,000
150	5,200
100	6,000

shown that the dose per fraction is a key and critical factor in renal tolerance in mice irradiated locally to both kidneys in an unanesthetized, but tightly restrained condition. These authors subjected the animals to irradiation using a single fraction up to 64 fractions, varying the dose per fraction, but keeping the overall treatment time constant at 3 weeks. They were able to demonstrate not only dose, but time-dependence as well, with respect to changes in urination frequency (events/24 h) and in glomerular function as assessed by residual ^{51}Cr-EDTA activity 1 h after intraperitoneal injection. From their data, it is clear that the isoeffective dose can be markedly increased by decreasing the dose per fraction and using hyperfractionation techniques. Table V gives data abstracted from their study. Also from the data of Stewart et al. [18], it would appear that irradiation at 200–300 cGy/fraction exhibits very little change in total isoeffective dose, and that may account for the data observed in our dog study, if mouse data can be used to describe the situation in the canine model.

These authors were also able to derive the a/β-ratio by plotting the reciprocal of total isoeffective dose against dose per fraction. The a/β-ratios thus derived were 2.9 ± 0.4 to 3.4 ± 0.4 Gy using the EDTA clearance assay and 2.7 ± 0.4 to 3.2 ± 0.2 Gy using the urinary frequency assay. These ratios are typical for late-responding normal tissues [19].

Conclusions

The animal and clinical data presented would appear to indicate that renal tolerance to radiation therapy administered under clinically compatible regimens may not be as limiting as previously thought. However, it is prudent at this time to retain a conservative dose limitation with respect to renal irradiation. We still, therefore, recommend doses not to exceed 2,500–2,800 cGy within 4–5 weeks.

The data also suggest that the renal function can be altered without the development of a clinically significant syndrome consistent with acute or chronic nephropathy and that hypertension or azotemia is not a necessary consequence of such altered renal function.

In reporting any results, clinical or experimental, regarding the effects of renal irradiation, it would be advisable to document not only the total dose delivered, but also the dose per fraction and the total time over which the dose has been delivered.

Additional animal studies must be performed to fully document the effects of renal irradiation on structural changes, functional changes, and the development of nephropathic syndromes with respect to total dose and fractionation considerations before any consideration be given to alteration of recommended tolerance doses in adults. It must always be acknowledged that children will exhibit a greater sensitivity than adults.

References

1 Åsheim, Å.; Persson, F.; Persson, S.: Renal clearance in dogs with regard to variations according to age and sex. Acta physiol. scand. *51:* 150–152 (1961).

2 Avioli, L. V.; Lazor, M. Z.; Cotlove, E.; Brace, K. C.; Andrews, J. R.: Early effects of radiation on renal function in man. Am. J. Med. *34:* 329–337 (1963).

3 Dean, A. L.; Abels, J. C.: Study by newer renal function tests of unusual case of hypertension following irradiation of one kidney and relief of patient by nephrectomy. J. Urol. *52:* 497–501 (1944).

4 Doub, H. P.; Hartman, F. W.; Bolliger, A.: Relative sensitivity of kidney to irradiation. Radiology *8:* 142–148 (1927).

5 Fajardo, L. F.: *Pathology of radiation injury*, chapter 8: urinary system (Masson, New York, 1982).

6 Fajardo, L. F.; Brown, J. M.; Glatstein, E.: Glomerular and juxta-glomerular lesions in radiation nephropathy. Radiat. Res. *68:* 177–183 (1976).

7 Hamada, K.: Studies on renal clearance. II. Changes of kidney and renal clearance following X-ray irradiation to the kidney in rabbits. Acta urol. jap. *10:* 3–26 (1964).

8 Holliday, M. A.; Egan, T. J.: Renal function in man, dog and rat. Nature *193:* 748–750 (1962).

9 Kapur, S.; Chandra, R.; Antonovych, T.: Acute radiation nephritis. Light and electron microscopic observations. Archs Pathol. Lab. Med. *101:* 469–473 (1977).

10 Keane, W.; Crosson, J. T.; Staley, N. A.; Anderson, W. R.; Shapiro, F. L.: Radiation-induced renal disease: a clinicopathologic study. Am. J. Med. *60:* 127–137 (1976).

11 Kim, T. H.; Freeman, C. R.; Webster, J. H.: The significance of unilateral radiation nephropathy. Int. J. Radiat. Oncol. Biol. Phys. *6:* 1567–1571 (1980).

12 Kunkler, P. B.; Farr, R. F.; Luxton, R. W.: Limit of renal tolerance of X-rays: in-

vestigation into renal damage occurring following treatment of tumours of testis by abdominal baths. Br. J. Radiol. *25:* 190–201 (1952).

13 Luxton, R. W.; Kunkler, P. B.: Radiation nephritis. Acta radiol. *2:* 169–178 (1964).

14 Madrazo, A.; Schwarz, G.; Churg, J.: Radiation nephritis: a review. J. Urol. *114:* 822–827 (1975).

15 Maier, J. G.: Effects of radiation on kidney, bladder and prostate. Front. Radiat. Ther. Onc., vol. 6, pp. 196–227 (Karger, Basel 1972).

16 Mendelsohn, M. L.; Caceres, E.: Effects of X-ray to the kidney on the renal function of dogs. Am. J. Physiol. *173:* 351–354 (1954).

17 Redd, B. L.: Radiation nephritis. Review, report and animal studies. Am. J. Roentg. *83:* 88–106 (1960).

18 Stewart, F. A.; Soranson, J. A.; Alpen, E. L.; Williams, M. V.; Denekamp, J.: Radiation-induced renal damage: the effects of hyperfractionation. Radiat. Res. *98:* 407–420 (1984).

19 Thames, H. D.; Hendry, J. H.: *Fractionation in radiotherapy* (Taylor & Francis, Philadelphia 1987).

20 Warthin, A. S.: Changes produced in kidney by roentgen irradiation. Am. J. med. Sci. *133:* 737–746 (1907).

Arnold M. Markoe, MD, Department of Radiation Oncology,
Hahnemann University Hospital, Philadelphia, PA 19102 (USA).

Vaeth JM, Meyer JL (eds): Radiation Tolerance of Normal Tissues.
Front Radiat Ther Oncol. Basel, Karger, 1989, vol 23, pp 323–337

Bladder, Testicle, and Prostate Irradiation Injury

A. Robert Kagan[1]

University of California, Department of Oncology, Kaiser Permanente Hospital, Los Angeles, Calif., USA

If you make a mistake, make a new one each time!

Bladder

We have chosen to explore severe radiation injury, rather than *all* injury, as a marker of tolerance[1]. We would propose that mild radiation injury is too variable and subjective, depending weakly, if at all, on dose-time relationships. If a dose-time relationship exists, we think it will be for severe injury. In practice, if a radiation therapist has *one* patient who is severely injured sufficiently to require surgery, it may seriously erode his medical stature. The patient is presented and discussed at multiple subspecialty meetings in the hospital; and even if surgery is successful, usually the quality of life is poor. Severe morbidity (2 to 4%) for each pelvic organ may be a potential disaster amongst unsympathetic colleagues. The possibility that doses causing a 2–4% injury per organ may be necessary to cure the greatest number of cancers must be contemplated by all of us, but is not the subject of this paper.

In many series, a *predictable* injury rate for a *single* organ, such as the bladder, does not begin before the dose-time level at which 15% injury occurs. For the bladder, for example, patients who sustain injury at the dose-time level below the 15% injury point do so in a sporadic fashion. We think that the 15% injury rate is excessive for early disease, although it may be allowable for irradiation of advanced cancer. In our practice in early disease, we treat to the dose which indicates a threshold for injury of 2–4%. For more advanced disease, we would consider treating to the dose which causes 10–15% injury.

[1] I am grateful to Dr. Brace Hintz for his additions and corrections.

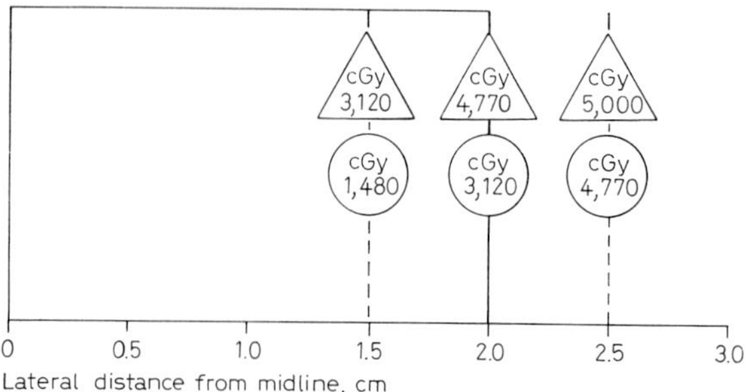

Fig. 1. Effect of misplacement of midline block on delivered dose (5,000 cGy AP/PA pelvis, midplane depth 10 cm, 4-cm midline block). Shifts in the midline block can alter the dose to point A from external beam radiations by 10% (7–14%). Circles represent ideal placement of the midline block; triangles show midline block misplaced by 0.5 cm. Contributed by Mr. John Bellotti.

Long-term bladder symptomatology following radiation therapy for cervical carcinoma may be more frequent than realized [2]. The recorded evidence of serious radiation injury to the bladder depends on whether the *denominator* is the *initial* number of patients or *surviving* patients. For groups of patients with predominantly early cancers wherein survival is 70%, little change in incidence occurs; in advanced stages, where the survival is less than 50%, the incidence will depend largely on which denominator is chosen.

Overall, the percentage of serious radiation injury to patients irradiated for pelvic neoplasms is 10%, and about one-third of these will undergo an operative procedure. The organs injured depend on the dose of external radiations, and whether curietherapy is used. Although ureteral and urethral injuries occur, most of these occur in concert with bladder injury which may share morbidity with rectum, rectosigmoid, and small intestine [3]. The percent of bladder injury *alone*, to which the question of normal tissue tolerance must be addressed, is small, 2–4%. The most satisfactory grading system for injury, for us, depends on full recovery or not, and if irreparably injured, whether a surgical procedure was initiated or not [4]. Unfortunately for us, the Gynecologic Oncology Group, Radiation Therapy Oncology Group, and European Organization for Research on Treatment of Cancer grading systems leave much room for subjectivity and ambiguity. Severe injury for Gynecologic Oncology Group, Radiation Therapy Oncology Group, and European Organization for Research on Treatment of Cancer does not necessarily mean an operative procedure, which to us is the most objective indication of sever-

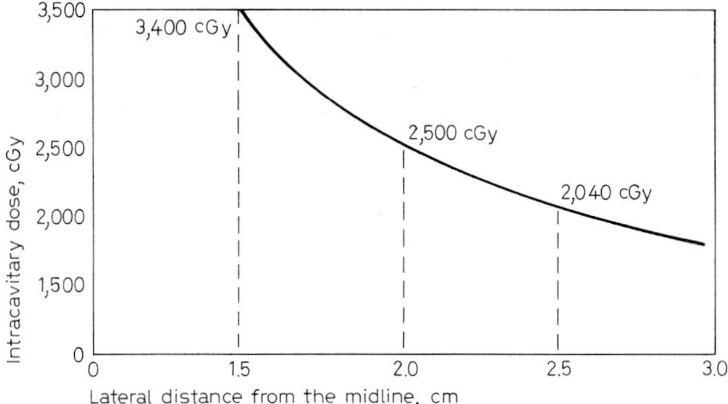

Fig. 2. Intracavitary dose profile (Fletcher tandem and ovoids, 0.5-cm changes in the cesium position can change the dose by 20%–36%). Contributed by Mr. John Bellotti.

ity. We will try to keep you, the reader, aware of the grading system being used.

Neither point A nor the dose to the posterior Foley catheter are *good* predictors of radiation injury to the bladder. Which portions of the bladder receive the largest dose (the maximum bladder dose may *not* be in the midline), the position(s) of the patient during curietherapy, accuracy of the placement of the midline shield when used, and more than one intracavitary application may all lead to hot spots in some patients and cancel out potential hot spots in others, without our awareness of the changes. With intracavitary curietherapy, a difference of 0.5 cm at 2 cm lateral to the cervix can *easily* amount to a difference of 1,000 rad, and most investigators agree that the difference between injury and noninjury to the bladder with external irradiation combined with curietherapy is only *500 rad*. Theoretically, the most accurate dose data to the bladder should be in patients with external irradiation, one intracavitary application, no midline shield, and no parametrial boost (figs. 1, 2).

The applicator is important. Mini ovoids, tandem and plaque, and a protruding source without ovoids are all accepted treatment techniques, but the internal shielding protecting the bladder is *missing*. Internal shielding which is not accounted for in computer programs may, if in proper alignment, reduce bladder doses by as much as 10% for radium or 20% for cesium (table I). Probe measurements by virtue of the size of the probe record integral doses, not peak doses. Peak doses may be missed if the computer printout is not in the plane of the peak dose.

Orton and Wolf-Rosenblum [5] reported 410 treated stage II_B–III

Table I. Effect of shielding in colpostats on bladder dose (4 mm Tungsten)

Isotope	Percent dose reduction	
	2 mm above cervical os	8 mm below cervical os
Cesium	27	34
Iridium	43	55
Radium/cobalt	19	25

Dose reduction to the bladder that can be obtained with 4 mm tungsten filtration in the colpostats. *The dose reduction is not taken into account in the computer printout.* The percent contribution to the bladder dose at a point 8 mm below the cervical os from the colpostats is 70% and 2 mm above the cervical os is 54%. Thus, the closer the bladder is to the colpostats, the more significant is the dose reduction from the colpostat with filtration. For cesium, the dose reduction is 50%, i.e. 70–34% 8 mm below the os and 54–27% 2 mm above the os. These generalizations apply only when the bladder is midway between the colpostats (contributed by Dr. Art Olch).

Table II. Cancer of the cervix irradiation regimes [6]

	Technique I	Technique II	Technique III (recommended for early lesions)
Whole pelvis, rad	6,000	6,000	5,000
Midline shield	1/3	2/3	3/5
Curietherapy, mgh	6,000	8,000	2,000–6,000 for 1–3 linear sources

patients with carcinoma of the cervix; 156 were alive at 5 years, 48 had moderate to severe complications, and 33 were evaluable. Complications were coded as: 2 = necrosis, stenosis, ulcer; 3 = bladder fistula, colostomy for rectal stenosis, and 4 = rectal fistula. Bladder complications were, in general, not as severe as rectal complications. A 10% complication rate, including all three grades of bladder injury, was noted at a Time Dose Fractionation Factor (TDF[2]) of 150. A TDF of 170 is 5,000 rad in 6 weeks TDF (80) plus 4,500 gamma rad at 60 rad TDF (90), and a TDF of 152 is 5,000 rad in 6 weeks TDF (80) plus 3,600 rad at 60 rad TDF (72).

Perez [6] prefers to maximize the central shield in early cancer (stages I and II_A) of the cervix. 7,200 combined rad to point A may be delivered by the techniques shown in table II. In technique II, compared to technique I, 2,000 less rad is delivered to the bladder. Perez [6] evaluated 785

[2] $\text{TDF} = \text{Numbers of fractions} \times \text{daily dose}^{1.538} \times \left(\frac{\text{time in days}}{\text{number of fractions}}\right)^{0.169} \times 10^{-3}.$

Table III. Cancer of the cervix – dose and complications [6]

Number of patients	Combined dose to bladder rad	Grade 2 and 3 complications %
199	6,000 and below	2
457	7,000–8,000	4
125	8,000–9,000	12
37	9,000>–10,000+	8

patients, 50% of whom were stages I and II_A. Grade 2 complications, cystitis, ureteral stricture and incontinence, were noted in 16 patients (4 in I and II_A). Grade 3 complications of cystitis, ulcer, fistula, ureteral stricture and miscellaneous were noted in 25 (12 in I and II_A). Overall, a 3–4% incidence of grade 2–3 complication was found unrelated to dose (table III). Perez [6] concluded that bladder tolerance occurred with combined doses of 7,500–8,000 rad.

Crook et al. [7] studied 348 patients with cervical carcinoma, 50% were treated by tandem and protruding sources. Fourteen of 348 (4%) had bladder complications. Two patients had grade 3 reactions consisting of death or fistula requiring surgery. The threshold dose was 7,500 combined rad. Eleven patients needed constant medical treatment (grade 2). The threshold combined dose was 5,900 rad.

Pourquier et al. [8] investigated 79 urinary complications in 624 patients for a complication rate of 2%. These authors used external beam, two cesium applications, and parametrial boost in many of their patients. Grade 3 complications consisted of hemorrhagic bladder mucosa and decreased bladder capacity. Grade 4 complications consisted of disabling symptoms, fistula, or ureteral stenosis. The conclusions of Pourquier et al. [8] are somewhat difficult to memorize, since these authors believe that the threshold dose required to cause complications cannot be defined as a single number. Nine patients had grade 3 and 4 complications, and their doses are as shown in table IV. Evaluating grades 1–4 bladder complications together, a 25% complication rate occurs at a combined dose of 7,500 rad (table V). In general [8], complications are associated if a large portion of one's treatment is curietherapy or if one's external beam doses approach 6,500–7,000 rad. Both of these conditions Pourquier et al. [8] admit, tend to occur with the more advanced stages.

It appears that a combined dose of 7,500 rad and greater is *above* bladder tolerance. Hunter et al. [9] understand the problems of dose determination in the bladder during irradiation for cancer of the cervix.

These authors suggest that the use of intracavitary transvesical ultrasound and simultaneous radiography will give a more accurate anatomy of the bladder and, therefore, result in a more accurate dose determination. These findings indicate a lower threshold dose than 7,500 combined rad. Hunter et al. [9] recommend 7,000 combined rad, the external beam

Table IV. Dose to the bladder in patients severely injured by irradiation [8]

Combined dose to the bladder rad	External beam rad	Curietherapy rad
6,100	4,000	2,100
6,900	4,300	2,600
8,800	4,200	4,600
8,400	4,900	3,500
8,500	5,000	3,500
9,000	4,800	4,200
9,000	5,000	4,000
9,000	5,000	4,000
9,000	5,000	4,000

Table V. Percent of patients with any bladder injury and dose [8]

Grades 1–4 bladder complications, combined dose	%
5,500–6,000	5
6,000–7,500	10
7,500–9,000	22
9,000 plus	48

Table VI. TDF approximating 108[1]

700 × 5 = 3,500	
520 × 8 = 4,160	
440 × 10 = 4,400	
400 × 12 = 4,800	
360 × 14 = 5,040	
300 × 18 = 5,400	
275 × 20 = 5,500	
230 × 28 = 6,440	
200 × 35 = 7,000	
180 × 40 = 7,200	
170 × 40 = 6,800	
150 × 40 = 6,000	(TDF 85)

[1] Elimination of 2–5 fractions will result in a TDF of 85.

being 4,600 rad in 23 fractions with 2,400 rad at 80 rad/h as bladder tolerance. Kagan et al. [4] are in agreement with the lower threshold dose: 5,000 rad in 25 fractions external beam (TDF 80) plus 1,800 rad delivered at 43 rad/h (TDF 31) for a total of 7,000 rad or a TDF of 111. Bladder complications necessitating surgery at this dose are 5% in surviving patients.

In the management of cancer of the bladder and prostate, external beam irradiation alone is used. Duncan and Quilty [10] and Quilty et al. [11] reported 963 patients treated with a 10 × 10 field formed by two posterior obliques and one anterior port. One hundred and two patients suffered complications, of which 90 were bladder only, with 2 cystectomies, 2 urinary diversions and 4 deaths giving a grade 2–4 (grade 2 = severe frequency, dysuria, hematuria and reduction in bladder capacity; grade 3 = contracted bladder, severe hemorrhage, cystitis; grad 4 = death related to irradiation injury) bladder complication rate of 10% and an operative complication rate of 1%. Duncan [10] concludes that 5,500 rad, 20 fractions daily dose 275, for a TDF of 108 is the level where maximum cure rate can be obtained with a grade 3–4 complication rate of 20%. In a study designed to establish maximum cure at minimum morbidity, Duncan and Quilty [10] treated patients with regimens of 5,750, 5,250, and 5,000 rad at 20 fractions, 5 equal fractions per week. He concluded that 5,500 rad at 20 fractions of 275, TDF 108, was the optimum dose and has been using this regimen since 1975. In his series, a TDF [11] of 108 gave a grade 3–4 morbidity of 20% which may be considered too high, but in deference to Duncan's extensive experience, we add the list of TDF approximating 108 (table VI). Nussbaum et al. [12] found tolerance at 10–20% injury to be a TDF of 111, but suggested that after recent major surgery, the dose should be reduced to a TDF of 84, and added, regarding biological equivalent doses, that one should not deviate much from 180–250 rad/fraction/day. To avoid morbidity, Nussbaum et al. [12], Duncan and Quilty [10], and Quilty et al. [11] agree, means keeping to a TDF of 85.

Sack et al. [13] reported on 204 patients with adenocarcinoma of the prostate treated at 900–1,000 rad/week in five equal fractions to 4,400–5,000 rad with large opposed fields, rest, and then a rotation boost; 92 patients received 6,500 rad or greater. Fifteen patients suffered from chronic cystitis, stricture, incontinence, or fibrosis of the bladder or urethra. Four severe complications occurred necessitating a bypass or cystectomy. Therefore, 7% of the patients needed constant medical supervision, and 2% demanded surgery; these are applicable percentages to grade 1 wherein the 5-year survival is 80%, but the complication rate may be higher in grade 3 patients whose survival at 5 years is 40%.

Pilepich et al. [14] writing on the Radiation Therapy Oncology Group experience in 453 patients with adenocarcinoma of the prostate found no dose response for genitourinary morbidity; 15% primarily nonoperative injuries consisting of cystitis, hematuria, and stricture occurred at doses of 6,250 to 7,000 rad. A major surgical intervention or prolonged hospitalization was the outcome in 2 patients. Rounsaville et al. [15] reported 251 patients treated for adenocarcinoma of the prostate 6,500–7,500 rad range with a minimum follow-up of 3 years. Four patients had severe genitourinary complications consisting of fistula or fatal sepsis for a 3% serious complication rate in patients *surviving* 5 years. Complications were more frequent when one port of opposed ports was treated per day.

Yu et al. [13] reviewed a series of 356 patients with carcinoma of the bladder treated with 60–66 Gy over 6–7 weeks. After 45–50 Gy, a reduced bladder 10 × 10 cm port was employed by 360° rotation. Disease-free survival at 5 years was 9–31%, depending on stage. Excluding 47 salvage cystectomy patients, 7 patients of 309 (2%) had serious complications comprising of cystitis requiring transfusions or cystectomy and contracted bladder.

Many radiation oncologists get the opportunity to treat cancer of the bladder only after this organ has been 'flogged' by many transurethral resections or a partial cystectomy, or by intravesical chemotherapy or immunotherapy. In this setting, there is no or little ideal bladder mucosa and thus little organ reserve for any added physical injury; clearly, the tolerance dose in this situation is less. In fact, curative doses may never be reached, and the treating physician must be satisfied with 5,000 rad in 25 fractions. Palliation with 2,000 rad in 5 fractions may even be too intense.

Antonakopoulos et al. [16] studied the pathology of the bladder wall after 30 biopsies of the bladder wall in 25 patients. All tissues of the bladder were damaged to some degree after irradiation. Fourteen of the 30 biopsies had 3+ changes. The most common severe change was a fibrosis which was most prevalent around the blood vessels and associated with collagen, and occurred at doses of 6,000 rad or greater. Fibrosis was not confined to the lamina propria, but extended *throughout* the bladder wall. Moderate to severe damage to the endothelial cells of blood vessels was observed in all but 3 patients. Antonakopoulos et al. [16] concluded that 'primary damage to the endothelial cells of the blood vessels leads to a stasis and ischemia, that permanent alteration and stimulation of fibroblasts is the underlying cause of the fibrosis, and that there is damage and loss of individual muscle cells.'

In summary, using external beam and curietherapy, the threshold is a combined dose of 6,500 rads at which *sporadic* injury occurs. Between 7,500 and 8,000 rad, a *predictable* injury of 20% can be expected. In patients with cancer of the bladder and prostate, a predictable injury of 10% begins to occur at 6,000 rad. After multiple transurethral resections of the prostate or of the bladder or bulky tumor compromising bladder function, normal bladder tolerance is often decreased. Weekly dose rates exceeding 1,000 rad or large fractions will necessitate total doses below 6,000 rad.

Testicle

The testicle is an exquisitely radiosensitive organ. With modern super-voltage equipment the dose 2.5–3 cm outside the light port is 10% and at 5 cm is less than 1%; *but* only 100 rad received by the testicle can result in azoospermia for 1 year, and as little as 15 rad will depress spermatogenesis for over 2 months [17–19]. In a large series [20] of cancer patients who received radiation therapy directed below the diaphragm with the intent of excluding the testicle(s), fertility was depressed by 25%. Parenthetically this doubled when chemotherapy was added [20]. Gritz et al. [21] evaluating 88 long-term survivors of cancer (39 seminoma, 49 carcinoma) of the testicle noted that only 1% had severe erectile dysfunction before the diagnosis, and 6% after the treatment at the time of interview.

Erectile dysfunction has been reported in two-thirds of men irradiated for cancer of the prostate [22]. Studies such as these must be corrected for hypertension, diabetes mellitus, hypercholesterolemia, and cigarette smoking, all of which predispose to impotency. Our experience with patients referred for radiation therapy for cancer of the prostate is that 50%, prior to treatment, are impotent or nearly so. Of the 50% that remain, over half have had some major decrease in potency over the preceding years. The remaining 25% of the patients remain sexually active, but most have to cope with a 'dry' or small ejaculation.

Much less than 10% of the tumor dose should reach the testicle from any port designed for irradiating patients with cancer which in practical terms may be translated as shown in table VII. At dosages of 400–600 rad given in a single fraction, germinal epithelium, as demonstrated by serial biopsy, will begin to reappear by 8 months, but complete recovery of the spermatogonia takes 5 or more years [19]. Some sperm may appear in the semen by 24 months; however, quality and quantity for fertilization may take 5–7 years. Spermatogonal failure and recovery after radiation can be predicted by an elevated and then declining level of follicle-stimulating hormone. This is not inhibited by testosterone; its regulation is by a hormone, inhibin, which depends on the integrity of spermatogonia B which

Table VII. Dose to unshielded testicle after irradiation to primary site

Primary site	Tumor dose rad	10% [1] dose to the testicle in 15–33 fractions rad
Hodgkin's lymphoma	4,000	400
Wilms' tumor	3,000	300
Seminoma	3,000	300
Prostate	6,600	660
Rectum	5,000	500

[1] Measured doses to the testicle are 3–5% of the tumor dose depending on size of port and whether fields are stationary or rotation. Added shielding against the direct beam and testicular cups to reduce scatter from the thighs can reduce the dose to less than 1% [Chan, personal commun.].

is the radiosensitive cell in the testis. In two groups of cancer patients that have been most widely studied, those with Hodgkin's disease and testicular tumors, subfertile sperm counts have been observed *before* any treatment, as demonstrated by attempts at cryopreservation [23, 24]. It is unfair, in our opinion, that radiation is always blamed for impotency or infertility when the cancer itself or other factors such as hypertensive medication or birth control measures are ignored, even in more complex epidemiological studies. The well-known sensitivity of the testicle to low doses of radiation, even though recovery eventually occurs, seems to be the main reason for incriminating radiation therapy as the sole cause for permanent sterility.

Alkylating agents, such as nitrogen mustard and procarbazine and high-dose cyclophosphamide used in bone marrow transplantation of patients with aplastic anemia, have produced permanent oligozoospermia without hypotestosteronemia. All patients who receive prednisone, vincristine, methotrexate and 6-mercaptopurine develop reversible oligozoospermia [18, 25]. In most bone marrow transplant patients undergoing irradiation of 7–10 Gy plus intensive chemotherapy, azoospermia and elevated levels of follicle-stimulating hormone are common. Failure to enter puberty because of inadequate levels of testosterone can be treated with androgen [26, 27]. Failure to enter male puberty, which may occur in patients undergoing bone marrow transplantation, results from lack of testosterone. It is well accepted that radiations can destroy seminiferous spermatogenesis, the exocrine function of the testicle; but completely destroying the endocrine function of Leydig cells to secrete testosterone is not known in the adult. On the contrary, in adult patients libido may be intact despite the presence of azoospermia. Recent studies [28] of patients after irradiation for cancer of the prostate have demonstrated decreased levels (as much as a 50% decrease of baseline) of testosterone and elevated gonadotrophin levels which have returned to pretreatment levels within 18 months. The *highest* estimated dose to the testicles after irradiation for carcinoma of the prostate in this study would approximate 1,000 rad in 30 fractions [28].

In the prepubertal leukemic male in complete remission, the testicle has been given 24 Gy in 12 fractions as an elective measure to prevent leukemic relapse in the testicle, which is thought to be a sanctuary site. These patients may produce enough testosterone to enter puberty. (The adrenal gland may secrete enough testosterone to initiate puberty, i.e. phallic development and hair growth. However, in practice, if the pace of pubertal development is too slow, then testosterone is usually given.) However, children who relapse in the testicles and who receive 24 Gy in 12 fractions for active leukemia may not have sufficient testosterone to enter puberty [29]. Since the leukemic cells are found in the interstitium and not in the seminiferous tubules, we would propose that the leukemic cells are the prime cause for the hypotestosterone state. For completeness, children who have received 2,400 rad in 12 fractions to the pituitary-hypothalamus as a part of elective brain irradiation for leukemia, do not show deficits in gonadotrophic hormones [30].

Concerning offspring of long-term survivors, Mulvihill and Byrne [22] collected data from 719 male and female cancer survivors with 1,515 pregnancies: 4% had major birth defects, 7% were electively aborted, and 13% underwent spontaneous abortions. These percentage rates are no greater than those of a 'normal' population. This large series of pregnancies in and by survivors of cancer consists of patients with adolescent and childhood cancer which includes Hodgkin's disease, neuroblastoma, Wilms' tumor, leukemia, trophoblastic disease, and malignancy developing in pregnancy. Management of these patients usually consisted of a conglomeration of radiation and chemotherapy.

In summary, adults who received radiations 'nearby' to the testicles as defined as 10% of the tumor dose (a very high estimate) may undergo oligospermia with recovery at 5 years or recovery at 1 year with smaller doses. In children receiving 20 Gy of fractionated radiations or patients treated with alkylating drugs, permanent oligospermia should be anticipated. Inadequate levels of testosterone may be found in survivors of total body irradiation and bone marrow transplantation, as well as those irradiated for testicular leukemia. Impotency depends on many factors, most of which interact; implicating radiations as the sole cause is not justified in our present state of knowledge.

Prostate

The radiosensitivity of the normal prostate gland has not been studied vigorously which means that this part of the discussion is especially susceptible to vague opinions, shaky judgments, and more than just a few wild guesses. In our patients, having had transperineal biopsies only, who have been irradiated for adenocarcinoma of the prostate and who are sexually active, dry or almost dry ejaculations are common following 6,600–7,400 rad at 800 rad, 4 fractions/week. This observation may be documented 3 months after irradiation. Exactly when during the course of radiation the prostate gland begins to dry up, we do not know. In a series of 40 patients who were irradiated for adenocarcinoma of the prostate, 30 of whom received 7,000–7,500 rad in 7–8 weeks and 10 patients who received radiations to the prostate for other pelvic cancers, atrophy of glandular epithelium as evidenced by the disappearance of nonneoplastic prostate glands was noted as the single hallmark of radiation injury [32]. This disappearance of glandular epithelium has also been observed with 4,000 rad preoperative irradiation for cancer of the bladder. Gill et al. [33] noted severe changes in the prostate after 3,000 rad in 3 weeks, consisting of atrophy of normal glands. Also noted was disruption of the epithelium of the vas deferens and seminal vesicles.

Strictures are increased fourfold and incontinence threefold following a transurethral resection [34–37]. Urethral stricture secondary to gonorrheal urethritis necessitating regular dilatation influences us to recommend treatment other than irradiation for curable lesions. Postirradiation strictures are often lengthy and more difficult to correct surgically than postgonorrheal strictures. The urethra itself may be assumed to be quite radioresistant, since injury from intraluminal curietherapy (radium), commonly applied in the past, did not produce excessive morbidity, as did intracavitary curietherapy of the bladder. Therefore, operative procedures such as transurethral resection must, to a large degree, cause the necessary ischemic vascular damage and functional cell injury that impedes recovery after radiations.

As expected, histologic evidence of significant radiation injury occurs after ^{125}iodine implantation; doses of 8,000 rad in 300 days, 1 cm outside the perimeter of the seeds, are usual [34]; however, much larger doses occur in the center of the gland. One should be very cautious when interpreting tumor doses from curietherapy without seeing the isodose curves. For example, the 100% isodose line describing doses of 9,000–15,000 rad with ^{198}Au in 14 days may not encompass the entire gland, but merely the lobe or nodule. In this context, interpretation of tolerance is not meaningful, since a portion of the prostate gland has received a much lower dose.

To summarize, normal prostate epithelium is very radiosensitive to 3,000 rad in 3 weeks. Recovery after this dose is undetermined, but after 6,600 rad, no recovery of normal glandular epithelium may be anticipated.

References

1 Barendsen, G. W.: Dose fractionation, dose rate and iso-effect relationships for normal tissue responses. Int J. Radiat. Oncol. Biol. Phys. 1982; *8:* 1981–1997.

2 Parkin, D. E.; Davis, J. A.; Symonds, R. P.: Long-term bladder symptomatology following radiotherapy for cervical carcinoma. Radiother. Oncol. 1987; *9:* 195–199.

3 Kontturi, M.; Kauppila, A.: Ureteric complications following treatment of gynaecological cancer. Ann. Chir. Gynaecol. 1982; *71:* 232–238.

4 Kagan, A. R.; Nussbaum, H.; Gilbert, H., et al.: A new staging system for irradiation injuries following treatment for cancer of the cervix uteri. Gynecol. Oncol. 1979; *7:* 166–175.

5 Orton, C. G.; Wolf-Rosenblum, S.: Dose dependence of complication rates in cervix cancer radiotherapy. Int. J. Radiat. Oncol. Biol. Phys. 1986; *12:* 37–44.

6 Perez, C. A.: Carcinoma of the uterine cervix; in Perez, C. A.; Brady, L. W. (eds): Principles and Practice of Radiation Oncology. Philadelphia, Lippincott, 1987, pp 919–955.

7 Crook, J. M.; Esche, B. A.; Chaplain, G., et al.: Dose-volume analysis and the prevention of radiation sequelae in cervical cancer. Radiother. Oncol. 1987; *8:* 321–332.

8 Pourquier, H.; Delard, R.; Achille, E., et al.: A quantified approach to the analysis and prevention of urinary complications in radiotherapeutic treatment of cancer of the cervix. Int. J. Radiat. Oncol. Biol. Phys. 1987; *13:* 1025–1033.

9 Hunter, R. D.; Wong, F.; Moore, C., et al.: Bladder base dosage in patients undergoing intracavitary therapy. Radiother. Oncol. 1986; *7:* 189–197.

10 Duncan, W.; Quilty, P. M.: The results of 936 patients with transitional cell carcinoma of the urinary bladder primarily treated by radical megavoltage X-ray therapy. Radiother. Oncol. 1986; *7:* 299–310.

11 Quilty, P. M.; Duncan, W.; Kerr, G. R.: Results of a randomised study to evaluate influence of dose on morbidity in radiotherapy for bladder cancer. Clin. Radiol. 1985; *36:* 615–618.

12 Nussbaum, H.; Kagan, A. R.; Wollin, M., et al.: Guidelines for radiation injury to bowel and bladder from external irradiation alone. Cancer Clin. Trials 1981; *4:* 295–299.

13 Sack, H.; Nosbuesch, Stuetzer, H.: Radiotherapy of prostate carcinoma. Results of treatment and complications. Radiother. Oncol. 1987; *10:* 7–15.

14 Pilepich, M. V.; Asbell, S. O.; Krall, J. M., et al.: Correlation of radiotherapeutic parameters and treatment related morbidity. Analysis of RTOG study 77–06. Int. J. Radiat. Oncol. Biol. Phys. 1987; *13:* 1007–1012.

15 Rounsaville, M. C.; Green, J. P.; Vaeth, J. M., et al.: Prostatic carcinoma. Limited field irradiation. Int. J. Radiat. Oncol. Biol. Phys. 1987; *13:* 1013–1020.

16 Antonakopoulos, G. N.; Nicks, R. M.; Berry R. J.: The subcellular basis of damage to the human urinary bladder induced by irradiation. J. Pathol. 1984; *143:* 103–116.

17 Clifton, D. K.; Bremner, W. J.: The effect of testicular X-irradiation on spermatogenesis in man. J. Androl. 1983; *4:* 387–392.

18 Meistrich, M. L.: Relationship between spermatogonial stem cell survival and testis function after cytotoxic therapy. Br. J. Cancer 1968; *53:* 89–101.

19 Rowley, M. J.; Leach, D. R.; Warner, G. A., et al.: Effect of graded doses of ionizing radiation on the human testis. Radiat. Res. 1974; *59:* 665–678.

20 Bryne, J.; Mulvihill, J. J.; Myers, M. H., et al.: Effects of treatment on fertility in long-term survivors of childhood or adolescent cancer. N. Engl. J. Med. 1987; *317:* 1315–1321.

21 Gritx, E. R.; Wellisch, D. K.; Landsverk, J. A.: Psychosocial sequelae in long-term survivors of testicular cancer. Psychosoc. Oncol., in press.

22 Goldstein, I.; Feldman, M. I.; Deckers, P. M.: Radiation-associated impotence. JAMA 1984; *251:* 903–910.

23 Brenner, J.; Vugrin, D.; Whitmore, W. F. Jr.: Effect of treatment on fertility and sexual function in males with metastatic nonseminomatous germ cell tumors of testis. Am. J. Clin. Oncol. 1985; *8:* 178–182.

24 White, R. D.; Krane, R. J.: Iatrogenic causes of infertility; in White, R. D. (ed): International Aspects of Male Infertility. Baltimore, Williams & Wilkins, 1982, pp 174–185.

25 Clarke, S. J.; Resnick, M. I.: Infertility following radiation and chemotherapy. Urol. Clin. North Am. 1978; *5:* 531–535.

26 Leiper, A. D.; Grant, D. B.; Chessels, J. M.: Gonadal function after testicular radiation for acute lymphoblastic leukaemia. Arch. Dis. Child 1986; *61:* 53–56.

27 Sklar, C. A.; Ramsay, N. K. C.: Endocrine dysfunction after successful bone marrow transplantation; in Nesbit, M. E. Jr. (ed): Clinics in Oncology. London, Saunders, 1985, vol 4, No 2, pp 345–352.

28 Bergman, B.; Dambeer, J. E.; Littbrand B., et al.: Sexual function in prostatic cancer patients treated with radiotherapy, orchiectomy or oestrogens. Br. J. Urol. 1984; *56:* 64–69.

29 Shalet, S. M.; Horner, A.; Ahmed, S. R., et al.: Leydig cell damage after testicular irradiation for lymphoblastic leukaemia. Med. Pediatr. Oncol. 1985; *13:* 65–68.

30 Shalet, S. M.: The effects of cancer treatment on growth and sexual development; in Nesbit, M. E. Jr. (ed): Clinics in Oncology. London, Saunders, 1985, vol 4, No 2, pp 223–238.

31 Mulvihill, J. J.; Byrne, J.: Offspring of long-term survivors of childhood cancer; in Nesbit, M. E. Jr. (ed): Clinics in Oncology. London, Saunders, 1985, vol 4, No 2, pp 333–343.

32 Bostwick, D. G.; Egbert, B. M.; Fajardo, L. F.: Radiation injury of the normal and neoplastic prostate. Am. J. Surg. Pathol. 1982; *6:* 541–551.

33 Gill, W. B.; Schoenberg, H. W.; Banno, J. J., et al.: Sandwich radiotherapy (3,000 and 4,500 rad) around radical retropubic prostatectomy for stage C prostatic carcinoma. Urology 1980; *16:* 470–475.

34 Green, N.; Goldberg, H.: Severe rectal injury following radiation for prostatic cancer. J. Urol. 1984; *131:* 701.

35 Jacobson, G. M.; Smith, J. A. Jr.; Stewart, J. R.: Postoperative radiation therapy for pathologic stage C prostate cancer. Int. J. Radiat. Oncol. Biol. Phys. 1987; *13:* 1021–1024.

36 Kaufman, J. J.; Smith, R. B.; Raz, S.: Radiation therapy in carcinoma of the prostate: A contributing cause of urinary incontinence. J. Urol. 1984; *132:* 998–999.

37 Perez, C. A.; Walz, B. T.: Irradiation of carcinoma of the prostate localized to the pelvis. Analysis of tumor response and prognosis. Int. J. Radiat. Oncol. Biol. Phys. 1980; *6:* 923.

38 Schellhammer, P. F.; Ladaga, L. E.; El-Mahdi, A.: Histological characteristics of prostatic biopsies after ^{125}iodine implantation. J. Urol. 1980; *123:* 700–705.

39 Yu, W. S.; Sagerman, R. H.; Chung, C. T., et al.: Bladder carcinoma. Experience with radical and preoperative radiotherapy in 421 patients. Cancer 1985; *56:* 1293–1299.

A. Robert Kagan, MD; Department of Radiation Oncology,
Kaiser Permanente Hospital, Los Angeles, CA 90027 (USA)

Vaeth JM, Meyer JL (eds): Radiation Tolerance of Normal Tissues.
Front Radiat Ther Oncol. Basel, Karger, 1989, vol 23, pp 338–340

Discussion

Dr. Tralins: Dr. Vaeth, in today's climate where coronary artery bypass surgery is quite common, is there any concern from a radiation therapeutic standpoint regarding damage?

Dr. Vaeth: I wouldn't know how to answer that. Obviously you have an answer in mind. What do you think?

Dr. Tralins: Very often we see patients who require lung irradiation, for, e.g., lung carcinoma, and these are patients who've had multiple surgeries including coronary artery surgery. Often they can't undergo cancer surgery. We're called upon to treat these people. I have been treating more and more of these types of patients, I guess without much concern, and I personally have not seen any complications from it. I was wondering if anyone on the panel or in the audience cares to comment on it.

Dr. Vaeth: Without an answer from the audience, and since you're talking about heart, I would like to comment on Bob Stewart's paper, because when I finished my training, I cast aside the dose of 1,000 rad a week being holy and started irradiating patients, particularly with large fields, with lesser doses, e.g., 900 rad/week in four or five fractions. We have never had cardiac difficulties. I presented a paper ages ago about 20 patients studying them with serial ECGs before, during, and after heart irradiation and with SGOT studies. We found no cardiac damage in those patients.

Dr. Vaeth: A question about prostate and impotence. As radiation oncologists, we are constantly having to defend external beam radiation therapy on prostate cancer versus radioactive implants. Now, a 'new' operation where they spare a sympathetic nerve on the posterior prostate (and call it cancer surgery), and we're having to defend against this inadequate operation. It's having to be defended on the basis of impotence. Recently, I came across very interesting urological data from the University of California. A urologist, Dr. Finkel, has written some very startling data that we as irradiation therapists should keep in mind. His data show that 60% of the men over 65 and nearing 70 years are impotent. These are healthy men. If the man has any urological disorder, and certainly I would say prostate cancer is an urological disorder, this moves up to 75%. Throw into the equation all the things that Dr. Kagen was talking about: hypertension, medications, and other illnesses along with this. What do you expect after radiation therapy, or anything, for that matter? Riding a MUNI bus in San Francisco, you're going to be impotent when you get off the bus, if you fall into that category. I think we should be getting back to reality and what we're doing in treating prostate cancer.

Dr. Pense: Dr. Kagen, first, I think it will help us in our interviewing technique if we don't use this modern terminology of being sexually active. I don't really think that's very indicative of anything. It certainly doesn't let us separate out things like dry ejaculates. I think we should be more specific about what we're talking about. On the question of impotence, you've talked about dry ejaculate, and saying all irradiated men get dry ejaculate, are these people impotent after full-dose irradiation? In treating seminomas, do you think that most of this dose, as you're talking about, comes from internal scatter? You say if you used a transmission shield, you got rid of that? I didn't quite understand that.

Dr. Kagen: Yes. What you're doing is you're double-blocking the edge of the beam, the penumbra. In other words, 10% comes to the testicle, 50% is the light field, and 10% occurs about 3 cm outside (you're blocking that away), and 5 cm away it's about 1%. With regard to impotence, you won't be able to get these details by a questionnaire, at least I can't. We tried to get the exact detail you're talking about with a questionnaire, after the first questionnaire just outlined the general field, and the questionnaires were left in the room, not filled out. As a matter of fact, we had a few nice epithets on some of them, as to what we could do with them. If you start out with 100 men that are sexually active and give them external beam irradiation therapy, then 40% of them aren't sexually active anymore. What is a surprise to me is that when you ask these patients about intercourse, ejaculations, success, erections, and so forth, you find that 75% of them are on their way down anyway. 50% of them aren't sexually active, and 25% are sort of in their male climacteric. You're not starting out with 100 active men anyway.

Dr. Pense: You're saying we don't know the answer to the question of whether after giving 6,500 rad to the prostate of a person potency is lost?

Dr. Kagen: We don't know.

Moderator: Certainly you know of patients, whom you have treated to 6,500 rad, who are quite potent.

Dr. Vaeth: I want to support what Dr. Kagen was saying about the interview process. I interview my patients, husband and wife, together in my office, and I ask them very leading questions that are sometimes a little embarrassing to both of them about their sexual activity. Frequently, an elderly man, will smile at his wife and say 'Well, we just aren't interested in sex anymore', and she'll smile and say 'No'. Once you get the patient back in the examining room alone, he'll say 'You know, doctor, I did want to chat with you a little bit. You know, I haven't been interested in sex with my wife for the last year, and she isn't either, but I've, well, I hate to say this, but I sort of fool around a little bit, and I can do very well, and in fact I'm doing very well, but please don't tell my wife this.' Now, how the devil are you going to write that up as a sexual interview? Your first thing says he's impotent, and the second says he's a liar. How do you rate that? To conduct a valid sexual interview is a very difficult thing.

Vaeth JM, Meyer JL (eds): Radiation Tolerance of Normal Tissues.
Front Radiat Ther Oncol. Basel, Karger, 1989, vol 23, pp 341–348

Normal-Tissue Tolerance in the Irradiation of Female Breast

Bernard Pierquin, Laval Grimard, Ginette Marinello
Centre Hospitalo-Universitaire Henri-Mondor, Créteil, France

Aside from lactation, the breast does not serve any essential physiological function. It is, however, pivotal in our image of feminity and, therefore, breast conservation in the management of breast cancer is an important objective. It can be accomplished in the majority of tumors using relatively high doses which will impair lactation but provide satisfactory cosmetic results. Consequently, radiotherapy, with or without limited surgery, is the main modality in the conservative management of breast cancer.

The organs and tissues included in the treatment volume are the mammary gland itself, adipose tissue (especially in patients with large breasts and in postmenopausal patients), skin, muscles (especially pectoralis major), bones (ribs, clavicle, scapula, humerus), pleura, lungs, heart and pericardium, nervous tissue (brachial plexus, sympathetic nervous tissue, spinal cord in some techniques), and esophagus (in some techniques).

The doses absorbed by these different structures depend on the techniques used. We will first described the technique used at Henri-Mondor Hospital [4] which, with minor modifications, are applied in many centers. For external irradiation the patient lies supine with her head turned to the opposite side and the arm abducted to 90° on an armrest. Two tangential portals are used to treat the breast itself. They cover the entire breast and the chest wall. These beams are not parallel opposed, but angled superiorly to decrease lung irradiation. The angles are determined after a computerized dosimetric study of a transverse section of the chest obtained at the level of the nipple with conventional tomography or tomodensitometry (CT scan). Wedges are used if required to achieve dose optimization. The dose is prescribed to a reference isodose covering the medial and lateral borders of this target volume (fig. 1). We minimize the amount of lungs included and limit the skin dose, especially at the nipple, to 120% of the reference isodose. In a standard situation, with a

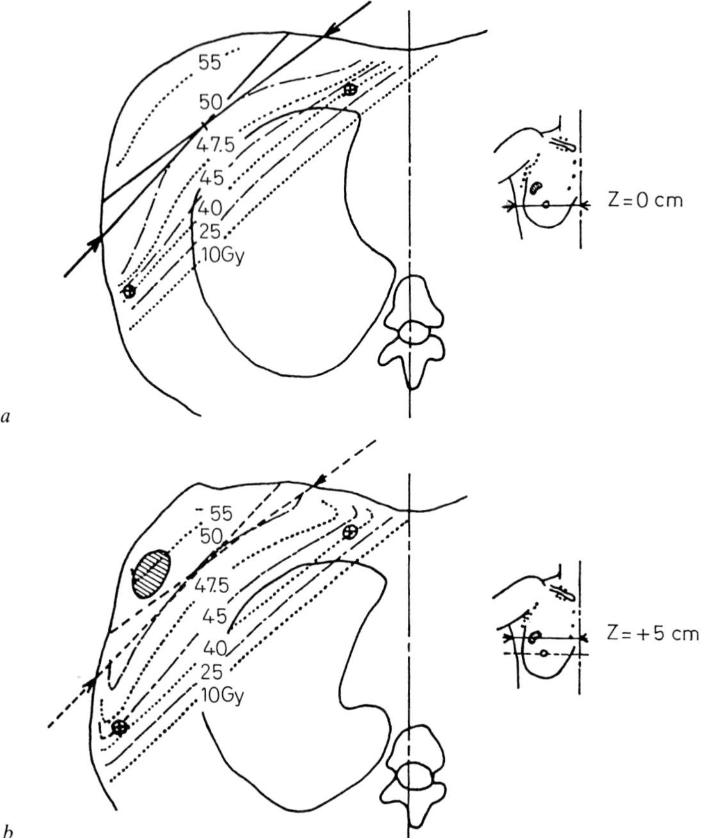

Fig. 1. Distribution of the dose at the nipple level *(a)* and at the tumor level *(b)*.

dose of 45 Gy prescribed at the reference isodose on the chest wall, we obtain around 50 Gy at the central axis and less than 55 Gy at the skin (nipple). At depth, the lung dose received can be important and frequently separate dosimetric studies are done above and below the nipple. In all cases a maximum thickness of 2.5 cm of lung can be included on the tangentials (taken from the 50% isodose). This is verified on port films.

The volume covered by the boost corresponds to the initial tumor volume and cannot be greater than 30% of the entire breast. The boost is given by an ^{192}Ir implant, and the dose is prescribed at the reference isodose corresponding to 85% of the basal dose rate according to the Paris System. The dose is 20 Gy for tumorectomized patients with a com-

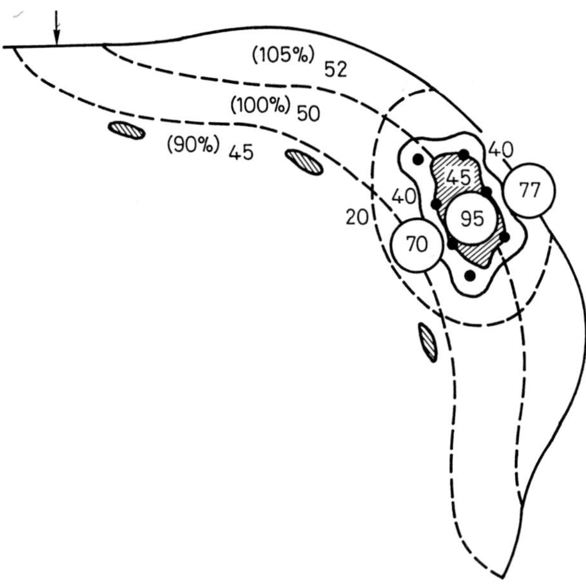

Fig. 2. Distribution of the dose. Basal irradiation (telecobalt) plus boost (^{192}Ir, 40 Gy).

plete excision and 35 Gy for residual tumors (with or without previous tumorectomy). The dose at the center of the target volume and at the level of the basal dose rate is 15–20% higher. For a reference isodose of 20 Gy, the dose at the center of the implant is 23–24 and 40–42 Gy when the dose prescribed is 35 Gy.

In summary, the entire mammary gland, taking into account the implant, receives a dose varying from 45 to less than 60 Gy. The tumor receives a dose varying from 70 to 75 Gy in patients with a satisfactory tumorectomy and from 85 to 95 Gy in patients without tumorectomy or in those with positive margins. The overdose or hyperdose sleeve surrounding the iridium wires is ignored – but not forgotten (fig. 2).

The lymph node bearing sites are irradiated by an anterior supraclavicular-axillary portal, a posterior axillary field to supplement the dose at midplane of the axilla, and an internal mammary field to cover the inferior internal mammary nodes. A dose of 45 Gy is given to these volumes, prescribed at 3 cm depth and midaxilla, which include ipisilateral ribs, pulmonary apex, shoulder, brachial plexus, and many muscles, the pectoralis major being the most important. The larynx and the humeral head are shielded. The anterior portals are angled 10–15° to avoid irradiating the spinal cord and most of the esophagus. The axilla is not treated if the patient had a negative axillary sampling (level I and II). For patients not having an axillary dissection, an electron boost of 24 Gy is given to the lower axilla, providing a total dose of 70 Gy. A direct portal is used. An electron boost of 15 Gy is given to the internal mammary chain systematically providing a total dose of 50–55 Gy to this node-bearing site.

^{60}Co or X-ray energies of 4–5 MV are used to treat these target volumes. The boosts are given with electrons of 10 and 13 MeV to cover a depth of 3–4 cm. We use a standard fractionation: 9 Gy/week in 5 fractions/week for the photons and 4 fractions/week for the electrons.

We will now present our observations, and those from other centers using the same techniques, on the effect of irradiation at 10 years and more on normal tissue. There is a moderate and diffuse sclerosis of the entire mammary gland which maintains an elastic consistency. Natural aging causes the untreated breast to fall, while the irradiated gland remains firm and gives a more youthful appearance: this appearance becomes evident after 10 years of follow-up. A few of our patients required cosmetic surgical repair of the nontreated breast. The skin appears normal. In the area of the boost, sclerosis is more pronounced, frequently this moderate fibrosis encompasses the volume covered by the reference isodose of the implantation. This area can be associated with skin changes: atrophy and the greater problem of telangiectasia which can be mild or diffuse. These radiation changes are directly proportionate to the total dose and the location of the implant volume in relation to the skin. In other words, the skin sequelae and telengiectasia in particular become more apparent as the radioactive lines, and particularly the overdose sleeve, approach the skin (fig. 3). Fat is an aggravating factor of radiation sclerosis. Using the same dose we found large and fatty breasts to incur more pronounced sequelae (diffuse edema, retracted skin, peau d'orange phenomenon and pseudoinflammatory episodes). It is possible that a more fragile and/or less abundant microvascular environment in these large breasts explains this greater radiosensitivity.

The other structures, including lung, pleura, bones, and nervous tissue, do not receive a dose above 45 Gy. Therefore, long-term radiation changes are minimal and free of major complications. The problems of matching the various fields with overlapping is well known, especially between the breast target volume and the lymph node bearing volume. The electron boost to the axilla and parasternal areas also potentiates the risk of exceeding normal-tissue tolerance. Some of the problems incurred include severe fibrosis at field junction, rib fractures, symptomatic pneumonitis, and parasternal fibrotic nodules.

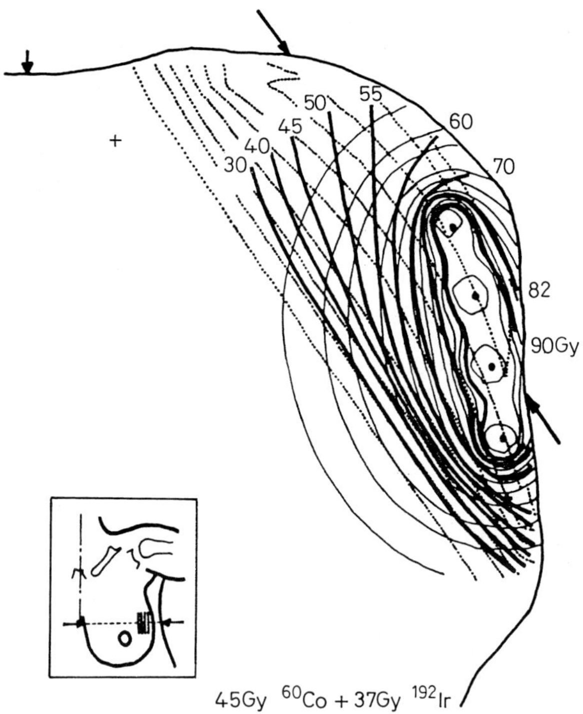

Fig. 3. Location of the implant volume (^{192}Ir) in relation to the skin.

Overall, the lesions caused by irradiation in a properly treated population of patients are minimal. The radiation sclerosis to the mammary gland does not cause any significant handicap. We frequently see some retraction of the pectoralis major muscle which decreases hyperabduction of the arm. This is the only noticeable limitation in the range of motion of the upper extremity. Physical therapy, wich does not cause excessive fatigue of scapular muscles, is indicated. Overzealous exercises are discouraged because of the possibility of severe myalgias and, rarely, a muscular rupture. Arm edema is rare without axillary dissection. Edema is found in 25–35% of the patients having an axillary sampling followed by 45 Gy. Neuralgias are common, occurring over the subclavicular area, the axilla, and the medial aspect of the upper arm. They are mild and transitory. We have never seen a clinically significant brachial plexopathy. The pulmonary complications consist of apical pulmonary fibrosis seen in almost every patient. In a few cases, where our treatment volume included more lung than intended, a symptomatic radiation pneumonitis occurred. The symptoms of fever, cough, and dyspnea lasted for a few weeks. This syndrome is associated with bronchoalveolar edema and simulates a pneumopathy which improves without functional defects. Rib fractures are incommon and heal spontaneously within a few weeks [1, 5, 6].

Major complications often result from faulty radiotherapy technique. The margin of error acceptable in the radiotherapy of the breast is narrow. Radical irradiation with curative intent does not allow a large therapeutic ratio. While 45 Gy is within tissue tolerance of the normal structures in the treatment volume, a 15 or 20% error in the dose received implies serious complications: major radiation sequelae of normal tissue or poor locoregional control. Under 40 Gy subclinical disease is not satisfactorily controlled. Above 50 Gy we see permanent nervous and muscular lesions. This may become a major problem if we exceed 55 Gy. Exceeding 60 Gy to the entire breast, we find massive radiation sclerosis and risk of necrosis (fig. 4). Consequently, radiotherapy of breast cancer requires sophisticated techniques with adequate support from the physics department, including a computerized treatment planning system and precise dosimetry. The medical staff and the radiotherapy personnel must be highly qualified.

Long-term results confirm this study of radiation effects and tolerance of normal tissue in breast cancer. A retrospective analysis of 245 patients with a minimum follow-up period of 13 years (and 435 patients with a minimum of follow-up period of 10 years) has demonstrated few complications (table I) and good cosmetic results (table II) [6, 7].

In conclusion, conservative treatment of breast cancer provides a high rate of local control with only 10% of locoregional failure at 13 years. This is accomplished within tolerance of normal tissue and allows 90% of women, apparently cured at 13 years, to conserve their breasts with a good cosmetic result.

Conclusions

Lactation is usually permanently suppressed after a total dose of 45–55 Gy. Fortunately, breast cancer is less common during the child-bearing years and very few women will 'risk' a pregnancy after being treated for breast cancer. The senior author had 3 patients who delivered healthy babies after conservative management. We advised against breast-feeding. None tried from the normal breast and none had lactation from the previously irradiated breast. Our experience with simultaneous use of irradiation and chemotherapy is limited. In the few cases we had

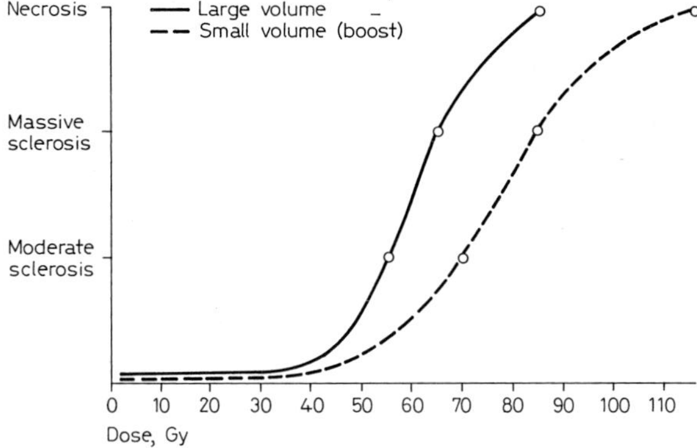

Fig. 4. Normal-tissue tolerance in relation to the dose in basal irradiation (large volume) and boost (small volume).

Table I. Breast cancer conservative treatment, 245 patients with a follow-up period of 13 years.

	Degree			
	1 (moderate complications)		2 (severe complications)	
	n	%	n	%
Arm edema	14	6	1	0.5
Surgery plus radiotherapy	5/20	25		
Radiotherapy only	9/225	4		
Brachial neuropathy	0		0	
Limitation of shoulder	15	6	0	
Rib fracture	4	1.5	0	
Inflammatory sclerosis	3	1	1	0.5

Table II. Cosmetic results at 10 years of follow-up

Stage	Excellent		Fair		Mediocre	
	n	%	n	%	n	%
T_1	65/77	84	10/77	13	2/77	2
T_2	69/113	61	36/113	35	7/113	4
T_3	9/24	37	10/24	42	5/24	21

(CMF), there was no significant enhancement of skin reaction. Based on some recently published data [2, 8], we will cautiously include in our treatment policy the simultaneous use of chemotherapy (CMF) and irradiation for patients at high risk of metastatic disease. Among the 1,500 patients treated over the past 27 years, we have encountered only on case of radiation-induced cancer (skin sarcoma at 8 years). This low rate of secondary malignancies is also found in the literature [3, 9].

References

1 Calitchi, E., et al.: Analyse rétrospective à 10 ans des séquelles du traitement loco-régional des cancers du sein. Bull. Cancer *71:* 100 (1984).

2 Hrafnkelsson, J., et al.: Tolerance of radiotherapy combined with adjuvant chemotherapy in breast cancer. Acta oncol. *26:* 269 (1987).

3 Otis, C. N., et al.: The rapid onset of cutaneous angiosarcoma after radiotherapy for breast carcinoma. Cancer *57:* 2130 (1986).

4 Pierquin, B.; Huart, J.: Experience with breast conserving approaches at the Hospital Henri-Mondor; in Primary management of breast cancer, p. 80. Tobias, Peckham, (Arnold, London 1985).

5 Pierquin, B., et al.: Conservative treatment of breast cancer in Europe. Report of the Groupe Européen de Curiethérapie (review). Radiother. Oncol. *6:* 187 (1986).

6 Pierquin, B., et al.: Conservative treatment for breast cancer: long-term results (13 years). Radiother. Oncol. (To be published, 1989).

7 Pierquin, B.; Grimard, L.: Radiation therapy as primary treatment; in Breast cancer (UICC). (Springer, Berlin. To be published, 1989).

8 Ray, G. R., et al.: Impact of adjuvant chemotherapy on cosmesis and complications in stage I and II carcinoma of the breast treated by biopsy and radiation therapy. Int. J. Radiat. Oncol. Biol. Phys. *10:* 837 (1984).

9 Souba W. W., et al.: Radiation-induced sarcomas of the chest wall. Cancer *57:* 610 (1986).

Bernard Pierquin, MD, Centre Hospitalo-Universitarie Henri-Mondor,
F-94010 Créteil (France)

Vaeth JM, Meyer JL (eds): Radiation Tolerance of Normal Tissues.
Front Radiat Ther Oncol. Basel, Karger, 1989, vol 23, pp 349–366

Radiation Damage of Normal Tissues in the Treatment of Gynecological Cancers

Marvin Rotman, Hassan Aziz, Kwang N. Choi

Department of Radiation Oncology, State University of New York,
Health Science Center at Brooklyn, New York, N.Y., USA

Introduction

In recent years there has been considerable progress in the management of gynecological cancers utilizing sophisticated radiotherapeutic techniques and multidisciplinary treatment. While modern approaches have rsulted in increased survival rates, there continues a need for refinements in treatment methods to prevent short- and long-term complications. Ideally, cure of malignant disease should be achieved with minimal structural and functional changes in normal tissues. This concept, although very desirable, is seldom achieved, as the doses necessary for tumor control and that which will produce complications are almost similar (fig. 1). Since the initial rectal reaction descriptions by Tod and Mere-

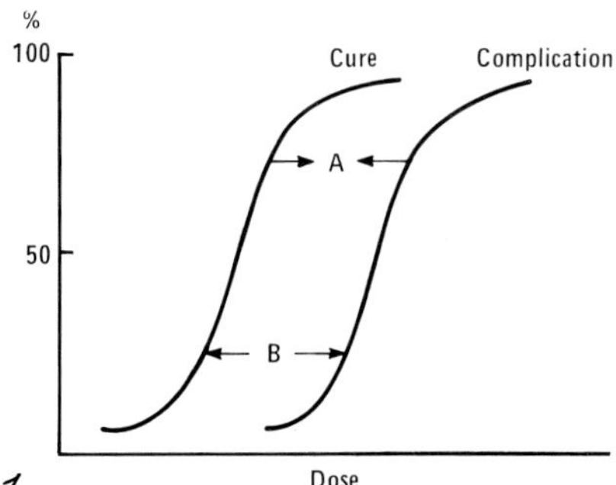

Fig. 1. Radiation damage of normal tissues in the treatment of gynecological cancers. Sigmoid curves for cure and complications. A = (1) Intrinsic factors: (a) diabetes, (b) hypertension, (c) old age, (d) diverticulitis, (e) anemia, (f) pelvic inflammatory disease, and (2) extrinsic factors: (a) brachytherapy: (i) compact system, (ii) protruding source, (iii) high dose rate, (iv) short source-surface distance; (b) external beam: (i) energy, (ii) edge effect, (iii) fraction size and number, (iv) chemotherapy, (v) surgery, (vi) socioeconomic state.

dith in 1938 [49] and subsequent classifications by Gray and Kottmeier [15] 2 decades later, there has been a spate of papers [1, 11, 31, 32, 36, 37] attempting to analyze the data related to normal tissue injury.

In these publications there have been described numerous techniques and schedules using a variety of equipments (extrinsic factors) and suboptimal brachytherapy procedures. Unreported have been contributing predisposing or intrinsic factors such as diabetes, hypertension, and inflammatory diseases which produce reduction in normal-tissue tolerance. The variability of the aforementioned factors have prevented any meaningful quantification, analysis, or comparisons of reported complications.

Types of Complications

Acute

Early reactions manifest themselves toward the end of the 3rd and 4th week of treatment and appear as a result of acute inflammatory changes in the bowel and bladder mucosa. Symptoms may range from abdominal cramps and tenesmus to watery diarrhea. Urinary symptoms include frequency, dysuria, and hematuria [7]. The urinary bladder is especially prone to develop infections and may produce symptoms at an earlier stage. Acute reactions are common and will generally respond to conservative management. Withers et al. [55] suggest that there is no relationship between severity of an early reaction and late complication. However, other authors, like Bourne et al. [4] and Kline et al. [22], have shown that the incidence of late complications in patients who had severe early reaction may be high. Bourne et al. [4]have shown that the incidence of chronic complications was 8.2% as compared to 3.0% in patients who were initially asymptomatic.

Chronic

Most late complications appear between 6 and 24 months after completion of radiation therapy [17]. Analysis of data, in fact, is incomplete before a minimum of 24 months and perhaps as much as 36 months. Bowel complications appear earlier than urinary complications and are also more common. Serious bowel complications range from chronic proctitis and slight thickening of bowel mucosa to complete obstruction and perforation, leading to colostomy. Late urogenital system complications may range from stenosis of the vagina to stenosis of ureters, hemorrhagic cystis, contracted bladder, and fistula formation as a result of bladder necrosis. Specific organ changes will be discussed later in this paper.

Late urinary and bowel complications are easily confused with recurrent disease. Often it is difficult to distinguish one from another by clinical or radiological means. Clinical history, time of appearance of the problem, and checking of the radiation techniques and dose given might be diagnostically helpful [7]. However, extreme caution is to be exercised in biopsying the suspected area which is to be avoided if at all possible after a course of radiation therapy. Indeed, fistula production in cervical carcinoma is most commonly iatrogenic in origin.

Pathogenesis

Cells lining the epithelium of bowel and urogenital system are mitotically active and are part of a rapid renewal system. The regeneration time of cells in the gastrointestinal tract mucosa is about 12–15 h [41]. These cells are radiosensitive, and their viability is essential for regeneration and repair. The sequence of events differs in the slow renewal system where the cells are not so radiosensitive and are found in mesenchymal subepithelial tissues, blood vessels, and muscles. Radiation produces most of the cell killing during the mitotic phase of the cell cycle in the cells of the epithelial lining. These cells may function until they attempt to divide again. This leads to an early radiation reaction which is due to depletion and denudation of the proliferative epithelium. There is also infiltration of the epithelial and subepithelial tissues with inflammatory cells associated with an increased vascular permeability. The gastrointestinal mucosa becomes thin, flat, and atrophic. The mucus-secreting cells have a higher survival rate, causing clinically an increased mucus production. If radiation is intense, the epithelium may slough, producing ulcers which may heal or progress according to dose. Late reaction is characterized by hyalinization of intima and media of arterial walls, with consequent hypertrophy and narrowing of the lumina. Late deposition of collagen in submucosa and subserosa becomes the chief feature of late-radiation injury. It is the late severe side effects the clinician and the patient both are concerned. Thickening of bowel may progress to obstruction, necrosis, or perforation with fistula formation.

Normal-tissue effects secondary to irradiation can induce a variety of changes, depending on the sensitivity of the cells of the tissue concerned. With the standard dose being given, i.e., 200 rad five times/week, Rubin and Casarett [41] and Rubin and Suman [42] have attempted to assign risk factors for each organ. The dose which will produce 5 and 50% severe complications is called $TD_{5/5}$ and $TD_{50/5}$, respectively. Admittedly, this provides a good indication concerning the susceptibility of each organ to irradiation, if the patient is treated in a standard time-dose schedule. However, caution should be exercised in cases where combined treatment is given, or some predisposing factors are present.

Patients receiving external irradiation may develop malabsorption, as reported by Lantz and Einhorn [25], to a rate of 22%. Treatment with external beam may also produce folate deficiency. Although malabsorption and folate deficiency syndromes are well documented, the mechanism of their occurrence is not understood.

Description of pathologic change and radiation complications do not take in account inherent differences in normal-tissue reactions that may relate to socioeconomic conditions.

Classification

The presence of many extrinsic and intrinsic factors, no doubt, influence rate and extent of complications. In an attempt to provide a measure of standardization in the description of these complications, Kottmeier in 1969 [24] graded the complications arising from bowel and urinary radiation damage according to severity of reaction. The classification of Kottmeier since then has been modified first by the WHO and later by European Organisation for Research in the Treatment of Cancer/Radiotherapy Oncology Group (EORTC/RTOG). The WHO classification, however, is more useful for grading acute and subacute effects only. The late toxic effects were related only to performance status of the patients. The EORTC/RTOG classification for late effects is beginning to be used more frequently and is essentially the same as that of Gray and Kottmeier [15] and Kottmeier [24], i.e., it provides a grading system for late complications. Grade I bowel complications include mild diarrhea, cramps, and slight discharge and bleeding, while grade II and III effects include excessive discharge, rectal bleeding or obstruction, and bleeding requiring surgery, respectively. The grade IV complications include more serious problems such as perforation of bowel and fistula formation.

Grade I urinary complications includce mild dysuria or slight hematuria. Cystoscopy may reveal a hyperemic bladder with a few telangiectatic spots. Grade II reaction include chronic or recurrent dysuria, infection, and hematuria. The bladder mucosa may be telangiectatic and atrophic. Grade III symptoms involve severe bladder spasm, gross hematuria, and incontinence, and cystoscopy may reveal contracted hemorrhagic cystitis. Grade IV complications include vesicovaginal fistulae, ureteral stenosis, or nonvisualization of the renal collecting system. It may be emphasized here that although a system for comparing the complications has emerged, many authors continue to use sometimes confusing and overlapping symptology for categorizing the effects of radiation on bowel or bladder [11, 36, 37].

Extrinsic Factors

The external radiation time-dose relationship must be considered as an important factor in assessing its effects on normal tissues. These include beam energy, number of ports and arrangement, and the size of the radiation portals. Using only anterior and posterior fields, especially with machines of less than 20 MeV, energy lateralization of dose or 'edge effect' may take place [13]. If only low-energy machines are available, patients should be treated with the multiple-field (four-field box) technique with all fields treated daily to avoid excessive doses to subcutaneous tissues, rectum, and bladder.

Beyond a total dose of 4,000–5,000 rad given within 4½–5½ weeks to the whole pelvis, the reported incidence of complications increases significantly. Delivering a higher dose, i.e., up to 7,000 rad in 7–7½ weeks, even when employing a shrinking-field technique, can give rise to severe rectosigmoiditis [17, 31, 32, 36].

When laparotomy is performed, either for exploration or for hysterectomy and pelvic node dissection, disruption of peritoneal lining occurs, increasing the chance of bowel adhesion and complications. Radical hysterectomy and lymphadenectomy, when combined with irradiation, have been reported to increase the complication rate by about four times [3]. Rotman et al. [39] have reported on a series of patients who either received irradiation alone for the treatment of carcinoma of the cervix or were treated with irradiation and surgery. The incidence of fistulae in patients who were treated with the combined modality was 15 as compared to 5% for those who received radiation only. It is advisable [13, 31] that if certain patients require both modalities, a compromise should be made in radiation dose and extent of surgery.

Para-Aortic Node Irradiation

The treatment of the para-aortic area with an extended field is associated with more high-grade small-bowel complications. The rate of complications depends on (1) total dose and fraction size; (2) the height of the para-aortic field for the ports approaching L2 and L1, possibly including large portions of stomach and small intestine, and (3) the number of fields treated daily. The presence and absence of surgical staging as a major contributing factor is still controversial. According to Rotman et al. [39] a total dose of 4,500 rad given at the rate of 160–180 rad/fraction through multiple fields can be easily tolerated. Senoussi et al. [43] reported that an additional 500–1,000 rad can be given as a boost dose via smaller and multiple ports without many complications, provided there was no previous surgical intervention. Potish et al. [35], after studying several series, categorized the complications according to the dose received and the presence and absence of staging surgery. In category I, complications were few, and the dose received was between 4,250 and 4,600 rad with no surgical staging. In category II, there was increased complication if the dose was increased to 5,500 rad, even without surgical staging. Category III and IV complications occurred as a result of delivering higher doses with surgical intervention. Complications are higher in patients who had surgical staging through the transperitoneal route as compared to retroperitoneal approach [2, 34]. However, the RTOG [40] thus far could not show surgery as a contributing factor in their prospective trial on over 360 patients.

Piver et al. [33, 34] reported a 25% complication rate in his series of patients who received para-aortic node irradiation with a dose ranging from 4,600 to 6,000 rad. Five of 20 patients developed eight serious complications, and there was a 15% mortality rate. Recently, RTOG trial 79–20 [40], a preliminary report, showed an increased rate of complications in patients who were randomized to receive prophylactic irradiation to the para-aortic area to a dose 4,500 rad within 5 weeks. Grade III and higher complications relating to large and small intestine were 8.9% as compared to 3.4% for pelvic irradiation only. In the same study, grade III and IV bladder complications were higher; 3.5% in the prophylactic para-aortic radiation group as compared to 1.1% in the group who received pelvic irradiation only.

Abdominal Irradiation

The common acute side effects as reported by various authors are related to the irradiated volume, the dose, and to the techniques of treatment such as open fields versus moving strips. In 1974, Fazekas and Meier [12], through a prospective randomized trial, had demonstrated that with the moving-strip technique there may be more gastrointestinal disturbance. However, other authors [14, 50] found no difference in gastrointestinal side effects. Approximately 55–75% of the patients have one or more symptoms of transient cramp, diarrhea, or nausea and vomiting.

Radiation cystitis and proctitis in whole abdominal irradiation are uncommon, and their range of occurrence may be 5–13%. In the series of Fuks [14] of 167 patients with ovarian cancer who received 4,500–6,000 rad to the lower abdomen, 78% had developed acute enteritis. A substantial number of patient showed weight loss. 14 of 70 of the patients of Smith et al. [46] showed >10% loss of weight.

Reports of hematologic toxicity secondary to abdominal irradiation vary. Fazekas and Meier [12] showed that the treatment of ovarian carcinoma with the moving-strip technique produces less hematological side effects compared to open-field methods. However, as has been demonstrated by Perez et al. [30], this side effect is substantial. These authors reported that since a large volume of bone marrow (50–60%) is included, the bone marrow may be depressed in a majority of the patients. Fazekas and Meier [12] and Perez et al. [39] reported different figures, probably depending on the dose which they delivered. Perez et al. [30] reported 26% patients having their white blood cell count falling below 3,000 and 40% having it between 3,000 and 4,000. The remainder had their white blood cell count between 4,100 and 5,500. However, Townsend et al. [50] noted that 56% of their patients had the white blood cell count below 3,000, while 43.6% had their red blood cell count below 150,000. Smith et al. [46] emphasize the fact that, due to hematologic problems, the treatment may be either delayed or abandoned in about 10% of the patients.

Chronic Effects of Whole Abdominal Irradiation

The gastrointestinal tract is the most frequent site to exhibit the late effects of irradiation of abdomen and pelvis. Dembo et al. [8] and Dembo [9, 10] with both moving-strip and open-field techniques reported an overall rate of 3.1% of bowel obstructions with a 5% incidence using open-field technique. Smith et al. [46] reported an incidence of 10%, 7 of 70 patients with small-bowel injury requiring surgery following strip irradiation. These patients had received 2,600–2,800 rad to each strip within 2½ weeks and an additional boost dose of 2,000 rad within 2 weeks to the pelvis. Perez et al. [30] reported on a series of patients who were treated with both open-field technique receiving 2,500–3,000 rad or with moving-strip technique giving 2,500 rad and boost to the pelvis of 2,500 rad. Major complications occurred in 5 of 52 patients. The complications included osteonecrosis of pubic bone in 1 patient, cystitis and ureteral stricture in 1, small-bowel obstruction in 1, and rectal ulcer in 1 patient.

Radiation-induced nephritis and hepatitis are potentially fatal complications [53] associated with treatment of ovarian carcinoma. If proper shielding is applied to protect these vital organs, the tumor may be protected either in the form of peritoneal seedings or lymph nodes. Wharton et al. [54] reported that prior to 1965, the liver was not shielded at M.D. Anderson Hospital during the treatment of ovarian carcinoma when applying the moving-strip technique. 14 of 65 patients who received 2,450–2,920 rad within 12 days to the liver developed radiation hepatitis. Ascites, pleural effusion, and hepatomegaly were the most common symptoms. There was an unexplainable difference in the timing of the onset of symptoms following completion of therapy, ranging from 4 weeks to 44 months. Only 1 patient had prior chemotherapy, and none of them had previous liver disease. Percutaneous needle biopsy or biopsy at laparatomy showed hepatic congestion, occlusion of central vein, and hyaline thickening of the arterial wall with peripontal fibrosis. Since then, shielding of the liver with 1 and kidneys with 2 half-value layer blocks has virtually eliminated the risk of radiation hepatitis and nephritis. Dembo et al. [8] reported 4 cases of radiation hepatitis occurring in a group of 226 patients who were treated with the moving-strip technique with no liver block. None of the 221 patients treated with the open-field therapy developed radiation hepatitis.

Intracavitary Irradiation

While the dose distribution from external irradiation is usually homogenous, the same cannot be said about brachytherapy. Brachytherapy is more likely to produce 'hot spots', producing complications. Several factors may be responsible for producing 'hot spots' and complications. Most important of these are (1) total and combined doses from brachytherapy and external therapy, (2) the arrangement of sources, (3) the type of applicator used and its source-surface distance, and (4) calculation of dose at a predetermined point such as point A with suboptimal radium application.

Total Radium and Combined Dose

Maxima after combining the dose from radium and external therapy were established by Fletcher [13] to indicate the maximum dose desirable in each stage of cervical cancer which would achieve a good therapeutic ratio. Maximum mgh for radium only were also cited for the treatment of early-stage disease. Unal et al. [51] have reported the effect of increased dosage in early-stage disease, wherre more than 900 mgh of radium and parametrial irradiation of more than 3,500 rad were given. In late-stage disease, complications were more common in patients who received a total of 7,500 mgh of radium and more than 2,000 rad of external therapy to whole pelvis and a boost of 1,500 rad to parametria.

Arrangement of Radium System

Protruding Source. Strockbine et al. [48] and Hamberger et al. [17] both have reported on the cause-and-effect relationship of protruding vaginal sources to the development of rectal and vaginal complications. Strockbine et al. [48] showed that 13 of 16 patients with rectal ulcers and 19 of 32 patients with fistula formation were treated with a protruding vaginal source. While Hamberger et al. [17] showed that 5 of 11 patients who received a protruding vaginal source or vaginal cylinder in addition to 5,000 rad of external therapy to the pelvis developed vaginal fistula and rectal strictures.

Deviated Tandems. Deviation of tandem to one side may produce a hot spot at the uretrovesical junction, and area located at the angle formed by the laterally deviated tandem and colpostats [51]. Ureteral strictures, sigmoiditis, and fistulae have been reported to have been produced by deviated tandems. Tandems which are flexed anteriorly and posteriorly may also deliver a high dose to bladder and rectum, producing cystitis and sigmoiditis, respectively.

Compact System. An intracavitary system that lends itself to become a compact system is especially prone to deliver high dose to adjacent structures like vagina, rectum, and bladder. These structures may receive high doses, if high intensity sources are used to avoid lengthy insertions or when the dose is calculated at a predetermined reference point, such as point A [38].

Types of Applicators

The Ernst applicator was described in 1946 and was popular in this country for more than 2 decades. However, some inherent defects were pointed out by Rotman et al. [38] who demonstrated that design deficiencies like compact system and a short source-surface distance might have been responsible for fourfold increases in the incidence of fistula formation as compared to patients treated with the Fletcher-Suit afterloading system, with its greater source-surface distance. The shortcomings found in the use of mini-ovoids can produce similar problems.

Calculation of the Dose at Point A

The relationship between the dose to vaginal mucosa and the dose to point A in the paracervical area should bear a relationship so that the dose at the vaginal mucosa is not exceeded beyond tolerance before achieving the paracervical dose at point A. This relationship may be

Table I. Carcinoma of cervix: incidence of rectal complications according to rectal combined dose

Authors	Combined dose rad	Number of patients	% severe complications grade III and IV	Comment
Kottmeier and Gray [57]	<6,000	231	6.5	In vivo measurement
	6,000–8,000	115	19	
	>8,000	23	26	
Pourquier et al. [36]	<7,000	58	3	Radiographic measurement on amt. rectal wall (CMRD)
	7,000–8,000	113	12	
	>8,000	110	27	
Perez et al. [32]	<8,000	640	5	Radiographic measurement at point of maximum dose
	>8,000	170	12	
Orton [29] (combined total dose range)	80–115	–	7	In vivo measurement
	116–136	–	7.7	
	137–162	–	11	
	163	–	21	

altered in many ways delivering higher dose to vaginal mucosa. Sub-optimal radium placements like compact systems, protruding source, and the displacement of ovoids caudally in a coned shaped vagina increase the incidence of complications [13].

Effect of Low and High Dose on Complications

Low-dose brachytherapy usually delivers approximately 1 rad/min to point A and high-dose rates of 150–200 rad/min. Hall [16] described the radiobiological effects of low and high doses on normal and neoplastic tissues. Decreasing dose rate with the same total dose produces less cell killing. Repair of sublethal damage and repopulation in normal tissues are noticeable with dose rates such as 1–100 rad. Below and above this range, there may be no changes in these radiobiological processes. With a low-dose rate, such as occurs in conventional therapy, the cell-killing mechanism is due to single-hit events with greater repair of normal tissue damage. However, in high-dose brachytherapy the repair of sublethal damage and repopulation of normal tissues are lost, increasing the chance of normal-tissue damage. These radiobiologic observations were substantiated by Joslin et al. [20], Inoue et al. [19], and Utley et al. [52] who reported a 10–20% increase in the incidence of complications and led to a great deal of caution in this country in adopting this technology. In spite of the high complication rates reported from Japan, its use in that country has continued. Shigematsu et al. [44] in a randomized trial concluded that both local control and complication rates were higher in the high-dose group. Most of the complications were related to rectal bleeding, as only 10 patients developed hematuria. Nori et al. [28], Utley et al. [52], Newman et al. [27], and recently Koga et al. [23] have reported no increase in serious complications by fractionating the high-dose applications. Nori et al. [28] pointed out that for both high- and low-dose brachytherapy, there is a linear relationship between the total dose received at point A and the number of insertions regarding tumor control and complications. Thus adjustments in brachytherapy insertions and total dose can be expected to decrease the complication rate without affecting tumor control rates. Orton [29] suggested a reduction of 20–50% of the total dose at point A and modification of fractionation in high-dose brachytherapy in order to obtain complication rates similar to that resulting from low-dose brachytherapy.

Organ Radiation Tolerance

Rectum

As indicated [9, 27], the rate of complications arising in the rectum depends on the total combined dose. Table I shows that if the combined dose to the rectum is greater than 7,000–8,000 rad, there is a high incidence of complications. In 1982, Pourquier et al. [36] described in detail dosimetric considerations for the rectum in the treatment of cervical cancer. The rectal surface dose was analyzed for intracavitary treatment (using Fletcher-Suit applicator) and for external therapy (20 MeV) for both the groups of patients with or without complications. The rectal surface dose was defined as occurring on a line drawn from the junction of S1 and S2 and passing inferiorly 5 mm below the ovoids to the anterior margin of the anus. The relationship of developing or not developing complications was drawn according to mean and maximum dose on the anterior surface of rectum with or without external irradiation. When a combined dose of external therapy and intracavitary irradiation is defined as maximal cumulative rectal dose exceeding 7,000 rad, complications were observed to increase. Whole pelvic external irradiation in excess of 4,500 rad seems to increase the incidence of complications. In general, patients who had developed rectal complications had received 400–600 rad more (external therapy) as compared to patients without complications. Patients receiving 7,000 rad as maximal cumulative rectal dose have only 10–15% chance of developing complications, while patients receiving 7,500–8,000 rad may have a 23% chance of developing complications. Grey and Kottmeier [15] had reported similar observations before by direct measurement of rectal dose. Critical doses from intracavitary therapy increase, as the dose from external therapy decreases with no reciprocal relationship. As such, there is no fixed relationship between the two types of treatment, and proportional changes in the dose from intracavitary treatment must be considered according to the dose of external therapy to avoid major complications.

Bladder and Ureter

In the treatment of carcinoma of the cervix, the incidence of complications arising in bladder and ureter is considerably less in frequency as compared to complications arising in the lower intestinal tract. Pourquier et al. [37] have recently reported an incidence of serious complications of only 2.2% in a group of 624 patients. Urinary complications usually occur late and are more difficult to manage. These complications are more likely to occur with combined treatment with irradiation and surgery. Hemorrhagic cystitis, contracted bladder, ureteral stenosis, and vesicovaginal fistula are severe grade III–IV complications.

Several authors [11, 32, 37] have found a correlation between the dose to the bladder and complications (table II). Perez et al. [32] have described the critical dose of bladder below 7,000 rad which produces the least number of complications; however, a high rate of complications may be produced if the bladder dose is increased up to 8,000 rad. These authors have also described a close relationship between large intracavitary doses and increased bladder complication. Patients who receive only 2,000 rad of external therapy and a large intracavitary dose in the range of 5,400–7,200 mgh may develop a higher rate of bladder complications. Kagan et al. [21], in addition to show the relationship high dose-bladder complications, have also described the anatomical differences, such as a narrow vagina, which may increase the rate of complications.

As in the case of rectosigmoid, Pourquier et al. [37] have recently described the relationship between cumulative bladder dose obtained at the most posterior part of the balloon filled up with 7 cm^3 of contrast medium and bladder complications. These authors observed that if the maximal cumulative bladder dose was kept under 6,500–7,000 rad, very few complications occurred. They also observed a significant contribution of an intracavitary dose to bladder to the development of complications. If the pelvis received external therapy of up to 4,000 rad or less, and the contribution from intracavitary dose was higher, there was a greater

Table II. Carcinoma of cervix: incidence of bladder complications according to combined dose

Authors	Combined dose	Number of patients	% complications	Comments
Kottmeier and Gray [57][a]	<8,000	329	5.5	In vivo measurement
	8,000–9,000	21	10	
	>9,000	17	29	
Perez et al. [32][b]	<8,000	648	4	Radiographic measurement at the point of maximum dose
	>8,000	162	11	
Pourquier et al. [37][c]	7,000 or less	370	7.5	Radiographic measurement at the most post point of balloon
	>7,000	254	20	

[a] Grades II and III.
[b] All Grades I–IV (EORTC/RTOG).
[c] Grade III and IV complications only (2.2%).

chance of developing bladder complications. On the contrary, if the total cumulative dose was largely from external therapy, a dose of 6,500–7,000 rad was tolerated easily.

Gynecologic surgery is responsible for the major incidence of ureteral injuries. The periureteral arterial plexus runs longitudinally down each ureter. It is recognized that without previous irradiation the ureteral blood supply can be sacrificed. Radiation therapy and surgery can have a profound effect on ureteral tone. The autonomic nerve supply which envelops the pelvic ureter from the hypogastric and sacral plexus adds to ureteral dysfunction when disturbed by surgery and irradiation. Radiation therapy can affect nerves directly or by fibrous enlargement.

Anatomically, the part of the ureter which receives higher doses of radiation lies within 1.5 cm of the lateral fornices of the vagina. As such, the distal 4.5 cm of the ureters are especially vulnerable to higher brachytherapy doses. In young patients with roomy vaginas the intravaginal colpostats can be pushed up high, closer to the ureterovesical junction.

Rotman et al. [39], after reviewing his own series and the world literature, showed considerably increased rates of obstructive uropathy, as demonstrated by pyelogram only. These authors estimated that, in fact, the combined physiological and mechanical obstructive uropathy rate may be as high as 30%. A physiological obstruction may occur soon after surgery, as a result of ligating the ureteral plexus and blood vessels with resultant atony of ureter and pooling of urine in the proximal part of the ureter, producing hydronephrosis and infection. Ureteral obstruction due to development of fibrosis in the pelvis can cause obstruction. From the rate of production of mechanical obstruction, it would appear that ureters are not very radiosensitive structures. A paracervical dose of more than 8,000 rad or hot spots from a suboptimal radium system can produce ureteral damage [45]. The dose delivered to ureter and parametrium is very important and should be kept within the above limits. Chau et al. [6] have reported ureteral strictures at lower doses.

Endometrium

Uterine complications are rare in the treatment of endometrial carcinoma, since total abdominal hysterectomy and bilateral salpingo-oophorectomy most commonly are part of the treatment; chronic effects of radiations on corpus, upper vagina, and Fallopian tubes are not observed. However, if radiation therapy has been used preoperatively, certain acute changes at the time of total abdominal hysterectomy and bilateral salpingo-oophorectomy are observed. Changes are most apparent in the endometrial lining, with development of superficial ulceration and considerable inflammatory component. Some of the ulcerations are large and sharply demarcated. These ulcers are finally replaced by dense collagenous scar. Microscopically there may be foci of hemorrhage, fibroblasts, and telengiectatic blood vessels [5].

Stokes et al. [47] described various combinations of adjuvant irradiation and their complications in endometrial carcinoma. In their series 12 of 304 patients developed serious complications including bowel obstruction (n = 5), rectal ulcers (n = 2), and urinary complications, (n = 4). One patient developed malabsorption syndrome.

Combinations of preoperative radium and postoperative external irradiation produced a high complication rate of 20%. Preoperative external therapy alone or postoperative radium alone reduce the overall complication rate to 12% or less. Stokes et al. [47] showed that increasing the dose to the vaginal apex can increase the complication rate. A dose of less than 5,500 rad gives a complication rate of 3%. If the total dose to the apex is increased to more than 10,000 rad, the complication rate increases to 15%.

Vagina

Hintz et al. [18], by studying the development of necrosis of vaginal mucosa in the treatment of carcinoma of the vagina, showed a relationship between vaginal mucosal tolerance and radiation dose. According to their study, the tolerance of the distal vagina was considerably lower than that of the upper vagina. The distal part of the vagina was shown to tolerate up to 9,800 rad delivered by combined brachytherapy and external therapy, while the upper part of the vagina tolerated up to 14,000 rad. The posterior wall appears to be more radiosensitive as compared to anterior and lateral walls, since all episodes of necrosis in the series of Hintz et al. [18] occurred on the posterior wall, irrespective of the location of the tumor.

Perez et al. [31] reported a 7% complication rate for treatment of stage O and I disease and one of 15% for stage II patients. Due to the short survival of stage III and IV patients, no complications were reported. The most common complications were fibrosis of the vagina and patches of mucosal necrosis. Two percent to the patients had proctitis, and 1% developed rectovaginal fistula.

Ovary

The radiosensitivity of ovarian structures varies considerably. The ovum in the young follicle is more radiosensitive than the ovum in the mature follicle. In contrast, the granulosa cells which line the follicles become more radiosensitive as they mature. The cells derived from the corpora lutea are radiosensitive. The exact dose required to permanently cause cessation of ovulation is unknown, although patients near the menopause require a smaller dose than younger women. A single dose of 400–500 rad to the ovaries of older women may produce complete cessation of menses, while in younger patients a comparative result may be achieved when 1,200–2,000 rad are given within 10–12 days [26]. Zukerman [56] showed that in women 35–39 years of age only 11 of 51 patients resumed menstruation after receiving a single dose of 400–500 rad, while in a group of 30- to 34-year-old women 10 of 15 resumed menstruation.

The ovaries that receive 3,000–4,000 rad become smaller and smooth, mainly because of loss of germinal epithelium and disappearance of follicles. Blood vessels are damaged in the ovarian stroma, and there is a dense proliferation of fibrous tissues with the microscopic picture resembling that in old females.

References

1 Alert, J.; Jiminez, J.; Beldarrain, L.; Montalave, J.; Cora, C.: Complications from irradiation of carcinoma of uterine cervix. Acta radiol. (Oncol.) *19:* 13–15 (1980).

2 Berman, M. L.; Lagasse, L. D.: The operative evaluation of patients with cervical carcinoma by an extraperitoneal approach. Obstet. Gynec. *50:* 658 (1977).

3 Boronow, R. C.: Vesico-vaginal fistula, radiation and gynecologic cancer. Am. J. Obstet. Gynec. *111:* 85–90 (1971).

4 Bourne, R. G.; Kearsley, J. H.; Grove, W. D.; Roberts, S. J.: The relationship between early and late gastrointestinal complications of radiation therapy for carcinoma of cervix. Int. J. Radiat. Oncol. Biol. Phys. *9:* 1445–1450 (1983).

5 Brady, L. B.; Marko, A. M.; DeEulis, T.; and Lewis, G. C.: Combined radiotherapy and chemotherapy in gynecologic oncology (in press).

6 Chau, P. M.; Fletcher, G. H.; Rutledge, F. N.; Dodd, G. D.: Complications in high dose, whole pelvis irradiation in femoral pelvic cancer. Am. J. Roentg. Rad. Ther. nucl. Med. *87:* 22–40 (1962).

7 Choi, K.; Aziz, H.; Rotman, M.: Complications in the radiotherapeutic management of gynecological cancers; in Nori, Hilaris, Radiation therapy of gynecological cancer, pp. 239–249 (Liss, New York 1957).

8 Dembo, A. J.; Bush, R. S.; Beale, F. A.; Bean, H. A.; Pringle, J. F.; Sturgeon, J.; Reid, J. G.: Ovarian carcinoma. Improved survival following abdominopelvic irradiation in patients with a completed pelvic operation. Am. J. Obstet. Gynec. *134:* 793 (1979).

9 Dembo, A. J.: Post-operative abdominopelvic irradiation in patients with epithelial cancer of ovary. J. Cancer. Res. clin. Oncol. *10:* 91–93 (1984).

10 Dembo, A. J.: Abdominopelvic radiotherapy in ovarian cancer: a 10-year experience. Cancer *55:* 2285–2290 (1985).

11 Esche, B. A.; Crook, J. M.; Horiot, J. C.: Dosimetric methods in the optimization of radiotherapy for carcinoma of the cervix. Int. J. Radiat. Oncol. Biol. Phys. *13:* 1183–1192 (1987).

12 Fazekas, J. T.; Meier, J. G.: Irradiation of ovarian carcinomas: a prospective comparison of the open field and moving strip technique. Am. J. Roentg. Rad. Ther. nucl. Med. *120:* 118–123 (1974).

13 Fletcher, G. H.: Squamous cell carcinoma of uterine cervix; in Fletcher, Textbook of radiotherapy, pp. 720–772 (Lea & Febiger, Philadelphia 1980).

14 Fuks, Z.: External radiotherapy of ovarian cancer standard approaches and new frontiers. Semin. Oncol. *2:* 253 (1975).

15 Grey, M. J.; Kottmeier, H. L.: Rectal and bladder injuries following radiation therapy for carcinoma of cervix. Am. J. Obstet. Gynec. *74:* 1294–1303 (1957).

16 Hall, E. J.: Radiation dose rate, a factor of importance in radiobiology and radiotherapy. Br. J. Radiol. *45:* 81–97 (1972).

17 Hamberger, A. D.; Unal, A., et al.: Analysis of severe complications of irradiation of carcinoma of the cervix: whole pelvis irradiation and intracavitary radium. Int. J. Radiat. Oncol. Biol. Phys. *9:* 367–371 (1983).

18 Hintz, B. L.; Kagan, A. R.; Chan, P.; Gilbert, H. A.; Nussbaum, H.; Rao, A. R.; Wollins, M.: Radiation tolerance of the vaginal mucosa. Int. J. Radiat. Oncol. Biol. Phys. *6:* 711–716 (1980).

19 Inoue, T.; Hori, S.; Miyata, Y.; Ozeki, S.; Shigematsu, Y.: High versus low dose rate intracavitary irradiation of carcinoma of the uterine cervix. A preliminary report. Acta radiol. (Oncol.) *17:* 277–282 (1978).

20 Joslin, C. A. F.; Smith, C. W.; Mallik, A.: The treatment of cervix cancer using high activity Co60 sources. Br. J. Radiol. *45:* 257–270 (1972).

21 Kagan, A. R.; DiSaia, P. J.; Wollin, M.; Nussbaum, H.; Tawa, K.: The narrow vagina, the enigma for radiation injury. Gynecol. Oncol. *14:* 291–298 (1976).

22 Kline, J. C.; Buchler, D. A.; Boone, M. L.; Peckham, B. M.; Carr, W. F.: The relationship of reactions to complications in the radiation therapy of cancer of the cervix. Radiology *105:* 413–416 (1972).

23 Koga, K.; Watanabe, K.; Kawano, M.; Kusumoto, S.; Nishikawa, K.; Kawano, K.; Kuroki, T.; Mori, N.: Radiotherapy of the uterine cervix by remotely controlled afterloading intracavitary system with high dose rate. Int. J. Radiat. Oncol. Biol. Phys. *13:* 615–618 (1987).

24 Kottmeier, H. L.: Complications following radiation therapy in carcinoma of cervix and their treatment. Am. J. Obstet. Gynec. *88:* 854 (1969).

25 Lantz, B.; Einhorn, N.: Intestinal damage and malabsorption after treatment for cervical carcinoma. Acta radiol. (Oncol.) *23:* 33–36 (1984).

26 Moss, W. T.; Brand, W. N.; Bathfora, H.: The ovary. Response of the normal ovary to irradiation; in radiation oncology: rationale, techniques and results; 5th ed., pp. 505–518 (Mosby, St. Louis 1979).

27 Newman, H.; Jur, B.; James, K. W.; Smith, C. W.: Treatment of cancer of the cervix with a high dose rate afterloading machine (the cathetron). Int. J. Radiat. Oncol. Biol. Phys. *9:* 931–937 (1983).

28 Nori, D.; Hilaris, B. S.; Batata, M. A.: Remote afterloading in cancer management. II. Clinical applications of remote afterloaders; in Hilaris, Batata, Brachytherapy oncology, pp. 101–118 (Memorial Sloan Kettering Cancer Center, New York 1981).

29 Orton, C. G.: Radiobiological dose rate considerations with remote afterloading; in Shearear, Recent advances in brachytherapy physics, pp. 109–200 (American Institute of Physics, New York 1981).

30 Perez, C. A.; Walz, B. J.; Jacobson, P. L.: Radiation therapy in the management of carcinoma of ovary. Nat. Cancer Inst. Monogr. *42:* 119 (1975).

31 Perez, C. A.; Camel, H. M.; Kao, M. S.; Askin, F.: Randomized study of preoperative radiation and surgery or irradiation alone in the treatment of stage IB and IIA carcinomas of uterine cervix. Preliminary analysis of failures and complications. Cancer *45:* 2759–2768 (1980).

32 Perez, C. A.; Breaux, S.; Bedwineck, J. M.; Madoc-Jones, H.; Camel, H. M.; Purdy, J. A.; Walt, B. J.: Radiation therapy alone in the treatment of carcinoma of the uterine cervix. II. Analysis of complications. Cancer *54:* 235–246 (1984).

33 Piver, M. S.; Vongtama, V.; Barlow, J. J.: Para-aortic lymph node irradiation for carcinoma of uterine cervix, using split course technique. Gynecol. Oncol. *3:* 168–175 (1975).

34 Piver, M. S.; Barlow, J. J.; Krishnamsetty, R.: Five-year survival (with no evidence of disease) in patients with biopsy confirmed aortic node metastasis from cervical carcinoma. Am. J. Obstet. Gynec. *139:* 575 (1981).

35 Potish, R.; Adcock, L.; Jones, T.; Levitt, S.; Prem, K.; Savage, J.; Twiggs, L.: The morbidity and utility of periaortic radiotherapy in cervical carcinoma. Gynecol. Oncol. *15:* 1–9 (1983).

36 Pourquier, H.; Dubois, J. B.; Delard, R.: Cancer of the uterine cervix. Dosimetric guidelines for prevention of late rectal and rectosigmoid complications as a result of radiotherapeutic treatment. Int. J. Radiat. Oncol. Biol. Phys. *8:* 1887–1895 (1982).

37 Pourquier, H.; Delard, R.; Achille, E.; Daly, N. J.; Horiot, J. C.; Kéiling, R.; Pigneux, J.; Rozan, R.; Schraub, S.; Vrousos, C.: A quantified approach to the analysis and prevention of urinary complications in radiotherapeutic treatment of cancer of the cervix. Int. J. Radiat. Oncol. Biol. Phys. *13:* 1025–1033 (1987).

38 Rotman, M.; John, M. J.; Roussis, K.; Moon, S. H.; Choi, K. N.; Syed, M.; Chan, B.; Sall, S.; Stone, M.: The intracavitary applicator in relation to complications of pelvic radiation: the Ernst System. Int. J. Radiat. Oncol. Biol. Phys. *4:* 951 (1978).

39 Rotman, M.; John, M. J.; Moon, S. H.; Choi, K. N.; Stowe, S. M.; Abitbol, A.; Herkovic, T.; Sall, S.: Limitations of adjunctive surgery in carcinoma of the cervix. Int. J. Radiat. Oncol. Biol. Phys. *5:* 327–332 (1979).

40 RTOG Trial 79–20: Prophylactic irradiation of para-aortic nodes vs. pelvic irradiation only in the treatment of carcinoma of cervix.
41 Rubin, P.; Casarett, G. W.: Clinical radiation pathology, vol. 1 (Saunders, Philadelphia 1968).
42 Rubin, P.; Suman, D.: Principles of radiation oncology and cancer radiotherapy; in Rubin, Clinical oncology: a multidisciplinary approach; 6th ed., pp. 58–71 (Rochester 1983).
43 Senoussi, M. A. E.; Fletcher, G. H.; Borlace, B. C.: Correlation of radiation and surgical parameters in complications in the extended field technique for carcinoma of the cervix. Int. J. Radiat. Oncol. Biol. Phys. *5:* 927–934 (1979).
44 Shigematsu, Y.; Nishiyama, K.; Masaki, N.; Inoue, T.; Miyata, Y.; Ikeda, H.; Ozeki, S.; Kawamura, Y.; Yurachi, K.: Treatment of carcinoma of uterine cervix by remotely controlled afterloading intracavitary radiotherapy with high dose rate. A comparative study with a low dose rate system. Int. J. Radiat. Oncol. Biol. Phys. *9:* 351–356 (1983).
45 Slater, J. M.; Fletcher, G. H.: Urethral strictures after radiation therapy of carcinoma of cervix. Am. J. Roentg. Rad. Ther. nucl. Med. *121:* 269–272 (1971).
46 Smith, J. P.; Rutledge, F. N.; Delclos, L.: Post-operative treatment of early cancer of the ovary. A random trial between post-operative irradiation and chemotherapy. Natn. Cancer Inst. Monogr. *42:* 149–153 (1975).
47 Strokes, S.; Bedwinek, J.; Breaux, S.; Kao, M.; Camel, M.; Perez, C.: Treatment of stage I adenocarcinoma of the endometrium by hysterectomy and irradiation. Analysis of complications. Obstet. Gynec. *65:* 86–92 (1985).
48 Strockbine, M. F.; Hancock, J. E.; Fletcher, G. H.: Complications in 831 patients with squamous cell carcinoma of the intact uterine cervix treated with 3,000 rad or more whole pelvis radiation. Am. J. Roentg. Rad. Ther. nucl. Med. *108:* 293–304 (1970).
49 Tod, M. C.; Meredith, W. J.: Dosage system for use in the reatment of cancer of uterine cervix. Br. J. Radiol. *11:* 809 (1938).
50 Townsend, R.; Glanssburn, J. R.; Brady, L. W.; Rowland, J.: Whole abdominal irradiation for carcinoma of the ovary. Cancer clin. Trials *2:* 351–358 (1979).
51 Unal, A.; Hamberger, A. D.; Seski, J. C.; Fletcher, G. H.: An analysis of severe complications of irradiation of carcinoma of cervix. Treatment with intracavitary radium and parametrial radiation. Int. J. Radiat. Oncol. Biol. Phys. *7:* 999 (1981).
52 Utley, J. F.; Essen, C. F. von; Horn, R. A.; Moeller, J. H.: High dose afterloading brachytherapy in carcinoma of uterine cervix. Int. J. Radiat. Oncol. Biol. Phys. *10:* 2259–2263 (1984).
53 Essen, C. F. von; Seay, D. G.; Moeller, J.; Hilbert, J. W.: Fractionated intracavitary radiation therapy with the brachytron. General techniques and preliminary results in the treatment of cervix. Am. J. Roentg. *120:* 101–110 (1974).
54 Wharton, T.; Delclos, L.; Gallager, S.; Smith, J.: Radiation hepatitis by abdominal irradiation with the cobalt 60 moving strip technique.
55 Withers, H. R.; Thames, H. D.; Peters, L. J.: Differences in fractionation response of acutely and late responding tissues; in Karcher, K. H., Progress in radiation oncology, vol. 2, pp. 287–296. (Raven Press, New York 1982).
56 Zukerman, S.: The sensitivity of gonads to radiation. Clin. Radiol. *19:* 1–15 (1965).
57 Kottmeier, H. L.; Gray, M. J.: Rectal and bladder injuries in relation to radiation dosage in carcinoma of the cervix. Am. J. Obstet. Gynec. *82:* 79–82 (1981).

M. Rotman, M. D.: Department of Radiation Oncology,
State University of New York, Health Science Center at Brooklyn,
New York, NY 11203 (USA)

Vaeth JM, Meyer JL (eds): Radiation Tolerance of Normal Tissues.
Front Radiat Ther Oncol. Basel, Karger, 1989, vol 23, pp 367–389

Clinical Radiation Tolerance of Brain, Spinal Cord, and Peripheral Nerves Laboratory and Patient Data as Clinical Guides

Melvin L. Griem

Department of Radiation Oncology University of Chicago, Chicago, Ill., USA

Perspective

In preparation for this symposium the author has made an extensive survey of the literature including the older citations. These citations are included in toto in the reference section [11, 85]. At the time of the last normal-tissue symposium, there was a small number of reports on radiation injury of the nervous system [5, 6, 8, 12, 13, 16, 18, 28, 39, 41, 52, 69, 71, 75, 77, 82, 93, 106, 121, 129, 130]. The editor of this symposium, in fact, was one of the early pioneers in the field of documenting injury to the nervous system in humans [129].

The specific aims of this review article are to provide an introduction into the biology of the injury processes and to provide detailed quantitative data on the injury of the nervous system in animals and humans which would be of use to guide the practicing radiation oncologist.

The problem of defining normal-tissue tolerance in humans was clearly defined by Mendelsohn [90] at a symposium in Carmel. The basic problem is the determination of a dose-response curve for a tissue such as the central nervous system for large animals and humans in this litigious society. Few people report complications in the framework of the total population so managed.

When the last symposium on this subject was published as volume 6 of the 'Frontiers of Radiation Therapy and Oncology' in 1972, the data presented by Kramer et al. [70] on the sensitivity of the nervous system documented 56 pathologically confirmed cases of cerebral necrosis in the literature. The denominator of the number of patients at risk was not available. There have been several attempts to add to this data base by Salazar et al. [109] in 1979, Gilbert and Kagan [46] in 1980, Sheline et al. [114] in 1980, Mark and Wong [86] in 1981, and by Cohen and Creditor

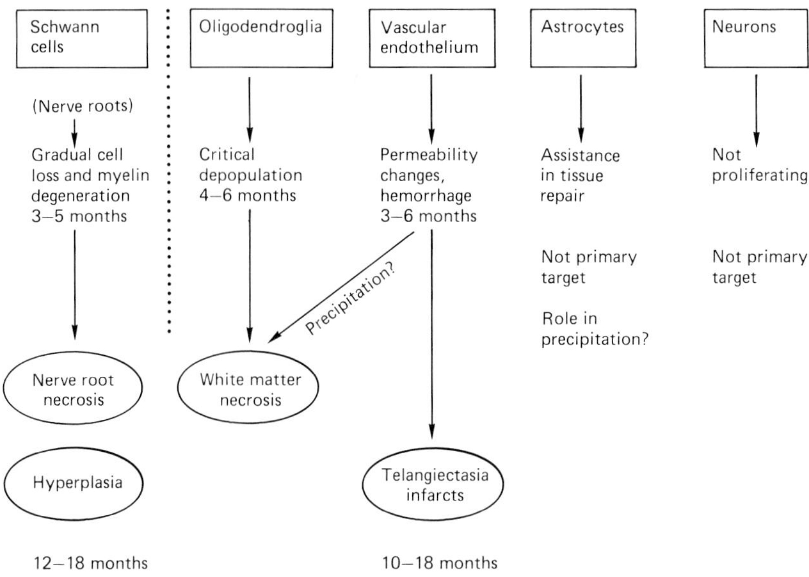

Fig. 1. Major tissue types of the central nervous system and the radiation-induced lesions. [From ref. 125, with permission.]

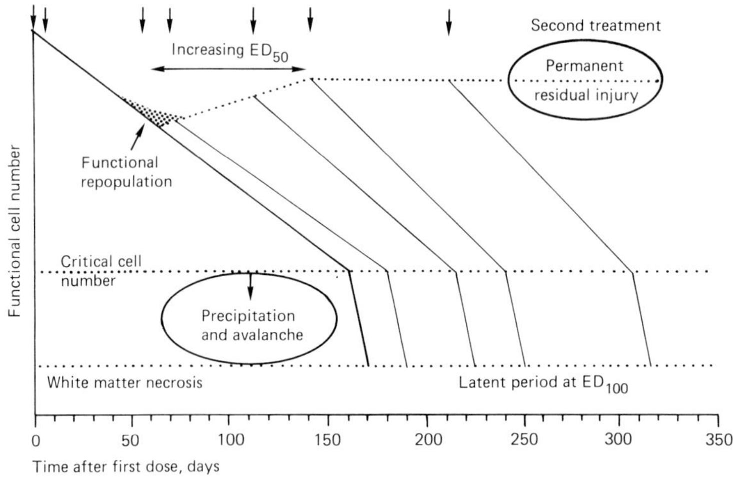

Fig. 2. Representation of the development of white matter necrosis, as derived from split-dose experiments. [From ref. 125, with permission.]

[29] in 1981 for spinal cord. Most of these reports are with standard fractionation (SF; 2 Gy/day, 5 days/week). Coupled with this pure photon data is the problem of the effect of surgery on tolerance and more importantly the effects of cytotoxic chemotherapy on the nervous tissues involved, as pointed out by Rubin [107] and discussed by Byfield [24] and Davis [35].

These modifying factors make the quantitation of injury more difficult. There are a number of in vitro experiments on tissue culture and rodent studies on cells and tissues of the nervous system, which provide clues to possible effects, and a few large-animal studies on monkeys, dogs, and burrows which are useful [20, 26, 59, 61, 95]. For the spinal cord, data on injury are more extensive and well summarized by Cohen and Creditor [29] in 1981. Data on spinal cord injury from the laboratory are very helpful, particularly for fractionation studies [2, 57, 81, 130–132, 134, 135, 139, 141]. Recent patient data concerning spinal cord injury are now available from clinical experience to guide us [1, 5, 65, 97, 127, 130, 137]. Data on cranial nerve injury and peripheral nerve injury are also available [6, 66, 117, 123]. Neutron data are available for both brain and spinal cord [25, 30, 78, 79, 83, 96].

Biology

Many classical articles and reviews present information on how ionizing in radiation causes nervous system demage [1, 32, 39, 44, 114, 132]. The complex interaction of nervous tissue has been further refined by van der Kogel [134] and by Thames and Hendry [125], as shown in figure 1. From this the functional cell number can be estimated in figure 2 and the different types of injury quantitiated, as shown in table I. The blood-brain barrier is changed by modest doses of radiation, and the drug permeability of nervous tissue is changed and is influenced by drug concentration, time of delivery, duration of drug exposure, as well as such factor as frequency and recall phenomena [39, 49, 52, 102]. The vascular effects have been extensively discussed during this symposium.

In the analysis by Sheline et al. [114], which is very useful for the practicing radiation oncologist, various reactions are defined: (1) the acute reactions occurring promptly after treatment; (2) the early delayed reactions characterized by somnolence syndrome, transient postirradiation deterioration, and necrotizing leukoencephalopathy and mineralizing microangiopathy. [108] – these findings may be seen during the first several months following irradiation and are self-limited–, and (3) the late delayed reactions include cerebral necrosis [27, 88], effects on the

Table I. Types of delayed radiation damage observed in animal spinal cord experiments [from ref. 134, with permission]

	Cervical, early delayed damage	Cervical, late delayed damage	Lumbar, progressive radiculopathy
Type of lesion	white matter necrosis	telangiectasia, haemorrhage	nerve root necrosis
Possible target cell	oligodendrocyte	vascular endothelium	Schwann cell
Dose level (single dose), Gy	⩾20	~15–20	⩾20
Latency period, months	~6	8–18	~5
Repair (D_2–D_1), Gy	8	5.5	7.5
Start of regeneration after irradiation, weeks	8–10	16–20	1–4

hypothalmus and pituitary, injury of cranial nerves, and impaired intellectual ability. Radiation carcinogenesis will not be considered, since this subject is covered in a recent symposium on the topic [15].

Photon Dosimetry

For this review the author has taken any data where 250-KV or similar kilovoltage radiation was mentioned, a relative biological effectiveness (RBE) of 1.15 was used as suggested by Sheline et al. [114].

He also converted to R to rad [60], so as to consider all information in terms of a megavoltage dose. For this review the gray (Gy) is used throughout the article.

Fetal Nervous System Injury

The fetal nervous system is quite sensitive to ionizing radiations. Doses below 0.5 Gy have been reported to cause problems in the human [92]. In the atomic bomb studies, tests in Japan of children in grade school revealed lower scores in children exposed to the atomic radiation in utero [113]. From that same symposium tissues of the eye and certain CNS sites were shown to be sensitive to irradiation in the 0.01- to 0.1-Gy range [72]. This sensitivity may extend into the 1st year of life; however, the detailed dose-response curve is not available for humans.

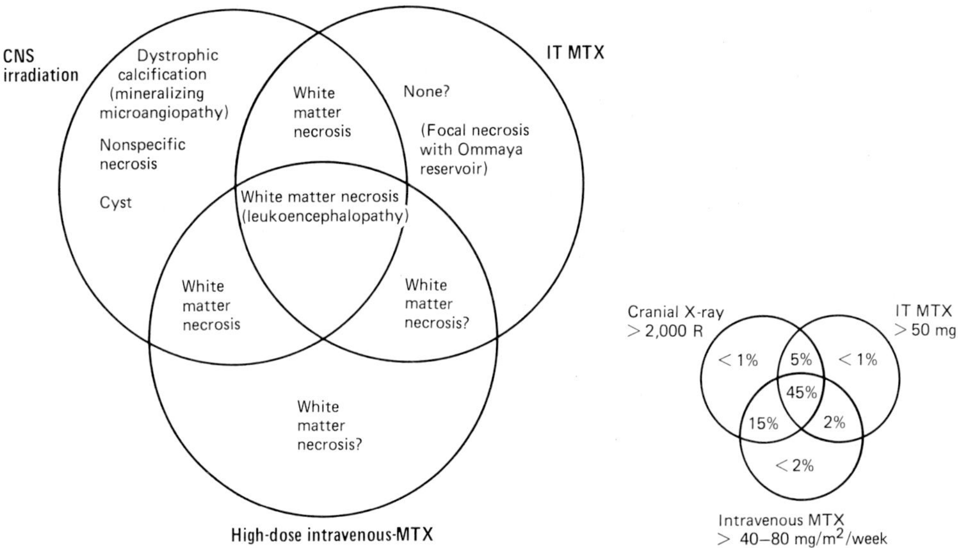

Fig. 3. Interaction of chemotherapy and radiation. IT = Intrathecal; MTX = methotrexate. [From ref. 107, with permission.]

Children Brain Data

For young patients data on CNS injury have been well documented by Danoff [32] in her review presented in 1983. In the early delayed reaction, somnolence has been reported [44]. For late reactions, children under the age of 2 are quite sensitive to radiations, when high-dose therapy for brain tumors is used [120]. There is significant loss of mental ability [34, 38, 40, 73, 89, 128]. Growth may be effected through endocrine factors [34, 63, 94]. Doses of X-ray above 24 Gy with SF have been reported to cause a decrease in head size and IQ and that the effect is more profound on girls than on boys and is age related [128].

These reactions are compounded by chemotherapy, especially methotrexate [10]. Bleyer and Giffin [10] found that the time of administration effects outcome and that this injury can be minimized by administration of the methotrexate before irradiation. The route of drug administration is also important in the injury process, as pointed out by Rubin [107] in figure 3, where the combination of intrathecal methotrexate and intravenous drug with irradiation compounds the injury. Somnolence syndrome may be seen without focal defects 4–8 weeks after prophylactic cranial irradiation of 18–24 Gy for acute lymphoblastic leukemia [98].

Table II. CNS late effects and chemotherapeutic agents [from ref. 107, with permission]

Acute encephalopathies	Mineralizing microangiopathy
IT MTX–XRT	XRT ± IT MTX
XRT ± IT MTX	Cerebral atrophy
HD MTX ('stroke-like')	IT MTS ± XRT
Asparaginases (early and late)	IT arabinoside C ± XRT
HMM/PMM	Pontine myelinolysis
Ftorafur (IV)	XRT ± IT MTX
Procarbazine	Neuropathies
BCNU (intracarotid)	Vincas (VCR, VDS, VBL; also cranial)
cis-DDP (intarcarotid)	*cis*-DDP (also cranial and VIII)
Cyclophosphamide (?)	HMM/PMM
5-Azacytidine	Procarbazine
PALA	5–Azacytidine
Spirogermanium	VP-16-213; VM-26
Misonidazole	Misonidazole (also VIII)
High-dose arabinoside C	Methyl-G
Chronic encephalopathies	
Necrotizing leukoencephalopathy	
XRT→ IT MTX	
IT or W MTX	
IT arabinoside C	

It = Intrathecal; MTX = methotrexate; XRT = X-ray therapy; HD = high-dose; HMM = hexamethyl melamine; VCR = vincristine; *cis*-DDP = cisplatin; VBL = vinblastine; VP-16-213, VM-26 = podophalotoxin compounds.

Disseminated necrotizing leukencephalopathy may occur in the treatment of leukemias and lymphomas [108].

Van der Kogel and Sissingh [133] have noted that arabinoside C will also potentiate injury of the CNS, and mitotane has been reported to cause injury to the CNS in rodents when combined with X-rays [48]. Arabinoside C causes acute cerebellar dysfunction in humans [110]. Vincristine with or without X-rays may result in CNS injury [35]. Byfield [24] has suggested that 5-fluorouracil and procarbazine may also interact with X-rays in the CNS. Rubin [107] expanded on this theme in his review of late effects, as shown in table II. Both Danoff [32] and Sheline et al. [124] suggested that surgery may increase the frequency of CNS injury associated with irradiation. In children there is also a disturbance of hormonal function associated with irradiation of the hypothalamus and pituitary [63, 103]. There is growth retardation and reduction in growth hormone production when brain tumors are treated in children [33, 94].

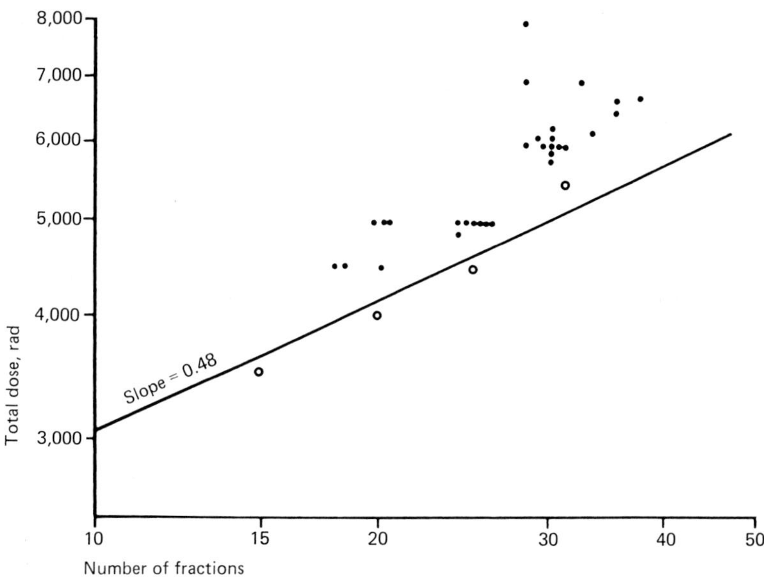

Fig. 4. Data for human brain tolerance. [From ref. 100, with permission.]

Adult Brain Data

Sheline et al. [114] and Kramer et al. [70] have done an excellent job of collecting the recorded injury in adult humans. Sheline et al. [114] analyzed their data using nominal standard dose and extended this to an analysis using the 'neuret', weighting the number of fractions [115]. Pezner and Archambeau [100] have taken some of these data and created the brain tolerance unit (fig. 4). The problem is that the absolute incidence cannot be determined, since the number of patients so treated is unknown. Marks et al. [84] and Marks and Griem [85] analyzed a population of patients treated with SF, where a change in dose resulted in reduction from a 5% incidence of cerebral necrosis to 0%.

These authors found that at a dose below 52.5 Gy there is no necrosis, at 55 Gy they had 1/66, at 60 Gy 4/100, at 65 Gy 1/4, and at 67.5 Gy 1/1 in their series of 371 patients. The brain near the pituitary may be somewhat more sensitive to irradiation [23, 28, 45, 53, 105]. Brain necrosis may be seen following the treatment of extracranial lesions and metastases [47, 74, 122].

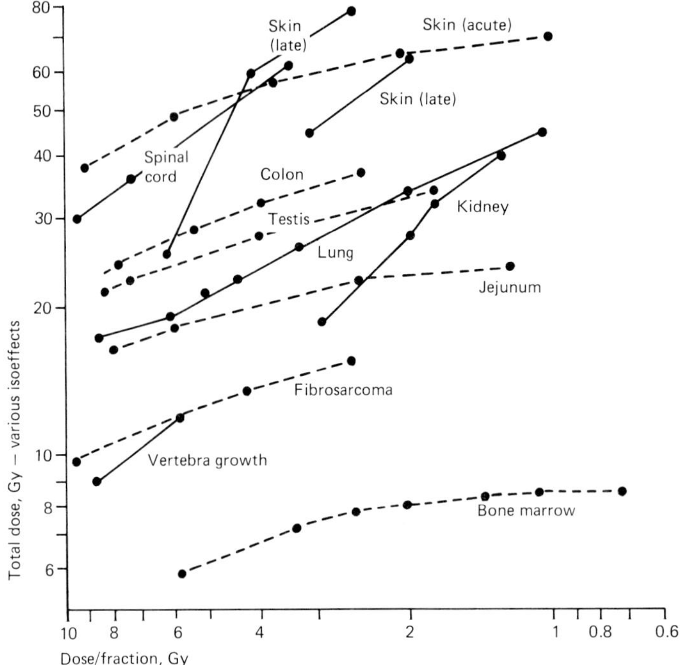

Fig. 5. Experimental tolerance data for a variety of tissues, indicating the difference between early- and late-responding tissues when the dose per fraction is considered. The solid lines representing the late-responding tissues show a steeper slope. [From ref. 125, with permission.]

Altered Fractionation

As would be predicted from the discussion of fractionation in this symposium and shown in figure 5 taken from the work of Thames and Hendry [125] and their collaborators at the M. D. Anderson Hospital, the nervous system is susceptible to late injury, particularly as the fraction size is increased. Experimental work by Hornsey and White [58] and Hornsey et al. [59] provides data for brain and for the comparison of brain and spinal cord (fig. 6). Large-animal experiments suggest increased injury with large fraction sizes [61].

In a patient treated for carcinoma of the nasopharynx, where the daily dose per fraction was 2.75 Gy, massive necrosis of the brain stem was found in regions receiving > 60 Gy and partial necrosis at sites receiv-

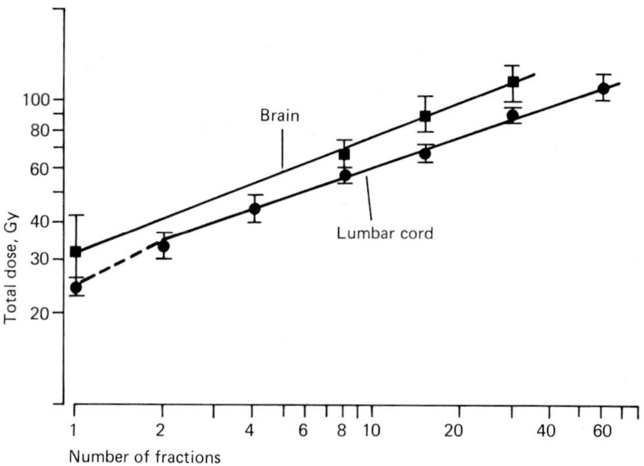

Fig. 6. Experimental animal data for CNS tolerance of brain and spinal cord. [From ref. 59, with permission.]

ing 58–60 Gy [9]. The study by Hindo et al. [56] of large single doses in humans suggests problems with the brain with single doses of 10 Gy. In burros a dose of 12 Gy in one fraction is lethal [20]. Kapp et al. [64], on the other hand, have used 6-Gy fractions with a radiation sensitizer without difficulty. In an RTOG study [17] a range of large fraction sizes was tested. Serious immediate reactions or early delayed reactions were not a problem; however, most patients were not observed for lated delayed reactions. Young et al. [143], on the other hand, found that rapid-course treatment resulted in problems. Analyzing these various series and the estimates of the late-effect factor of 1.66 for the alpha/beta ratio suggested by Withers [141], keeping the daily dose per fraction at 2 Gy and limiting the total dose to 55 Gy, as suggested by Marks and Wong [86], should not produce significant brain injury. Some late histologic tissue injury is reported by Salazar et al. [109] from the high-dose/high-grade glioma study where the total dose was 80 Gy. When other factors such as diabetes are considered, increased brain injury has been reported [119]. Hypertension and steroids also increase the sensitivity of the CNS to radiation [3]. Chemotherapeutic agents increase brain injury in adults [19, 22, 24, 101, 110, 112], as suggested by Breuer et al. [19], Davis [35], and Rubin [107]. Retreatment of the brain is also possible [37]. Further data are needed on the whole topic of retreatment.

Table III. Isoeffect table for radiation myelopathy: linear-quadratic model [from ref. 29, with permission]

Fraction	Schedule															
	continuous		2/day		daily		3/week		2/week		weekly		interval-2 weeks		monthly	
	Gy	days	Gy	days	Gy	days	Gy	days	Gy	days	Gy	days	Gy	days	Gy	days
2	16.09	1.2	16.09	1.5	16.09	2	16.09	3	16.59	5	16.59	8	17.59	15	18.59	29
3	18.84	1.4	18.84	2.0	19.34	4	19.34	6	19.84	8	20.84	15	22.34	29	24.84	57
4	21.59	1.6	21.59	2.5	21.59	5	22.09	8	22.59	12	24.09	22	26.59	43	31.59	85
5	23.34	1.8	23.34	3.0	23.84	6	24.84	10	25.34	15	27.34	29	30.84	57	37.34	113
6	25.09	2.0	25.59	3.5	26.09	7	26.59	12	27.59	19	30.59	36	35.09	71	43.59	141
7	26.84	2.2	26.84	4.0	27.84	9	28.84	15	29.84	22	33.34	43	39.34	85	49.84	169
8	28.09	2.4	28.59	4.5	29.59	10	30.59	17	32.09	26	36.09	50	43.59	99	54.59	197
9	29.34	2.6	29.84	5.0	30.84	11	32.34	19	34.34	29	38.84	57	47.84	113	58.34	225
10	30.59	2.8	31.09	5.5	32.59	13	34.09	22	36.09	33	42.09	64	52.09	127	60.59	253
15	35.34	3.8	36.34	8.0	38.84	19	41.84	33	45.34	50	55.34	99	69.84	197	72.34	393
20	38.59	4.8	40.09	10.5	44.09	26	49.09	45	54.59	68	69.09	134	80.09	267	81.59	533
25	41.34	5.8	43.84	13.0	49.34	32	55.34	56	62.84	85	82.34	169	87.84	337	89.34	673
30	44.09	6.8	46.59	15.5	53.59	39	62.09	68	71.59	103	90.59	204	94.09	407	96.09	813

Nominal standard dase equivalent: D = 1, 134; *(number of fractions in the total treatment **0.35) *(treatment time in days between the first and last treatment **0.07).
Response level: log S.Fr = 2.01; Eq.D1 = 11.6 Gy; probit = 3.3; probability 5%; Size = 10 cm.

Spinal Cord Data

As already pointed out, our editor [129] reported some of the early observations on injury of the spinal cord in patients. This analysis was expanded by Wara et al. [137] and Lambert [76]. Additional data for the cervical spinal cord in adults can be found in the paper by Kim and Fayos [65]. These analyses deal with standard fractionation. Since spinal cord injury is such a devastating problem, there are several excellent reviews of the data included in several chapters in the publication by Gilbert and Kagan [46]. Large-fraction irradiation has resulted in myelopathy [36, 54]. Cohen and Creditor [29] have collected the data and analyzed the material with a linear-quadratic as well as other models. The data for the spinal cord for the linear-quadratic fit are presented in table III from the analysis of spinal cord injury in humans made by Cohen and Creditor [29]. The work of Thames et al. [124] and the excellent experimental work by van der Kogel [132] show that the risk of cord injury increases with the dose per fraction, being a late-responding tissue. An alpha/beta ratio of 1.66 is suggested for spinal cord from the analysis of Withers et al. [142]. In the RSNA categorical course on treatment planning, Withers [141] pointed out the need for careful decision making in irradiation of the spinal cord even in palliative situations, data are shown in table IV as a guide in the treatment planning process. Wilson and Hall [140] discussed the need to treat all radiation fields every day to lessen normal-tissue effects, and such effects are also seen in table IV.

The known data on spinal cord injury from the laboratory and the clinic [1, 104] and the estimates by Hornsey et al. [59] that the brain is somewhat more resistant to observable injury, as shown in figure 6. One can make some projections on the tolerance of the brain with standard fractionation which fits with the reports of Marks et al. [84, 87], Marks and Wong [86], and Pezner and Archambeau [100].

Fractionation: Brain and Spinal Cord

Above 12 Gy one can expect major CNS injury in the immediate and early reaction time frame. Hindo et al. [56] found that a dose of 10 Gy was tolerated, and one of 6 Gy has been used in upper hemibody radiation without major difficulty. Kapp et al. [64] have reported that a dose of 6 Gy, given on a weekly basis for seven treatments, to the brain was possible without untoward side effects; however, the patients had high-grade astrocytomas, and long-term follow-up was not possible, so that some late effects may not have been observed. Large doses of radiations

Table IV. Dissociation between physical and biological doses [from ref. 141, with permission]

Regimen[a]	Physical dose[b]		Bio Gy-2[c]		Overall therapeutic ratio[d]
	spinal cord	tumor	spinal cord	tumor	
2 Gy AP-PA daily	2.06	2.00	2.09	2.00	0.96
2 Gy AP	1.62	2.00	1.44	2.00	0.93
2 Gy PA (on alternate days)	2.52	2.00	2.85	2.00	
3 Gy AP-PA daily	3.09	3.00	3.93	3.25	0.83
3 Gy AP	2.40	3.00	2.64	3.25	0.80
3 Gy PA (on alternate days)	3.78	3.00	5.46	3.25	
5 Gy AP-PA daily	5.15	5.00	9.20	6.25	0.68
5 Gy AP	4.00	5.00	6.00	6.25	0.66
5 Gy PA (on alternate days)	6.30	5.00	13.07	6.25	
6 Gy AP-PA daily	61.8	6.00	12.64	8.00	0.63
6 Gy AP	4.80	6.00	8.16	8.00	0.61
6 Gy PA (alternately)	7.56	6.00	18.06	8.00	

Although composite isodose curves for an AP-PA treatment prescription may show the dose to the spinal cord to be 103% of tumor dose regardless of dose-time factors, differences in fractionation patterns may produce vastly different isobieffective distributions. AP = Radiation beam directed from anterior to posterior; PA = radiation beam directed from posterior to anterior.

[a]Midline thoracic tumor at 11 cm depth; 10-MV X-rays, source-to-skin distance of 100 cm, and 20 × 10-cm field.

[b]Isodose curves show that midtumor = 100%; midspinal cord PA = 126%; AP = 80%.

[c]Bio Gy-2 = Equivalent in biological effect to a dose given in 2-Gy fractions.

[d]Average ratio = Bio Gy-2 tumor/bio Gy-2 spinal cord.

have been given in unusual fractionation patterns both in brain and spinal cord [5, 56, 62, 64, 114]. Kagan et al. [61] found brain necrosis in dogs so treated, and in patients with lung cancer, spinal cord injury is reported with large fraction sizes of 6 Gy/fraction [36].

Hyperfractionation

Two series [116, 118] have tested multiple-fraction/day treatment in high-grade gliomas, and there has been no evidence of late injury. If one considers the late-effect data from animal and human studies, a dose per fraction much above SF size of 2 Gy will lead to serious late side effects.

Table V. Late complications after irradiation of the breast [from refs. 93 and 125, with permission]

Complication	3,500–4,000 rad/4 weeks 5 × weekly (88 patients)		3,500–4,000 rad/4 weeks 3 × weekly (30 patients)	
	%	rad/fraction	%	rad/fraction
Severe chest wall fibrosis	2	200	20	>500
Rib fracture	7	200	10	>500
Severe pneumonitis	2	200	13	>500
Severe axillary fibrosis and frozen shoulder	2	200	20	333
Posterior scapular fibrosis	0	200	7	333
Arm edema	1	200	10	>500
Severe supraclavicular fibrosis	0	200	17	333
Brachial plexopathy	0	200	3	333

Acute responses were similar in all groups. Based on assessment of damage resulting primarily from either anterior–posterior supraclavicular fields (333 rad/fraction) or alternating tangential breast beams (500–600 rad/fraction).

The question of fractions sizes below SF or 1.8 Gy/fraction has been tested by Ang et al. [2], and no dose sparing was observed over SF; however, van der Schueren [135] has presented some data at this symposium which differ from those findings and may add to our understanding to tolerance of the spinal cord below 2 Gy/fraction. Since hyperfractionation and treatment with multiple fractions of radiations per day have become part of some treatment programs, information on small doses per fraction is needed to guide the radiation oncologist.

Cranial and Peripheral Nerves

The diagnosis of injury of the brachial plexus presents a dilemma between a metastatic lesion or radiation-induced injury [126]. The main feature of injury appears to be related to the dose per fraction. In the review by Kinsella et al. [66] the size of the dose per fraction became a critical factor when the dose was greater than 2 Gy/fraction. The reports by Aristizabal et al. [4], Harris and Levene [55], and Shukovsky and Fletcher [147] suggest that larger doses per fraction than 2 Gy increase injury of the optic pathways in the treatment of the pituitary region and

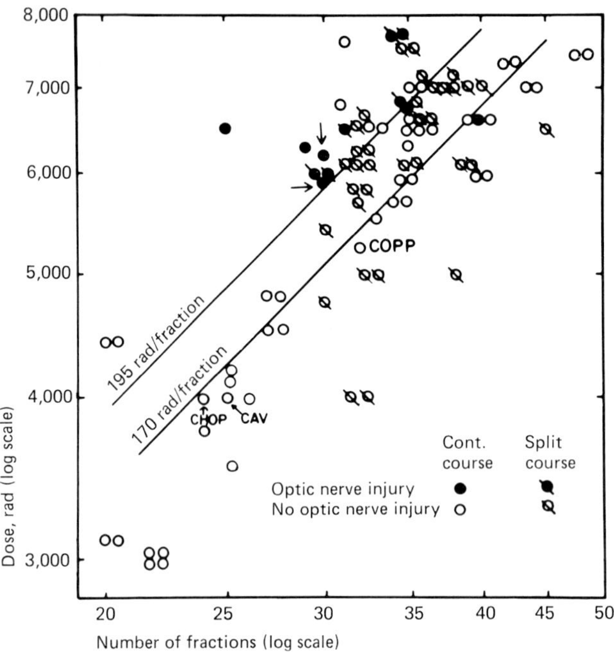

Fig. 7. Optic nerve injury. COPP = Cytoxan, Oncovin, prednisone, procarbazine; CHOP = Cytoxan; hydrodoxorubicin (Adriamycin), Oncovin; CAV = Cytoxan, Adriamycin, vincristine (Ducovin). [From ref. 99, with permission.]

that total doses over 50 Gy are not well tolerated. In the analysis of peripheral nerve injury by Montague [93], there was injury of the brachial plexus observed in this series when 333 Gy/fraction was used (Table V). With large doses per fraction peripheral nerve injury is seen [6, 121, 123, 138]. Kinsella [67] has reported on his experience with intraoperative radiation therapy of pelvic tumors where peripheral nerve injury has been observed. This author [67] has studied the problem of peripheral nerve injury recently and found that doses above 20 Gy in a single fraction produced late injury of the lumbosaccral plexus in dogs so treated. Since the fraction size appears to be the important factor, and the injury is a late reaction, fibrosis and possibly vascular injury are thought to be the principle mechanisms of injury.

In the analysis of a technique for treating tumors about the orbit, Parsons et al. [99] noted the frequency of optic nerve injuries and the critical factor of dose per fraction at the 2-Gy level, as shown in figure 7.

Bohne et al. [74] studied the inner ear, in particular the hair cells of the organ of Corti in a mammal with a long life: the chinchilla. Using SF and treatment 5 days/week to a total dose of 40–90 Gy, the number of hair cells was counted 2 years after treatment. The loss was 5% at 40 Gy and 25% at 90 Gy.

Interstitial Radiation and Tolerance

At the present time the type of implant and the methods of implantation are changing [50, 51, 111]. In the preliminary report [50] some necrosis is observed in those patients who are retreated for high-grade gliomas with implants following external therapy. As the series of patients so treated is expanded, and methods of implantation become standardized, the degree of necrosis seen should balance the ability to control the local lesion.

Neutron Radiation and Tolerance

There are several reports on spinal cord injury from neutron irradiation in clinical trials [25, 30, 78]. Cohen et al. [30] have reviewed the irradiation spinal cord injury from fast-neutron therapy. An RBE of 4 is suggested, and total doses below 11–12 Gy appear to be safe [30]. Since most of the brain tumor patients treated with neutrons have high-grade gliomas, the true incidence of late injury for the treatment situation is hard to predict; however, significant CNS injury was reported in the late time period in two series [79, 83].

Proton Irradiation and Tolerance

Fabricant et al. [42] and Fabricant [43] treated a larger series of patients to a very localized site with a proton beam directed to an arteriovenous malformation. The incidence of bleeding and other high-dose sequelae has been less than 5% [43]. Usually two doses of the proton beam are used with a total dose of 45 Gy.

Future of Nervous System Injury Analysis

Some changes are seen on X-ray and computerized tomography [68, 80, 91]. The addition of magnetic resonance imaging, to look at water content and provide vascular information, may increase our ability to detect early changes [31]. The ability to image oxygen and carbon-11-labeled glucose or the *D*-Glucose form provides a sensitive indicator of loss of brain substance. Immunological markers using monoclonal antibodies to test for myelin basic protein or similar nervous tissue markers may help in early detection of injury. Somatosensory evoked potentials, visual evoked potentials, and nerve conduction time measurements may identify early changes during the course of treatment. If detected, these indicators may guide the radiation oncologist to modify therapy, while the process is reversible.

References

1 Abbatucci, J. S.; Delozier, T.; Quint, R.; Roussel, A.; Brune, D.: Radiation myelopathy of the cervical spinal cord: time, dose, and volume factors. Int. J. Radiat. Oncol. Biol. Phys. *4:* 239–248 (1978).

2 Ang, K. K.; Thames, H. D.; Kogel, A. J. van der; Schueren, E. van der: Is the repair of radiation-induced sublethal damage in rat spinal cord dependent on the size of dose per fraction? Int. J. Radiat. Oncol. Biol. Phys. *13:* 557–562 (1987).

3 Aristizabal, S. A.; Boone, M. L. M.; Laguna, J. F.: Endocrine factors influencing radiation injury to central nervous system. Int. J. Radiat. Oncol. Biol. Phys. *5:* 349–353 (1979).

4 Aristizabal, S.; Caldwell, W. L.; Avila, J.: The relationship of time-dose fractionation factors to complications in the treatment of pituitary tumors by irradiation. Int. J. Radiat. Oncol. Biol. Phys. *2:* 667–673 (1977).

5 Atkins, H. L.; Tretter, P.: Time-dose considerations in radiation myelopathy. Acta radiol. (Ther.) *5:* 79–94 (1966).

6 Atkins, H. L.: Massive dose technique in radiation therapy of inoperable carcinoma of the breast. Am. J. Roentg. *91:* 80–89 (1964).

7 Barendsen, G. W.: Dose fractionation, dose rate and isoeffect relationships for normal tissue responses. Int. J. Radiat. Oncol. Biol. Phys. *8:* 1981–1997 (1982).

8 Berg, N. O.; Lindgren, M.: Time-dose relationship and morphology of delayed radiation lesions of the brain in rabbits. Acta radiol. *167:* suppl., pp. 1–118 (1958).

9 Berge, G.; Brun, A.; Hakansson, C. H.; Lindgren, M.; Nordberg, U. B.: Sensitivity to irradiation of the brain stem. Cancer *33:* 1263–1268 (1974).

10 Bleyer, W. A.; Giffin, T. W.: White matter necrosis, mineralizing microangiopathy and intellectual abilities in survivors of childhood leukemia: associations with central nervous system irradiation and methotrexate therapy; in Gilbert, Kagan, Radiation damage to the nervous system: a delayed therapeutic hazard, pp. 155–174. (Raven Press, New York 1980).

11 Bloom, H. J. G.: Intracranial tumors: response and resistance to therapeutic endeavors 1970–1980. Int. J. Radiat. Oncol. Biol. Phys. *8:* 1083–113 (1982).

12 Boden, G.: Radiation myelitis of the cervical spinal cord. Br. J. Radiol. *21:* 64 (1948).

13 Boden, B.: Radiation myelitis of brain stem. J. Fac. Radiol. *2:* 79 (1950).

14 Bohne, B. A.; Marks, J. E.; Glasgow, G. P.: Delayed effects of ionizing radiation on the ear. Laryngoscope *95:* 818–828 (1985).

15 Boice, J. D.; Fraumeni, J. F.: Radiation carcinogenesis (Raven Press, New York 1984).
16 Boldrey, E.; Sheline, G.: Delayed transitory clinical manifestation after radiation treatment of intracranial tumors. Acta radiol. (Ther. Phys. Biol.) *5:* 5–10 (1967).
17 Borgelt, B.; Gelber, R.; Larson, M.; Hendrickson, F.; Griffin, T.; Roth, R.: Ultrarapid high dose irradiation schedules for the palliation of brain metastases: final report of the first two studies by the Radiation Therapy Oncology Group. Int. J. Radiat. Oncol. Biol. Phys. *7:* 1633–1638 (1981).
18 Bouchard, J.: Radiobiologic effects on the central nervous system tissues and tumors; in Bouchard, Radiation therapy of tumors and diseases of the nervous system, pp. 29–48 (Lea & Febiger, Philadelphia 1966).
19 Breuer, A. C.; Blank, N. K.; Schoene, W. C.: Multifocal pontine lesions in cancer patients treated with chemotherapy and CNS radiotherapy. Cancer *42:* 2112–2170 (1978).
20 Brown, D. G.; Sasmore, D. P.; Jones, L. P.: Acute central nervous system syndrome in burros; in Haley, Snider, Response of the nervous system to ionizing radiation, pp. 503–512 (Academic Press, New York 1962).
21 Brown, W. J.; Kagan, A. R.: Comparison of myelopathy associated with megavoltage irradiation and remote cancer; in Gilbert, Kagan, Radiation damage to the nervous system: a delayed therapeutic hazard, pp. 191–206 (Raven Press, New York 1980).
22 Burger, P. C.; Kamenar, E.; Schold, S. C.; Fay, J. W.; Phillips, G. L.; Herzig, G. P.: Encephalomyelopathy following high-dose BCNU therapy. Cancer *48:* 1318–1327 (1981).
23 Burger, P. C.; Mahaley, M. S.; Dudka, L.; Wogel, F. S.: The morphologic effects of radiation administered therapeutically for intracranial gliomas: a postmortem study of 25 cases. Cancer *44:* 1256–1272 (1979).
24 Byfield, J. E.: Central nervous system toxicities from combined therapies; in Vaeth, Front. Radiat. Ther. Onc., vol. 13, pp. 228–240 (Karger, Basel 1979).
25 Catterall, M.; Bewley, D. K.; Fast neutrons in the treatment of cancer (Academic Press, London 1979).
26 Caveness, W. F.: Experimental observations: delayed necrosis in normal monkey; in Gilbert Kagan, Radiation damage to the nervous system: a delayed therapeutic hazard, pp. 1–38 (Raven Press, New York, 1980).
27 Cerella, R.; Geigin, I.; Newall, J.; Farina, A. T.: Histologic evidence of necrosis following radiotherapy for primary cerebral tumor. N. Y. St. J. Med. *78:* 1324–1327 (1978).
28 Crompton, M. R.; Layton, D. D.: Delayed radionecrosis of the brain following therapeutic X-radiation of the pituitary. Brain *84:* 85–101 (1961).
29 Cohen, L.; Creditor, M.; An iso-effect table for radiation tolerance of the human spinal cord. Int. J. Radiat. Oncol. Biol. Phys. *7:* 961–966 (1981).
30 Cohen, L.; Ten Haken, R. K.; Mansell, J.; Yalavarthi, S. D.; Hendrickson, F. R.; Awschalom, M.: Tolerance of the human spinal cord to high energy p(66)Be(49) neutrons, Int. J. Radiat. Oncol. Biol. Phys. *11:* 743–749 (1985).
31 Curran, C.; Hecht-Leavitt, C.; Schut, L.; Zimmerman, R. A.; Nelson, D. F.: Magnetic resonance imaging of cranial radiation lesions. Int. J. Radiat. Oncol. Biol. Phys. *13:* 1093–1098 (1987).
32 Danoff, B. F.: Complications and late effects of irradiation for brain tumors; in Marks, Griem, Syllabus: therapy of CNS tumors (Radiological Society of North America, Chicago 1983).
33 Danoff, B. F.: Cowchock, F. S.; Marquette, C.; Mulgrew, L.; Kramer, S.: Assessment

of the long-term effects of primary radiation therapy for brain tumros in children. Cancer *49:* 1580–1586 (1982).
34 Danoff, B. F.; Cowchock, F. S.; Kramer, S.: Childhood craniopharyngioma: survival, local control, endocrine and neurologic function following radiotherapy. Int. J. Radiat. Oncol. Biol. Phys. *9:* 171–175 (1983).
35 Davis, R. L.: Brain response to combined modality therapy; in Vaeth, Front. Radiat. Ther. Onc., vol. 13, pp. 58–66 (Karger, Basel 1979).
36 Dische, S.; Martin, W.; Anderson, P.: Radiation myelopathy in patients treated for carcinoma of bronchus using a six-fraction regime of radiotherapy. Br. J. Radiol. *54:* 29–35 (1981).
37 Dritschillo, A.; Bruckman, T. E.; Cassady, J. R.; Belli, J. A.: Tolerance of brain to multiple courses of radiation therapy. Br. J. Radiol. *54:* 782–786 (1981).
38 Duffner, P. K.; Cohen, M. E.; Thomas, P.: Late effects of treatment on the intelligence of children with posterior fossa tumors. Cancer *51:* 233–237 (1983).
39 Effects of ionizing radiation on the nervous system (International Atomic Energy Agency, Vienna 1962).
40 Eifel, P.; Cassady, J. R.; Belli, J. A.: Radiation therapy of tumors of the brain stem and midbrain in children: Experience of the JCRT and Children's Hospital Medical Center. Int. J. Radiat. Oncol. Biol. Phys. *13:* 847–852 (1987).
41 Eyster, E. F.; Nielsen, S. L.; Sheline, G. E.; Wilson, C. B.: Cerebral radionecrosis simulating a brain tumor. J. Neurosurg. *39:* 267–271 (1972).
42 Fabricant, J. I.; Lyman, J. T.; Frankel, K. A.: Heavy charged particle Bragg peak radiosurgery for intracranial vascular disorders. Radiat. Res. *104:* suppl., pp. 244–258 (1985).
43 Fabricant, J. I.: Personal commun. (1987).
44 Freeman, J. E.; Johnston, P. G. B.; Voke, J. M.: Somnolence after prophylactic cranial radiation in children with acute lymphoblastic leukemia. Br. med. J. *iv:* 523–525 (1973).
45 Ghatak, N. R.; White, B. E.: Delayed radiation necrosis of the hypothalamus. Archs Neurol. *21:* 425–430 (1969).
46 Gilbert, H. A.; Kagan, A. R.: Radiation damage to the nervous system (Raven Press, New York 1980).
47 Glass, J. P.; Hwang, T.-L.; Leavens, M. E.; Libshitz, H. I.: Cerebral radiation necrosis following treatment of extracranial malignancies. Cancer *54:* 1966–1972 (1984).
48 Glicksman, A. S.; Bliven, S. F.; Leith, J. T.: Modification of radiation damage in rat spinal cord by mitotane. Cancer Treat. Rep. *66:* 1545–1547 (1982).
49 Griffin, T. W.; Rasey, J. S.; Bleyer, W. A.: The effect of photon irradiation on blood-brain barrier permeability to methotrexate in mice. Cancer *40:* 1109–1111 (1977).
50 Gutin, P. H.; Leibel, S. A.: Stereotaxic interstitial irradiation of malignant brain tumors. Neurol. Clin. *3:* 883–893 (1985).
51 Gutin, P. H.; Phillips, T. L.; Hosobuchi, Y., et al.: Permanent and removable implants for the brachytherapy of brain tumors. Int. J. Radiat. Oncol. Biol. Phys. *7:* 137–138 (1981).
52 Haley, T. J.; Snider, R. S.: Response of the nervous system to ionizing radiation (Academic Press, New York 1962).
53 Harrop, J. S.; Davies, T. J.; Capra, L. G.; Marks, V.: Hypothalamic-pituitary function following successful treatment of intracranial tumors. Clin. Endocr. *5:* 313–321 (1976).
54 Hatlevoll, R.; Host, H.; Kaalhus, O.: Myelopathy following radiotherapy of bronchial carcinoma with large single fractions: a retrospective study. Int. J. Radiat. Oncol. Biol. Phys. *9:* 41–44 (1983).

55 Harris, J. R.; Levene, M. B.: Visual complications following irradiation for primary adenomas and craniopharyngiomas. Radiology *120:* 167–171 (1976).
56 Hindo, W. A.; De Trana, F. A.; Lee, M. S.; Hendrickson, F. R.: Large dose increment irradiation in treatment of cerebral metastases. Cancer *26:* 138–141 (1970).
57 Hopewell, J. W.; Wright, E. A.: The nature of latent cerebral irradiation damage and its modification by hypertension. Br. J. Radiol. *43:* 161–167 (1970).
58 Hornsey, S.; White, E.: Isoeffect curve for radiation myelopathy. Br. J. Radiol. *53:* 168–169 (1980).
59 Hornsey, S.; Morris, C. C.; Myers, R.: The relationship between fractionation and total dose for X-ray induced brain damage. Int. J. Radiat. Oncol. Biol. Phys. *7:* 393–396 (1981).
60 International Commission on Radiation Units and Measurements: Physical aspects of irradiation. ICRU Rep. 10b, Washington 1964.
61 Kagan, A. R.; Steckel, R. J.; Cancilla, P.; Juillard, G.; Patin, T.: The pathogenesis of brain necrosis: time and dose parameters. Int. J. Radiat. Oncol. Biol. Phys. *1:* 729–732 (1976).
62 Kagan, A. R.; Wollin, M.; Gilbert, H. A.; Nussbaum, H.; Hintz, B. L.; Rao, A.; Chan, P. Y. M.: Comparison of the tolerance of the brain and spinal cord to injury by radiations; in Gilbert, Kagan, Radiation damage to the nervous system: a delayed therapeutic hazard, pp. 183–190 (Raven Press, New York 1980).
63 Kaplan, S. L.: Effects of cancer treatment on hypothalamic and pituitary function in children. Proc. Conf. on Long-Term Normal-Tissue Effects of Cancer Treatment (American College of Radiology, Philadelphia 1981).
64 Kapp, D. S.; Wagner, F. C.; Lawrence, R.: Glioblastoma multiforme: treatment by large dose fraction irradiation and metronidazole. Int. J. Radiat. Oncol. Biol. Phys. *8:* 351–355 (1982).
65 Kim, Y. H.; Fayos, J. V.: Radiation injury of the cervical spinal cord. Int. J. Radiat. Oncol. Biol. Phys. *5:* suppl 2, p. 105 (1979).
66 Kinsella, T. J.; Weichselbaum, R.; Sheline, G. E.: Radiation injury of cranial and peripheral nerves; in Gilbert, Kagan, Radiation injury to the nervous system: a delayed therapeutic hazard, pp. 145–154 (Raven Press, New York 1980).
67 Kinsella, T. J.: Intra-operative X-ray therapy. Front. Radiat. Ther. Onc. (this volume).
68 Kingsley, D. P. E.; Kendall, B. E.: CT of the adverse effects of therapeutic radiation of the central nervous system. Am. J. Neuroradiol. *2:* 453–460 (1981).
69 Kramer, S.: The hazards of therapeutic irradiation of the central nervous system. Clin. Neurosurg. *15:* 301–318 (1967).
70 Kramer, S.; Southard, M. E.; Mansfield, C. M.: Radiation effects and tolerance of the central nervous system. Front. Radiat. Ther. Onc., vol. 6, pp. 332–345 (University Park Press, Baltimore 1972).
71 Kramer, S.; Lee, K. L.: Complications of radiation therapy: the central nervous system. Semin. Roentgenol. *9:* 75–83 (1974).
72 Kriegel, H.; Schmahl, W.; Gerber, G. B.; Stieve, F. E.: Radiation risks to the developing nervous system (Fischer, Stuttgart 1986).
73 Kun L. E.; Mulhern, R. K.; Crisco, J. J.: Quality of life in children treated for brain tumors: intellectual, emotional, and academic function. J. Neurosurg. *58:* 1–6 (1983).
74 Kusske, J. A.; Williams, J. P.; Garcia, J. H.; Pribram, H. W.: Radiation necrosis of the brain following radiotherapy of extracranial neoplasms. Surg. Neurol. *6:* 15–20 (1968).
75 Lambert, P. W.; Davis, R. L.: Delayed effects of radiation on the human central nervous system. 'Early' and 'late' delayed reactions. Neurology *14:* 912–917 (1964).

76 Lambert, P. M.: Radiation myelopathy of the thoracic spinal cord in long-term survivors treated with radical radiotherapy using conventional fractionation. Cancer *41:* 1751–1760 (1978).

77 Lampe, I.: Radiation tolerance of the central nervous system; in Buschke, Progress in radiation therapy, pp. 224–236 (Grune & Stratton, New York 1958).

78 Laramore, G. E.; Blasko, J. C.; Griffin, T. W.; Groudine, T. M.: Fast neutron teletherapy for advanced carcinomas of the oropharynx. Int. J. Radiat. Oncol. Biol. Phys. *5:* 1821–1827 (1979).

79 Laramore, G. E.; Griffin, T. W.; Gerdes, A. J.; Parker, R. G.: Fast neutron and mixed neutron/photon beam teletherapy for grade III and IV astrocytomas. Cancer *42:* 96–103 (1978).

80 Lee, K. F.; Suh, J. H.: CT evidence of gray matter calcification secondary to radiation therapy. Comput. Tomogr. *1:* 103–110 (1977).

81 Leith, J. T.; De Wyngaert, J. K.; Glicksman, A. S.: Radiation myelopathy in the rat: an interpretation of dose-effect relationships. Int. J. Radiat. Oncol. Biol. Phys. *7:* 1673–1677 (1981).

82 Lindgren, M.: Tolerance of brain tissue and sensitivity of brain tumors to irradiation. Acta radiol. *170:* 1–73 (1958).

83 Manz, H. J.; Woolley, P. V.; Ornitz, R. D.: Delayed radiation necrosis of brain stem related to fast neutron beam irradiation. Cancer *44:* 473–479 (1979).

84 Marks, J. E.; Baglan, R. J.; Prasad, S. C.; Blank, W. A.: Cerebral radionecrosis: incidence and risk in relation to dose, time, fractionation and volume. Int. J. Radiat. Oncol. Biol. Phys. *7:* 243–252 (1981).

85 Marks, J. E.; Griem, M. L.: Categorical course in therapy of CNS tumors (Radiological Society North America, Chicago 1983).

86 Marks, J. E.; Wong, J.: The risk of cerebral radionecrosis in relation to dose, time and fractionation. Prog. exp. Tumor Res., vol. 29, pp. 210–218 (Karger, Basel 1985).

87 Marks, J. E.; Baglan, R. J.; Wong, J.: Radiation damage to brain and cranial soft tissues: outcome and incidence before and after reduction in dose; in Walker, Thomas, Biology of brain tumor (Nijhoff, Boston 1986).

88 Martins, A. N.; Johnson, J. S.; Hendry, J. E.; Stoffel, T. L.; Di Chiro, G.: Delayed radiation necrosis of brain. J. Neurosurg. *47:* 336–345 (1977).

89 Meadows, A. T.; Massari, D. J.; Fergusson, J.; Gordon, J.; Littman, P.; Moss, K.: Declines in IQ scores and cognitive dysfunction in children with acute lymphoblastic leukemia treated with cranial irradiation. Lancet *ii:* 1015–1018 (1981).

90 Mendelsohn, M. L.: The biology of dose limiting tissues; in Time and dose relationships in radiation biology as applied to radiotherapy, pp. 154–160. Brookhaven National Laboratory Publication No. 50203 [C57] (National laboratory, Brookhaven, 1970).

91 Mikhael, M. A.: Radiation necrosis of the brain: correlation between computed tomography, pathology and dose distribution. J. Comput. assist. Tomogr. *2:* 71–80 (1978).

92 Mole, R. H.: Problems related to prenatal exposure of the nervous system: history and perspective; in Kriegel et al., Radiation risks to the developing nervous system (Fischer, Stuttgart 1986).

93 Montague, E. D.: Experience with altered fractionation in radiation therapy for breast cancer. Radiology *90:* 962–966 (1968).

94 Morris-Jones, P. H.: The effect of varying doses of cerebral irradiation on growth hormone production in childhood. Clin Endocr., *5:* 287–290 (1976).

95 Nakagaki, H.; Brunhart, G.; Kemper, T. L.; Caveness, W. F.: Monkey brain damage from radiation in the therapeutic range. J. Neurosurg. *44:* 3–11 (1976).
96 Ornitz, R.; Herskovic, A.; Bradley, E.; Deye, J. A.; Rogers, C. C.: Clinical observations of early and late normal tissue injury and tumor control in patients receiving fast neutron irradiation; in High LET radiations in clinical radiotherapy, pp. 43–50 (Pergamon Press, Oxford 1979).
97 Pallis, C. A.; Louis, S.; Morgan, R. L.: Radiation myelopathy. Brain *84:* 460 (1961).
98 Parker, D.; Malpas, J. S.; Sandland, R.; Sheaff, P. C.; Freeman, J. E.; Paxton, A.: Outlook following somnolence syndrome after prophylactic cranial irradiation. Br. med. J. *iv:* 554 (1978).
99 Parsons, J. F.; Fitzgerald, C. R.; Hood, C. I.; Ellingwood, K. E.; Bova, F. L.; Million, R. R.: The effects of irradiation on the eye and optic nerve. Int. J. Radiat. Oncol. Biol. Phys. *9:* 609–622 (1983).
100 Pezner, R. D.; Archambeau, J. O.: Brain tolerance unit: a method to estimate risk of radiation brain injury for various dose schedules. Int. J. Radiat. Oncol. Biol. Phys. *7:* 397–402 (1981).
101 Pratt, R. A.; Di Chiro, G.; Weed, J. D.: Cerebral necrosis following irradiation and chemotherapy for metastatic choriocarcinoma. Surg. Neurol. *7:* 117–120 (1977).
102 Rall, D. P.; Zubrod, C. G.: Mechanism of drug absorption and excretion: passage of drugs in and out of the central nervous system. A. Rev. Pharmacol. *2:* 109–128 (1962).
103 Rappaport, R.; Brauner, R.; Czernichou, P.; Thibaud, E.; Renier, D.; Zucker, J. M.; Lemerle, L.: Effect of hypothalamic and pituitary irradiation on pubertal development in children with cranial tumors. J. clin. Endocr. Metab. *54:* 1164–1168 (1982).
104 Reinhold, H. S.; Kaalen, J. G. A. H.; Unger-Gils, K.: Radiation myelopathy of the thoracic spinal cord. Int. J. Radiat. Oncol. Biol. Phys. *1:* 651–657 (1976).
105 Richards, G. E.: Effects of irradiation on the hypothalamic pituitary regions; in Gilbert, Kagan, Radiation damage to the nervous system: a delayed therapeutic hazard, pp. 175–180 (Raven Press, New York 1980).
106 Rider, W. D.: Radiation damage to the brain. A new syndrome. J. Can. Ass. Radiol. *14:* 67 (1963).
107 Rubin, P.: The Franz Buschke Lecture: late effects of chemotherapy and radiation therapy: a new hypothesis. Int. J. Radiat. Oncol. Biol. Phys. *10:* 5–34 (1984).
108 Rubinstein, L. J.; Herman, M. M.; Long, T. F.; Wilbur, J. R.: Disseminated necrotizing leukencephalopathy: a complication of treated central nervous system leukemia and lymphoma. Cancer *35:* 291–305 (1975).
109 Salazar, O. M.; Rubin, P.; Feldstein, M. L.; Pizzutiello, R.: High-dose radiation therapy in the treatment of malignant gliomas: final report. Int. J. Radiat. Oncol. Biol. Phys. *5:* 1733–1740 (1979).
110 Salinsky, M. C.; Levine, R. L.; Aubuchon, J. P.; Schutta, H. S.: Acute cerebellar dysfunction with high-dose Ara-C therapy. Cancer *51:* 426–429 (1983).
111 Sapozink, M. D.; Moeller, J. M.; McDonald, P. N.; Heilbrun, M. P.: Improved precision of interstitial brain tumor irradiation using BRW CT stereotaxic guidance system. Int. J. Radiat. Oncol. Biol. Phys. *13:* 1753–1760 (1987).
112 Schiffer, D.; Giordana, M. T.; Soffietti, R.; Tarenzi, L.; Milani, R.; Vasario, E.; Paoletti, P.: Radio- and chemotherapy of malignant gliomas: pathological changes in the normal nervous tissue. Acta neurol. *58:* 37–58 (1981).
113 Schull, W. J.; Otake, M.: Neurological deficit among the survivors exposed in utero to the atomic bombing in Hiroshima and Nagasaki: a reassessment and new directions; in Kriegel, Radiation risks to the developing nervous system (Fischer, Stuttgart 1986).

114 Sheline, G. E.; Wara, W. M.; Smith, V.: Therapeutic irradiation and brain injury. Int. J. Radiat. Oncol. Biol. Phys. *6:* 1215–1228 (1980).

115 Sheline, G. E.: Irradiation injury of the human brain: a review of clinical experience; in Gilbert, Kagan, Radiation damage to the nervous system, pp. 39–58 (Raven Press, New York 1980).

116 Shin, K. H.; Muller, P. L.; Geggie, P. H. S.: Superfractionation radiation therapy in the treatment of malignant astrocytoma. Cancer *52:* 2040–2043 (1983).

117 Shukovsky, L. J.; Fletcher, G. H.: Retinal and optic nerve complications in a high dose irradiation technique of ethmoid sinus and nasal cavity. Radiology *104:* 629–634 (1972).

118 Simpson, W. J.; Platt, M. E.: Fractionation study in the treatment of glioblastoma multiforme. Int. J. Radiat. Oncol. Biol. Phys. *1:* 639–644 (1976).

119 Smith, B. M.; McGinnis, W.; Cook, J.; Latourette, H.: Central nervous system changes complicating the use of radiotherapy for the treatment of a nasopharyngeal neoplasm in a diabetic patient. Cancer *43:* 2239–2242 (1979).

120 Spunberg, J. J.; Chang, C. W.; Goldman, M.; Auricchio, E.; Bell, J. J.: Quality of long-term survival following irradiation for intracranial tumors in children under the age of two. Int. J. Radiat. Oncol. Biol. Phys. *7:* 727–736 (1981).

121 Stoll, B. A.; Andrews, J. T.: Radiation-induced peripheral neuropathy. Br. med. J. *i:* 834–837 (1966).

122 Sundaresan, N.; Galicich, J. H.; Deck, M. D.; Tornita, T.: Radiation necrosis after treatment of solitary intracranial metastases. Neurosurgery *8:* 329–333 (1981).

123 Svensson, L. J.; Westling, P.; Larson, L. G.: Radiation-induced lesions of the brachial plexus correlated to the dose-time-fractionation schedule. Acta radiol. ther. phys. biol. *14:* 228–238 (1975).

124 Thames, H. D.; Withers, H. R.; Peters, L. J.; Fletcher, G. H.: Changes in early and late radiation responses with altered dose fractionation: implications for dose-survival relationships. Int. J. Radiat. Oncol. Biol. Phys. *8:* 219–226 (1982).

125 Thames, H. D.; Hendry, J. H.: Fractionation in radiotherapy (Taylor & Frances, London 1987).

126 Thomas, J. E.; Colby, M. Y.: Radiation induced or metastatic brachial plexopathy? A diagnostic dilemma. J. Am. med. Ass. *222:* 1392–1395 (1972).

127 Tokars, R. P.; Griem, M. L.: Carcinoma of the nasopharynx and optimization of radiotherapeutic management for tumor control and spinal cord injury. Int. J. Radiat. Oncol. Biol. Phys. *5:* 1741–1748 (1979).

128 Urion, D. K.; Waber, D.; Sallan, S.; Sollee, N.: Microcephaly and impaired cognitive function among survivors of acute leukemia who received prophylactic cranial irradiation. Ann. Neurol. *22:* 448 (1987).

129 Vaeth, J. M.: Radiation-induced myelitis; in Buschke, Progress in radiation therapy, vol. 3, pp. 16–26 (Grune & Stratton, New York 1965).

130 Brenk, H. A. S. van der; Richter, W.; Hurley, R. H.: Radiosensitivity of the human oxygenated spinal cord based on analysis of 357 cases receiving 4 MeV X-rays in hyperbaric oxygen. Br. J. Radiol. *41:* 205–214 (1968).

131 Kogel, A. J. van der: Radiation tolerance of the rat spinal cord: time-dose relationships. Radiology *122:* 505–509 (1977).

132 Kogel, A. J. van der: Late effects of radiation on the spinal cord: dose-effect relationship and pathogenesis, pp. 1–160 (Radiological Institute TNO, Rijswik 1979).

133 Kogel, A. J. van der; Sissingh, H. A.: Effects of intrathecal methotrexate and cytosine arabinoside on the radiation tolerance of the rat spinal cord. Radiother. Oncol. *4:* 239–251 (1985).

134 Kogel, A. J. van der: The cellular basis of radiation-induced damage in the central nervous system; in Potten, Hendry, Cytotoxic insult to tissue (Churchill Livingstone, Edinburgh 1983).
135 Schueren, E. van der: Repair kinetics in irradiation of lip mucosa and spinal cord: fractionation and low dose rate implications. Front. Radiat. Ther. Onc. (this volume)
136 Walker, M. D.; Strike, T. A.; Sheline, G. E.: An analysis of dose-effect relationship in the radiotherapy of malignant gliomas. Int. J. Radiat. Oncol. Biol. Phys. *5:* 1725–1731 (1979).
137 Wara, W. M.; Phillips, T. L.; Sheline, G. E.; Schwade, J. G.: Radiation tolerance of the spinal cord. Cancer *35:* 1558–1582 (1975).
138 Westling, P.; Svensson, H.; Hele, P.: Cervical plexus lesions following postoperative radiation therapy of mammary carcinoma. Acta radiol. ther. phys. biol. *11:* 209–216 (1972).
139 White, A.; Hornsey, S.; Radiation damage to the rat spinal cord: the effect of single and fractionated doses of X-rays. J. Radiol. *51:* 515–523 (1978).
140 Wilson, C. S.; Hall, E. J.: On the advisability of treating all fields at each radiotherapy session. Radiology *98:* 419 (1971).
141 Withers, H. R.: Fractionation in radiation therapy treatment planning; in Paliwal, Griem, Syllabus: a categorical course in radiation therapy treatment planning (Radiological Society of North America, Chicago 1986).
142 Withers, H. R., Thames, H. D., Jr.; Peters, L. J.: A new isoeffect curve for change in dose per fraction. Radiother. Oncol. *1:* 187–191 (1983).
143 Young, D. F.; Posner, J. B.; Chu, F.; Nisce, L.: Rapid-course radiation oncology of cerebral metastases: results and complications. Cancer *34:* 1069–1076 (1974).

Melvin L. Griem, MD, Department of Radiation Oncology, University of Chicago, 5841 S Maryland Avenue, Chicago, IL 60637 (USA)

Vaeth JM, Meyer JL (eds): Radiation Tolerance of Normal Tissues.
Front Radiat Ther Oncol. Basel, Karger, 1989, vol 23, pp 390–407

Pediatric Patients Tolerance Levels and Effects of Treatment

Sarah S. Donaldson

Department of Radiation Oncology, Stanford University Medical Center, Stanford, Calif., USA

Introduction

As a multidisciplinary approach to management of children with cancer has brought about increased numbers of long-term survivors, continual emphasis must be placed upon the effects of this treatment and the quality of life of these survivors. Improvements in survival have been demonstrated for each type of childhood cancer. Data comparing survival rates in 1950 with data up to and inclusive of 1984 reveal that currently 63% of children with cancer are being cured of their disease (fig. 1). However, there are numerous reports of early as well as late toxicity now being recognized in these survivors. As survival rates improve, even more reports can be expected.

Several factors must be recognized when addressing normal-tissue tolerance in children. By definition, children are undergoing maximal developmental changes when exposed to anticancer therapy. When cured, they have many years ahead in which to live with the impact of their therapy. Sufficient attention has not yet been paid to the physical, emotional, or psychosocial aspects of being a cancer survivor. In addition, the acute and/or long-term sequelae of treatment appear more pronounced and severe when occurring in a child as opposed to the effects seen in adults [1]. These important sequelae area (1) disturbances in growth and development; (2) physiologic impairment of organ function; (3) induction of genetic mutation, and (4) secondary oncogenesis.

The hypothesis advanced regarding radiosensitivity and radioresistance in children relates to the periods of active proliferation and differentiation and eventual maturation. There are specific phases of tissue proliferation during infancy and during the rapid growth spurts of childhood which determine radiosensitivity. Radiosensitivity of a tissue/organ is highest prior to and at the time of onset of proliferative activity in each

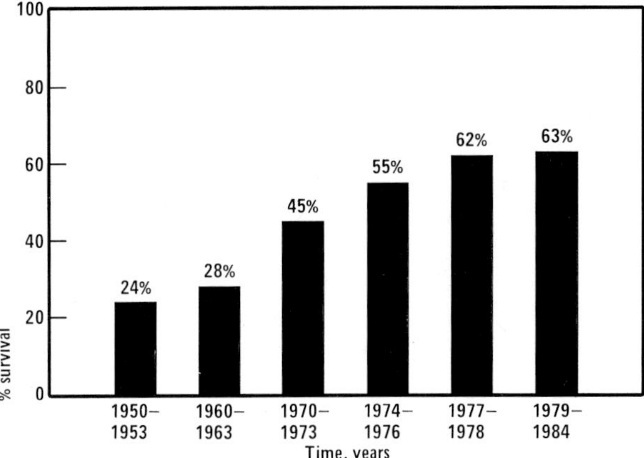

Fig. 1. Improvements in survival for children with cancer, age less than 15 years, from 1950 to the most current time span, 1979–1984, revealing a 63% relative 5-year survival.

organ system. The model advanced by Rubin *et al.* [2] suggests that radiosensitivity is determined by the growth rate and maturation of each tissue or organ individually. It has been thought that growth effects related to radiation are most pronounced when a child's treatment is delivered during periods of active growth, i.e., when less than 6 years of age and during puberty [3, 4]. Alternatively, it has been suggested that the effects of radiation are *not* observed until there is a call to proliferation. For example, skeletal changes secondary to radiotherapy given at a young age may not be observed until the child achieves his adolescent growth spurt. It is clear that radiation sensitivity varies for each organ and tissue irradiated.

Furthermore, the concept of radiosensitivity and radioresistance of normal tissues is completely modified by the uniform practice of multimodal therapy. Combined modality therapy is utilized in the management of virtually all children with cancer. The additive and/or synergistic effects of chemotherapy administered prior, during, or following a course of radiation therapy now demand new tolerance limits be set for virtually each organ system. There is no uniform quantitation of chemotherapy sensitization to irradiated tissues. The normal-tissue effects from combined modality therapy vary within the individual organ, drug utilized, dose and method of drug administration, radiation dose and volume, and timing of drug with irradiation. When dealing with children, it is not sufficient to discuss radiation effects alone, but rather one must consider the total effects from multimodal therapy. The following discussion addresses the effects and tolerance of a child with respect to growth and development, organ function, mutigenesis, and oncogenesis where data are available.

Growth

Skeletal System

Bone and soft tissue effects following megavoltage irradiation are well recognized to be directly related to irradiated volume and dose and inversely related to age at the time of treatment. Irradiation to bone may result in arrested chondrogenesis secondary to epiphyseal injury, deficient absorptive processes in calcified bone and cartilage due to metaphyseal injury, and altered periosteal activity and bone modeling from diaphyseal injury. Clinical studies of growth abnormalities related to radiotherapy have been best made among survivors of Hodgkin's disease, when afflicted during youth. Probert and Parker [3] and Probert et al. [5] were the first to demonstrate a disproportionate decrease in sitting height as compared to standing heigt among 22 youngsters who received total axial irradiation for Hodgkin's disease or medulloblastoma who were given high-dose therapy (3,500–4,400 cGy). They noted less deficit among those who received low doses (less than 2,500 cGy). The growth changes were thought to be most pronounced among those who were 6 years of age or less or in those in their adolescent growth spurt at the time of treatment. However, a more recent assessment of 112 children with Hodgkin's disease treated with high-dose irradiation to extended fields reveals that the age at the time of treatment is most critical. Children 13 years of age or less may be impaired by approximately 5% in both sitting and standing heights, while adolescents over the age of 13, even though they have not yet completed their growth, do not have a significant measurable deficit [6]. This relationship of dose with age supports the early classic study of Neuhauser et al. [7] who reported little, if any, growth disturbance with orthovoltage doses of 1,000 cGy given at any age, few changes when less than 2,000 cGy were administered, but pronounced changes seen with doses of greater than 2,000 cGy in children greater than 2 years of age at the time of treatment. Further evidence of the impact of spinal irradiation on overall growth is an assessment of leg length minus sitting height standard deviation score as compared to controls. Using this scoring system, a significant difference has been demonstrated as a function of age between those receiving spinal irradiation and measured using leg length minus sitting height standard deviation scores as compared to those receiving cranial irradiation alone. The younger the child when given irradiation, the greater the subsequent skeletal disproportion. Shalet *et al.* [8] estimated an eventual loss in height of 9 cm irradiation was given at age 1 year, 7 cm when given at 5 years, and 5.5 cm when given at 10 years.

Other than the standing/sitting height ratio of axial skeletal growth, we lack precise standards from which to measure bone growth abnormalities. Absence of symmetry has been noted, particularly in facial structures and leg length discrepancies, when unilateral treatment has been delivered. The severity of these changes has been poorly quantitated as a function of dose, volume, and age.

Organ Function

Hypothalmic-Pituitary Axis

The best understood central effect responsible for growth abnormalities is that of growth hormone (GH) deficiency. This has been described among children with brain tumors treated by surgery, radiotherapy, and occasionally chemotherapy or those with tumors which require central nervous system prophylaxis for prevention of central nervous system disease. Of the modalities utilized, cranial irradiation is the major contributor to the subsequent deficit.

Shalet [9] studied the relationship between radiation dose delivered to the hypothalmic-pituitary region and GH secretion among 56 children receiving cranial radiotherapy. He demonstrated an inverse correlation between dose of radiation and maximal GH response (fig. 2). Shalet [9] reported that 37 of 56 (66%) children had an impaired GH response (peak <20 mU/l), all but 1 of whom received doses of 2,900 cGy/3 weeks or greater. Supporting studies have since shown that doses of 2,700 or greater per 3 weeks to the hypothalamic-pituitary axis result in impaired GH responses [10]. Radiation fraction size is important as well as dose. It is believed that the younger the child, and the larger the radiation fraction, the more likely is the observation of impaired GH response. Children receiving prophylactic cranial irradiation for acute lymphoblastic leukemia have been studied for GH function with differing results. When 2,500 cGy is given in ten 250-cGy fractions, 14 of 17 children (82%) had subnormal GH response [11]. However, when 2,400 cGy in 20 120-cGy fractions per 4 weeks was given, only 1 child of 9 (11%) showed impaired GH response. All children were receiving multiagent chemotherapy. Even though they had blunted GH responses to pharmacological stimuli, these children showed normal growth velocity, and normal serum soma-

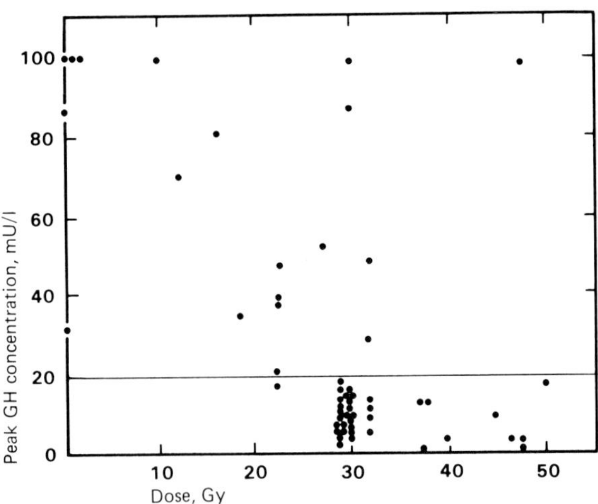

Fig. 2. Peak serum GH response as a function of radiation dose [modified from ref. 9].

tomedin activity, suggesting that normal physiologic requirements of GH had been met.

Shalet [9] has observed children with brain tumors treated by surgical excision and not subjected to radiotherapy, all of whom had normal GH responses to insulin tolerance test and a mean GH response not significantly different from control children. Thus, it appears that neither the presence of tumor in the brain nor neurosurgical intervention is responsible for the observed GH deficiency. Too few children with chemotherapy alone have been studied to know the additional impact it may present.

The major site of radiation-induced hypothalmic-pituitary axis damage is the hypothalmus. Although the pituitary gland may also be affected by radiation, there is strong evidence that the hypothalmus is more radiosensitive than the pituitary gland. Evidence for this includes raised serum prolactin levels [12], subnormal thyroid function in the presence of a normal but delayed rise of serum thyrotropin-stimulating hormone (TSH) after administration of thyrotropin-releasing hormone [12, 13], and an absent cortisol response to insulin hypoglycemia in a patient who showed a normal cortisol response to vasopressin injection [13]. Further evidence is demonstrated by a discordant GH response to different stimuli. The GH response to insulin hypoglycemia is affected by lower radiation doses of cranial irradiation. With increasing radiation dose the GH response to arginine stimulation is impaired [9]. There are several other adverse factors in addition to radiation-induced GH deficiency which may contribute to impaired growth. These include spinal irradiation and recurrent tumor and chemotherapy. Furthermore, commonly children have a poor appetite following definitive treatment with surgery and radiotherapy. The impact of growth impairment can be demonstrated within 1 year of completion of radiotherapy in the majority of children. It has been shown that 12 of 13 (92%) children grow poorly during the 1st year after radiotherapy, whether or not there was hormonal evidence of GH deficiency. GH therapy for radiation-induced GH deficiency is effective in resulting in increase in growth velocity for the children.

GH is the first anterior pituitary hormone to be affected by hypothalamic-pituitary radiotherapy. Doses in excess of 5,000 cGy to the hypothalamus and pituitary within 5–6 weeks have been associated with panhypopituitarism. It is generally concluded today that radiation doses of 2,400 cGy given in 150-, 180-, or 200-cGy fractions with concomitant chemotherapy will not result in impaired GH secretion. There is no convincing evidence that cytotoxic agents impair anterior pituitary function, although glucocortoids may affect many facets of hypothalamic-pituitary function.

Thyroid

Radiation-induced thyroid dysfunction was first described by the Stanford investigators [14], and is recognized to be dose dependent. Other factors such as previous lymphangiography and age at irradiation may also be important [15]. The lymphangiogram is implicated because the lymphangiographic contrast method uses ethiodal, a fat-soluble organic iodide which remains in the body for many months. It is thought that the iodide renders the thyroid gland increasingly radiosensitive, leading to a decrease in thyroxine production and a greater elevation of TSH. Since these early reports, others [16] have observed equivalent rates of thyroid dysfunction regardless of whether a lymphangiogram proceeded radiotherapy.

The Stanford studies [15] suggest a higher incidence of thyroid dysfunction following neck irradiation in young patients, with 48% incidence of TSH elevation in patients <20 years, but a 33% rate for other patients. Others feel that the age at irradiation is irrelevant. Data regarding dose of irradiation also suggest that in children there is a dose response. Constine *et al.* [17] have shown that among children receiving radiotherapy for Hodgkin's disease, doses in the range of 4,400 cGy carry a 73% incidence of hypothyroidism, as compared to 17% for those receiving less than 2,500 cGy along with chemotherapy. Furthermore, they showed an apparent reversal in the thyroid dysfunction with subsequent normalization of TSH and T_4, suggesting that the damage may not be complete.

Currently it is generally accepted that patients who are hypothyroid (raised TSH and decreased T_4), or those with compensated thyroid dysfunction (raised TSH, normal T_4) should receive T_4 replacement therapy. This policy is supported by the observation that an elevated TSH in the presence of radiation-damaged thyroidal tissue is known to be carcinogenic. Therefore, it is hoped that TSH suppression may lessen the potential for postirradiation thyroid carcinoma. Most data have, however, been accumulated in patients receiving high doses of irradiation for lymphoma or head and neck cancer. Rarely, Graves' ophthalmopathy and hyperthyroidism have been observed following radiotherapy to the thyroid gland. There are no convincing data that chemotherapy alone alters thyroid function. However, large numbers of children without additional radiotherapy have not been studied to clarify this point.

Gonads

When the ovaries of a young woman are irradiated, a fixed population of cells, when destroyed, cannot be replaced. Thus, effects on fertility are explained by a reduction in the fixed pool of oocytes. With increasing age, the pool of oocytes decreases such that ovarian ablation occurs following X-ray therapy and is recognized to be age dependent [18]. Conversely, preservation of ovarian function is also aided by a young age. While radiotherapy to the ovary in modest doses commonly causes ovarian failure in women in the perimenopausal age group, Stillman *et al.* [18] have shown that only 17 of 25 girls (68%) developed ovarian failure when both ovaries were exposed to a range of doses between 1,200 and 5,000 cGy (mean 3,200 cGy). It is known that amenorrhea, infertility, and high gonadotropin levels result when both ovaries are irradiated to doses of 2,000–3,000 cGy [19]. Among young girls undergoing oophoropexy, pelvic irradiation, and chemotherapy for Hodgkin's disease, the Stanford group [20] reported that 88% of the girls retain normal menstrual function. In these cases the radiation dose calculated to the transposed ovary ranged from 350 to 660 cGy [21]. However, with increasing age, the risk of ovarian dysfunction increases under the impact of chemotherapy, radiotherapy, and combined modality therapy [22].

No effect of chemotherapy on ovarian function in girls up to the age of 17 years was observed in one study of radiation effects on the ovary [18], while others [23] noted that 20% of prepubertal girls with leukemia treated with chemotherapy showed no follicle growth, and 80% had incomplete follicular development. Nicosia *et al.* [24] also found impaired follicular maturation as demonstrated by marked decreases in antral follicles as well as in primordial and primary follicles in prepubertal girls, most severe in malnourished patients who had received multiagent chemotherapy, with many *pre*pubertal patients classified as having failing ovaries when compared with age- and nutrition-matched controls.

It is important to attempt to preserve ovarian function whenever delivering pelvic radiation therapy in young children. Figure 3 demonstrates a computerized tomographic scan revealing a bulky pelvic Ewing's sarcoma in a young girl, the isodose distribution selected, and her radiotherapy treatment portal. The primary iliac tumor had an enormous intrapelvic component which involved one and abutted the contralateral ovary. This girl received combination chemotherapy of cytoxan, adriamycin, vincristine, and actinomycin D which caused a cessation of menses prior to the initiation of radiotherapy. By computerized tomography dosimetry, it was estimated that the right ovary would receive approximately 40% of the total tumor dose, or 2,220 cGy within 6 weeks, while the left ovary received a full radiation dose of 5,550 cGy within 6 weeks. Although this young woman became amenorrheic during induction chemotherapy and remained so throughout her treatment, she had return of normal menstrual function 1 month following cessation of therapy. She continues with normal menses, apparent fertility, and no evidence of disease, now 3 years following definitive therapy. This case demonstrates the importance of careful treatment planning with an aim of protecting normal tissues whenever possible. With an estimated left ovarian radiation dose of approximately 2,200 cGy in the setting of 50 weeks of high-dose alkylating agent chemotherapy, she has regained menstrual function and presumed fertility.

Cytotoxic drugs alone, most commonly the alkylating agents, are associated with sterility. The most completely studied drug is cyclophosphamide. This drug is associated with an absence of swelling or proliferation of thecal cells to form follicles, and high doses reduce the number of ova [25]. It is felt that the critical issue with respect to chemotherapy-induced sterility is the total dose of drug received. Susceptibility of cytotoxic-induced ovarian function is also age dependent. It has been predicted that ovarian failure should occur uncommonly in prepubertal and pubertal girls – although young girls have been reported to be affected by this therapy [26]. Recovery of menstrual function may appear after several years of presumed complete damage, thus close follow-up is warranted. Girls with ovarian failure should be offered sex steroid replacement containing estrogen and progesterone.

While effects of testicular irradiation are well described following single-fraction and fractionated radiation courses in adult men [27], the threshold dose of irradiation required to damage germinal epithelium in childhood is unknown. Among 10 males, age 17 to 36 years, irradiated for Wilms' tumor during childhood with estimated testicular doses ranging

a

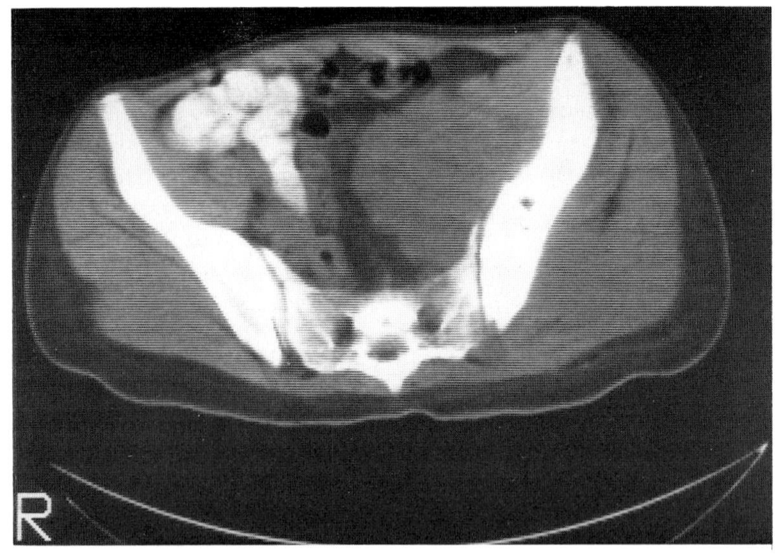

b

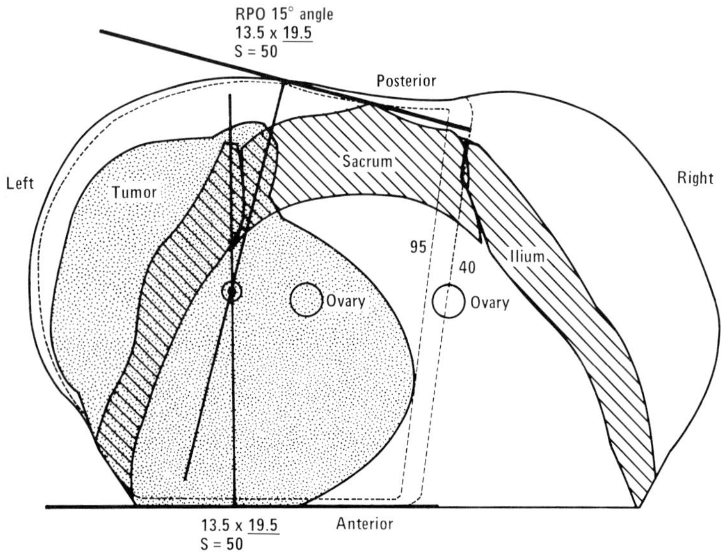

Fig. 3. Pelvic computerized tomographic scan revealing a bulky Ewing's sarcoma of the left ilium, with a large intrapelvic component obscuring the left ovary and abutting the region of the right ovary. *b* Isodose distribution from two unopposed evenly weighted fields, an anterior and a right posterior oblique (RPO) field, treated to the isocenter where the isodose values shown are a % of the dose to isocenter. Patient treated with 4MV, 80 cm SAD. The right ovary was estimated to receive approximately 40% of the tumor dose of 5,550 cGy or 2,220 cGy/6 weeks. *c* Radiotherapy portal film demonstrating the posterior field of the treatment plan displayed in *b*.

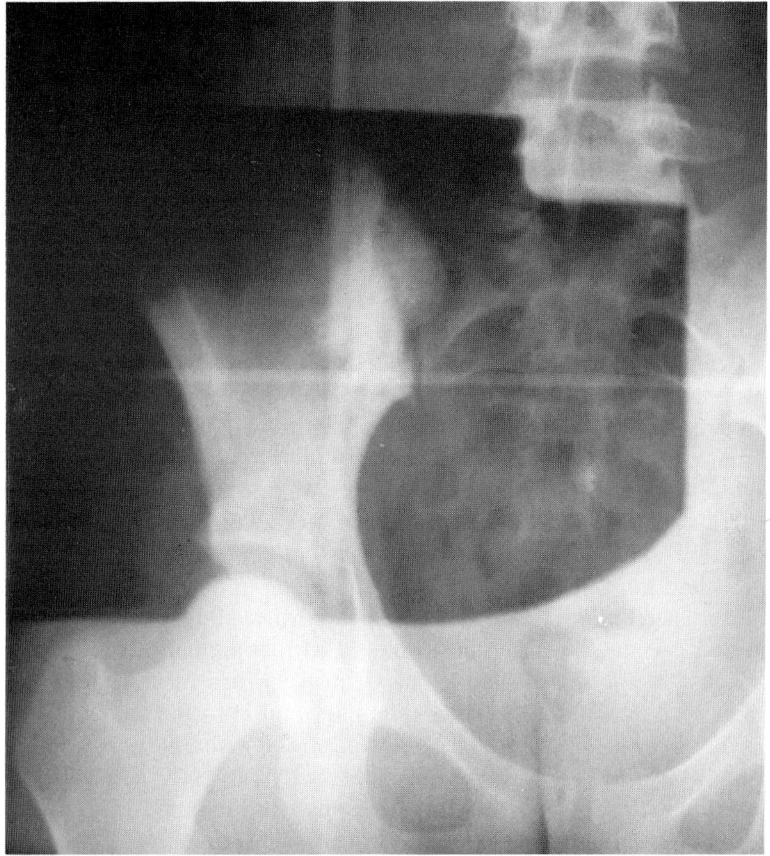

c

from 268 to 983 cGy/4 weeks, 8 of 10 (80%) were either oligo- or azoospermic when studied, and 7 had elevated follicle-stimulating hormone levels [28]. More recently, among young men with Hodgkin's disease irradiated using a gonadal shield in which the testicular radiation doses were limited to 28–135 cGy, 88% of men were fertile when tested 18–26 months following therapy [29].

Hormonal response, i.e., testosterone response to human chorionic gonadotrophin stimulation, has been evaluated among 6 boys given testicular radiation therapy for leukemic infiltration (2,400 cGy/3 weeks), demonstrating no testosterone response [30]. The contribution of the irradiation above the recognized chemotherapy effect in these boys is not known.

Cytotoxic-induced testicular injury is also dose dependent [31]. Data are quite convincing that adult males who receive 6 cycles of MOPP (nitrogen mustard, vincristine, procarbazine, and prednisone) chemotherapy are left with a complete azoospermia and germinal aplasia [32]. More recently, it has been suggested that only approximately 50% of adult patients will be so affected when only three cycles of drug are delivered [33]. It was hoped that prepubescent boys would be less affected than pubescent boys in whom virtually all (age 11–16 years) exposed to six cycles of MOPP developed gynecomastia and germinal aplasia on testicular biopsy, a tenfold rise in follicle-stimulating hormone, a twofold rise in luteinizing hormone, and a decrease in testosterone [34]. The gynecomastia is felt to be related to Leydig cell dysfunction. However, among prepubertal and pubertal boys with acute lymphoblastic leukemia, Leydig cell dysfunction was rarely demonstrated [35]. It is encouraging that among 14 boys with acute lymphoblastic leukemia treated with prednisone, vincristine, methotrexate, and 6-mercaptopurine, with 5-year follow-up, all had normal testicular function for their Tanner stage and normal gonadotropin and testosterone levels. Five of 6 boys tested had normal sperm counts. Similarly, Lendon et al. [36] found a reduced percentage of seminiferous tubules containing spermatogonia, but no germinal aplasia in boys treated with combination chemotherapy for acute lymphoblastic leukemia. The two drugs most responsible for testicular damage are cyclophosphamide and cytosine arabinoside (>1 g/m^2). Testicular tubular morphology improves with time, suggesting that, in many boys, spermatogenesis will recover by adulthood. Thus, it appears that even with a longer duration of therapy, the leukemic drugs, generally given to those of younger ages, are less injurious than those drugs used in the treatment of Hodgkin's disease. However, precise data regarding the sensitivity of prepubertal testes are lacking. It has been shown that prepubertal patients with poor nutritional status treated with chemotherapy are at increased risk for tubular injury and reduced spermatogonia [37]. Thus, the prepubertal testis may not be as quiescent as previously believed.

Central Nervous System

Tolerance of the brain to irradiation and multiagent chemotherapy has been extensively studied in children with acute lymphoblastic leukemia who received 2,400 cGy/2½ weeks cranial or craniospinal irradiation given in combination with five to six doses of intrathecal methotrexate. In the earliest prospective study of 18 children treated for acute lymphoblastic leukemia who were reexamined 3–5 years after completion of therapy,

Meadows et al. [38] described a decline of 10 or more IQ points among 11 of the 18 patients (61%), with those younger than 5 years of age or those with IQs greater than 110 showing the greatest declines. Retrospective studies have shown that 2,400 cGy resulted in significantly lower IQ scores (mean 92–93) than treatment with intrathecal methotrexate alone, intrathecal methotrexate and other agents, intravenous methotrexate, or no central nervous system treatment at all [39, 40]. Further confirmation came from another study of children treated with 2,400 cGy cranial irradiation and six doses of intrathecal methotrexate, in which the average full-scale IQ was 95, consistent with the findings in the previous studies [41]. It now is appreciated that the timing of radiotherapy and methotrexate is critical. Whenever possible it is advisable to administer methotrexate before radiotherapy, so to optimize a decline of methotrexate from the plasma and spinal fluid, as a means of reducing toxicity. However, youngsters receiving radiation doses as low as 1,800 cGy to the cranium, given following methotrexate administration, have not yet been studied in sufficient detail to know if these doses are, indeed, within tolerance limits.

Many patients with malignant brain tumors have been treated with radiotherapy alone, with studies revealing a wide range of abilities, and some children quite capable of independent living [42, 43]. However, many long-term survivors have been shown to have overall low levels of functioning with limitations of short-term memory and inability to carry out premorbid activities. Among these children, it is difficult to differentiate the effects of the brain tumor itself, the associated increased intracranial pressure, and the surgical resection from the effects of the dose and volume of radiotherapy. Although precise data are lacking, it is recognized that younger children are at greater risk for resultant learning disabilities than are those in whom myelination is complete at the time of treatment.

Mutagenesis

Both chemotherapy and radiotherapy are known mutagens. Furthermore, both modalities are teratogenic. Deleterious effects and fetal malformations have been reported following both agents, particularly when administered during the 1st trimester of pregnancy [44–47]. However, the critical issue is one of cancer occurring in the offspring of a cured survivor. Most germ cell mutations which occur in patients treated for cancer lead to a small number of lethal dominant mutations which result in a spontaneous abortion and are never recognized. Autosomal recessive mutations may also occur, however, may be latent and not expressed for many subsequent generations. The precise risk of fetal abnormalities following antineoplastic therapy is thought to be very small, requiring many generations and large numbers of evaluated patients for accurate predictions to be made. Current data indicate that the vast majority of offspring carried to term are normal.

The National Cancer Institute investigators [48] studied the long-term survivors of childhood and adolescent cancer and identified 7 cases of cancer among 2,308 offspring (0.30%) of 2,283 survivors and 11 cases of cancer among 4,719 offspring (0.23%) of 3,604 control patients. Thus, there were no excess cancers detected as compared to the general population. Similarly, the Stanford investigators [22] have observed no fetal wastage and no birth defects in their series of offspring among women treated successfully with radiotherapy, chemotherapy, or combined modality therapy for Hodgkin's disease.

Cancer in offspring of childhood cancer survivors may occur in two ways: (1) the offspring may inherit the genes that caused the parent's cancer or (2) they may acquire a new genetic abnormality induced in the parental germ cells by their therapeutic agents. The first possibility, inheritance, is most likely in the offspring of children with genetic forms of embryonal tumors such as retinoblastoma, Wilms' tumor, and neuroblastoma [49]. The second risk, that of germ cell effects induced by therapy and subsequently to the offspring, may be related to chemotherapy or radiotherapy. The potential for mutagenesis may be suspected whenever the therapeutic modality, radiotherapy or chemotherapy, shows in vitro mutagenesis. The ultimate genetic effect, however, is determined by the sex and age of the exposed patient, since germ cells exist at different developmental stages in males and females between birth and puberty. Oogonial mitosis is complete in fetal life; the ova are, therefore, less vulnerable than spermatogonia to point mutations, but more susceptible to nondisjunction and resultant chromosomal aneuploidy. Likewise, the offspring of treated males will be more likely to sustain-single-gene mutations or structural rearrangement, but little or no aneuploidy.

For radiotherapy, it is possible to estimate the genetic effect of gonadal radiation by the concept of doubling dose and a known dose-response curve. A gonadal dose of 200 rem in childhood produces a genetic risk of about 1% [50]. For the offspring of irradiated males, there is a risk for dominant mutations and chromosome structural rearrangement. The offspring of an irradiated female are at greater risk for aneuploidy. As the radiation exposure increases up to 1,000 rem, there is a linear increase in genetic effects; exposure beyond 1,000 rem usually produces sterility, while the risk of genetic abnormality is 1–5%, depending on dosage. The effects of chemotherapeutic agents in producing genetic abnormalities in offspring have not been measured.

Secondary Oncogenesis

Incidence rates for secondary malignant neoplasms have ranged from 3 to 12% for children treated before 1971 and are approximately 8% when patients treated more recently had been included in the projections [51, 52]. This risk is 10–20 times greater than that of a first neoplasm in the general population of age-matched individuals. Among children, genetics adds to the risk generated from radiation therapy and chemotherapy.

With respect to genetic risks, children with genetic forms of embryonal tumors such as retinoblastoma are at greatest risk of developing a second malignant tumor. Other genetic conditions related to increased risk of second malignant neoplasms include neurofibromatosis, the nevoid basal cell carcinoma syndrome, and xeroderma pigmentosum. The most frequent solid tumors related to preceding radiotherapy are sarcomas. Tucker et al. [53] in the Late Effects Study Group evaluated 9,170 patients who had survived 2 or more years after the diagnosis of a cancer in childhood and found a 2.7-fold risk of a bone cancer among patients who had had previous radiotherapy when compared with nonirradiated matched controls. There was a sharp dose-response gradient reaching a 40-fold risk following radiation doses to the bone greater than 6,000 cGy (table I). The relative dose-response effect among those who had been treated for retinoblastoma was similar to those treated for all other tumors. Alkylating agent chemotherapy also increases the risk of subsequent bone cancer. The relative risk of bone sarcoma associated with alkylating agents alone was 4.2, which rose with increasing drug exposure (expressed as alkylator score), whether or not radiation therapy was given to the affected site (table II). The sarcoma risks increased with greater amounts of chemotherapy and were not confounded by the high rate of sarcomas associated with the genetic form of retinoblastoma. Several studies [54, 55] of patients with retinoblastoma and Ewing's sarcoma have suggested that cyclophosphamide may potentiate the effects of radiotherapy in the development of secondary osteosarcomas.

Low doses of radiations affect the thyroid gland in youngsters, with doses in the range of 120 cGy causing a 100-fold increase in the risk of thyroid cancer [56]. Furthermore, low doses of scalp irradiation given for tinea capitis have been shown to be associated with an increased risk of brain and salivary gland tumors, as well as thyroid tumors [57]. Most

Table I. Relative risk of bone cancer as a function of radiation dose, adjusted for alkylating agent chemotherapy [modified from ref. 53]

Radiation dose, cGy					
0	<1,000	1,000–2,999	3,000–3,999	4,000–5,999	≥6,000
1.0	0.6	0.6	16.9	21.2	38.3

Table II. Relative risk of bone sarcoma as a function of radiation dose and alkylating agent chemotherapy [modified from ref. 53]

Relative risk	Alkylator score		
	0	1 or 2	≥3
None	1.0	4.8	8.5
<1,000 cGy	1.3	0.4	1.3
≥1,000 cGy	37.4	14.2	59.2

Table III. Relative risk of leukemia as a function of alkylating agent chemotherapy, adjusted for radiation therapy [modified from ref. 59]

	Alkylator score				
	0	1–2	3–4	5–6	≥7
Relative risk	1	0.7	8.4	16.0	24.2
Relative risk adjusted for radiation	1	0.7	7.9	18.3	23.2

recently there has been shown to be an excess number of brain tumors in children given 2,000–2,500 cGy to the cranium for prevention of central nervous system leukemia [58]. A possible relationship between tumors of the central nervous system and hematopoietic system similar to that of genetic retinoblastoma and osteosarcoma has been suggested.

Among the chemotherapeutic agents, the alkylating agents are known to increase the risk of leukemia, as well as solid tumors. Tucker et al. [59] (Late Effects Study Group), reported an increased risk of developing leukemia of 0.8% 20 years after initial diagnosis of cancer among 9,170 patients studied. The risk was highest among children having previously been diagnosed with Hodgkin's disease and rose to 4.2% at 20 years of follow-up. The risk of leukemia increased with increasing dose of alkylating agent and with multidrug therapy (alyklator score of >3).

The risk is significant, rising to 24 in the highest category (table III). These leukemias are primarily acute nonlymphocytic leukemia. Previous radiation therapy does not enhance the risk [59]. It is important to identify children with increased predisposition to a second malignant tumor as well as to modify therapy, avoiding carcinogens when other equally effective therapies are available.

References

1 Martinez, A.; Donaldson, S. S.; Bagshaw, M. A.: Special set-up and treatment techniques for the radiotherapy of pediatric malignancies. Int. J. Radiat. Oncol. Biol. Phys. 1977;2:1007–1016.

2 Rubin, P.; Van Houtte, P.; Constine, L.: Radiation sensitivity and organ tolerances in pediatric oncology: A new hypothesis. Front. Radiat. Ther. Oncol. Basel, Karger, 1982, vol. 16, pp. 353–376.

3 Probert, J.; Parker, B.: The effects of radiation therapy on bone growth. Radiology 1975;114:155–162.

4 Tefft, M.: Radiation effect on growing bone and cartilage. Front. Radiat. Ther. Oncol. Basel, Karger, 1972, vol. 6, pp, 289–311.

5 Probert, J.; Parker, B.; Kaplan, H.: Growth retardation in children after megavoltage irradiation of the spine. Cancer 1973;32:634–639.

6 Donaldson, S.; Kleeberg, P.; Cox, R.: Growth abnormalities associated with radiation in children with Hodgkin's disease. Proc. Am. Soc. Cl. Onc., 1988; *7:* 224.

7 Neuhauser, E.; Wittenborg, M.; Berman, L., et al.: Irradiation effects of roentgen therapy on the growing spine. Radiology 1952;59:637–650.

8 Shalet, S.; Gibson, B.; Swindell, R. L., et al.: Effect of spinal irradiation on growth. Arch. Dis. Child. 1987;62:461–464.

9 Shalet, S.: Growth and hormonal status of children treated for brain tumours. Childs. Brain 1982;9:284–293.

10 Shalet, S.; Beardwell, C.; Aarons, B., et al.: Growth impairment of children treated for brain tumors. Arch. Dis. Child. 1978;53:491–494.

11 Shalet, S.; Price, D.; Beardwell, C., et al.: Normal growth despite abnormalities of growth hormone secretion in children treated for acute leukaemia. J. Pediatr. 1979;94:719–722.

12 Samaan, N.; Bakdash, M.; Caderao, J., et al.: Hypopituitarism after external irradiation. Ann. Intern. Med. 1975;83:771–777.

13 Larkins, R.; Martin, F.: Hypopituitarism after extracranial irradiation: Evidence for hypothalamic origin. Br. Med. J. 1973;*i:*152–153.

14 Fuks, Z.; Glatstein, E.; Marsa, G. W., et al.: Long-term effects of external radiation on the pituitary and thyroid glands. Cancer 1976;37:1152–1161.

15 Glatstein, E.; McHardy-Young, S.; Brast, N., et al.: Alterations in serum thyrotropin (TSH) and thyroid function following radiotherapy in patients with malignant lymphoma. J. Clin. Endocrinol. Metab. 1971;32:833–841.

16 Tamura, K.; Shimaoka, K.; Friedman, M.: Thyroid abnormalities associated with treatment of malignant lymphoma. Cancer 1981;47:2704–2711.

17 Constine L. S.; Donaldson, S. S.; McDougall, I. R., et al.: Thyroid dysfunction after radiotherapy in children with Hodgkin's disease. Cancer 1984;53:878–883.

18 Stillman, R.; Schinfeld, J.; Schiff, I.: Ovarian failure in long-term survivors of childhood malignancy. Am. J. Obstet. Gynecol. 1981;139:62–66.
19 Shalet, S.; Beardwell, C.; Morris-Jones, P., et al.: Ovarian failure following abdominal irradiation in childhood. Br. J. Cancer 1976;33:655–658.
20 Donaldson, S. S.; Kaplan, H. S.: Complications of treatment of Hodgkin's disease in children. Cancer Treat. Rep. 1982;66:977–989.
21 LeFloch, O.; Donaldson, S. S.; Kaplan, H. S.: Pregnancy following oophoropexy and total nodal irradiation in women with Hodgkin's disease. Cancer 1976;38:2263–2268.
22 Horning, S.; Hoppe, R.; Kaplan, H., et al.: Female reproductive potential after treatment for Hodgkin's disease. N. Engl. J. Med. 1981;304:1377–1382.
23 Himelstein-Braw, R.; Byskov, A.; Peters, H., et al.: Follicular atresia in the infant human ovary. J. Reprod. Fertil. 1976;46:55–59.
24 Nicosia, S. V.; Matus-Ridley, M.; Meadows, A. T.: Gonadal effects of cancer therapy in girls. Cancer 1985;55:2364–2372.
25 Warne, G. L.; Fairley, K. F.; Hobbs, J. B., et al.: Cyclophosphamide-induced ovarian failure. N Engl J Med 1973;289:1159–1162.
26 Himelstein-Braw, R.; Peters, H.; Faber, M.: Morphological study of the ovaries of leukemic children. Br. J. Cancer 1978;38:82–87.
27 Rowley, M. J.; Leach, D. R.; Warner, G. A., et al.: Effect of graded doses of ionizing radiation on the human testis. Radiat. Res. 1974;59:665–678.
28 Shalet, S.; Beardwell, C.; Jacobs, H. S., et al.: Testicular function following irradiation of the human prepubertal testis. Clin. Endocrinol. 1978;9:483–490.
29 Pedrick, T. J.; Hoppe, R. T.: Recovery of spermatogenesis following pelvic irradiation for Hodgkin's disease. Int. J. Radiat. Oncol. Biol. Phys. 1986;12:117–121.
30 Shalet, S.: Disorders of the endocrine system due to radiation and cytotoxic chemotherapy. Clin. Endocrinol. 1983;18:637–659.
31 Buchanan, J.; Fairley, K.; Barrie, J.: Return of spermatogenesis after stopping cyclophosphamide therapy. Lancet 1975;ii:156–157.
32 Sherins, R. J.; Devita V. T.: Studies of men in remission after therapy. Ann. Intern. Med. 1973;79:216–220.
33 daCuna, M. F.; Meistrich, M. L.; Fuller, L. M., et al.: Recovery of spermatogenesis after treatment for Hodgkin's disease: Limiting dose of MOPP chemotherapy. J. Clin. Oncol. 1984;2:571–577.
34 Sherins, R.; Olweny, C.; Ziegler, J.: Gynecomastia and gonadal dysfunction in adolescent boys treated with combination chemotherapy for Hodgkin's disease. N. Engl. J. Med. 1978;299:12–16.
35 Shalet, S.; Hann, I.; Lenden, M., et al.: Testicular function after combination chemotherapy in childhood for acute lymphoblastic leukemia. Arch. Dis. Child. 1981;56:275–278.
36 Lendon, M.; Hann, I. M.; Palmer, M. K., et al.: Testicular histology after combination chemotherapy in childhood for acute lymphoblastic leukemia. Lancet 1978;ii:439–441.
37 Matus-Ridley, M.; Nicosia, S.; Meadows, A.: Gonadal effects of cancer therapy in boys. Cancer 1985;55:2353–2363.
38 Meadows, A.; Gordon, J.; Massari, D., et al.: Declines in IQ scores and cognitive dysfunction in children with acute lymphocytic leukaemia treated with cranial irradiation. Lancet 1981;ii:1015–1018.
39 Rowland, J.; Glidewell, O., Sibley, R., et al.: Effects of different forms of central nervous system prophylaxis on neuropsychologic function in childhood leukemia. J. Clin. Oncol. 1984;2:1327–1335.

40 Copeland, D.; Fletcher, J.; Pfefferbaum-Levine, B., et al.: Neuropsychological sequelae of childhood cancer in long-term survivors. Pediatrics 1985;75:745–753.
41 Robinson, L.; Nesbit, M.; Sather, H., et al.: Factors associated with IQ scores in long-term survivors of childhood acute lymphoblastic leukemia. Am. J. Pediatr. Hematol. Oncol. 1984;66:115–121.
42 Danoff, B. F.; Cowchock, F. S.; Marquette, C., et al.: Assessment of the long-term effects of primary radiation therapy for brain tumors in children. Cancer 1982;49:1580–1586.
43 Li, F. P.; Winston, K. R.; Gimbrere, K.: Follow-up of children with brain tumors. Cancer 1984;54:135–138.
44 Byrd, R.: Late effects of treatment of cancer in children. Pediatr. Clin. North. Am. 1985;32:835–857.
45 Sweet, D.; Kinzie, J.: Consequences of radiotherapy and antineoplastic therapy for the fetus. J. Reprod. Med. 1976;17:151–155.
46 Sieber, S.; Adamson, R.: Toxicity of antineoplastic agents in man. Chromosomal aberration, antifertility effects, congenital malformations, and carcinogenic potential. Adv. Cancer Res. 1975;22:57–155.
47 Nicholson, H.: Cytotoxic drugs in pregnancy: Review of reported cases. Br. J. Obstet. Gynaecol. 1968;75:307–312.
48 Mulvihill, J.; Myers, M.; Connelly, R., et al.: Cancer in offspring of long-term survivors of childhood and adolescent cancer. Lancet. 1987;ii:813–817.
49 Knudson, A. G.; Jr.: Genetics and the etiology of childhood cancer. Pediatr. Res. 1976;10:513–517.
50 Meadows, A.; Silber, J.: Delayed consequences of therapy for childhood cancer. CA 1985;35:271–286.
51 Mike, V.; Meadows, A.; D'Angio, G.: Incidence of second malignant neoplasms: Results of an international study. Lancet 1982;ii:1326–1331.
52 Li, F.: Second malignant tumors after cancer in childhood. Cancer 1977;40:1899–1902.
53 Tucker, M.; D'Angio, G.; Boice, J., et al.: Bone sarcomas linked to radiotherapy and chemotherapy in children. N. Engl. J. Med. 1987;317:588–593.
54 Strong, L.; Herson, J.; Osborne, B., et al.: Risk of radiation-related subsequent malignant tumors in survivors of Ewing's sarcoma. J. Natl. Cancer Inst. 1979;62:1401–1406.
55 Draper, G.; Sanders, B.; Kingston, J.: Second primary neoplasms in patients with retinoblastoma. Br. J. Cancer 1986;53:661–671.
56 Hempelmann, L.; Hall, W.; Phillips, M., et al.: Neoplasms in persons treated with X-rays in infancy: Fourth survey in 20 years. J. Natl. Cancer Inst. 1975;55:519–530.
57 Modan, B.; Baidatz, D.; Mart, H., et al.: Radiation-induced head and neck tumours. Lancet 1974;i:277–279.
58 Rimm, I.; Li, F.; Tarbell, N., et al.: Brain tumors after cranial irradiation for childhood acute lymphoblastic leukemia. A 13-year experience from the Dana-Farber Canter Institute and the Children's Hospital. Cancer 1987;59:1506–1508.
59 Tucker, M.; Meadows, A.; Boice, J., et al.: Leukemia after therapy with alkylating agents for childhood cancer. J. Natl. Cancer Inst. 1987;78:459–464.

Sarah, S. Donaldson, MD, Department of Radiation Oncology,
Stanford University Medical Center, Stanford, CA 93405 (USA)

Vaeth JM, Meyer JL (eds): Radiation Tolerance of Normal Tissues.
Front Radiat Ther Oncol. Basel, Karger, 1989, vol 23, pp 408–416

Radiation Carcinogenesis

Seymour H. Levitt

Department of Therapeutic Radiology-Radiation Oncology, School of Medicine, University of Minnesota Hospital and Clinics, Minneapolis, Minn., USA

This paper will address the subject of radiation carcinogenesis from the viewpoint of the Clinician. This is not nor could not be an in-depth analysis. For a more complete analysis, the reader should consult the papers by Boice and Fraumeni [5], Fajardo [10], Hall [12], and Upton et al. [12].

There has been and continues to be a major concern regarding the effect of irradiation on humans and nonhuman life. In humans, this concern includes complications related to acute and chronic effects and the development of malignant neoplasms. This concern has in many instances been excessive in view of the actual incidence of malignant neoplasms induced by irradiation. However, the concern is not without basis, and the actual incidence of malignant neoplasms resulting from irradiation is a major concern. Of major interest to the physician and other professionals involved in patient care is the incidence of malignant neoplasms secondary to the use of irradiation in the healing arts.

On this subject it is important to first look at the estimates of radiation exposure to the United States population in general. Exposure comes from natural background, cosmic rays, and radionuclides (natural materials, etc.). Less than half comes from the exposure to the healing arts, the primary role of which is played by diagnostic radiology [18]. Insofar as radiation carcinogenesis is concerned, natural background is the most frequent cause. It is worth noting that fewer than 3% of total cancer mortality is estimated to be due to all forms of radiations. Less than 1.5% of total cancer is due to the healing arts. It is also important to note that radiation carcinogenesis is essentially a long-term effect of radiations and is one of the overall effects of radiations [18].

Factors that influence the risk of carcinogenesis include the age at the time of exposure, the length of observation of the population, the characteristics of the radiations (whether they are electromagnetic or particulate), the source and type of exposure (external vs. internal, single-dose vs. fractionated vs. continuous), the rate of exposure, the total dose, and the characteristics of the population; for example: racial, environmental risk of nonradiogeneic neoplasia, etc. [10].

Carcinogenesis is a somewhat complex process which can be simplified by looking at the development factors. Radiations and chemicals can exert harmful effects at different stages in the transformation of normal cells into malignant tumors. These stages of transformation are as follows: *Initiation* is the first phase in which a factor such as radiation or chemical causes a usually irreversable genetic mutation of the normal cell that primes it for uncontrolled growth. Some initiators are radiations, urethane, and the nitrosamines. *Promotion*, the second phase, occurs when a substance encourages the initiated cells to reproduce faster than normal ones which increases the probability of malignant transformation. The effects of promotion are often reversible. Some promoters are DDT, saccharin, phenobarbitol, many chemicals in cigarette smoke, and irradiation. The final phase is *progression*, during which some of the altered cells undergo a second genetic mutation that allows them to grow uncontrollably without the stimulus of promoters and progress to full malignancy. In the mechanism of radiation oncogenesis irradiation can act as an initiator or a promoter or both so that ionizing radiation is classified as a complete carcinogen. Experimental data appear to indicate that it may play each of these roles, depending upon the neoplasm.

Fajardo [10] has defined factors which are necessary to be present in order to determine that irradiation has induced a human neoplasm. These include the following categories: (1) *possible radiation induction:* tumors that occur in the tissues exposed to ionizing radiation and are different from any local neoplasm present prior to radiation exposure and appear after a period of latency, probably more than 2 years for leukemias and 6 years for solid tumors – there are enough observable cases available to suggest a causal relationship; (2) *satisfactory evidence of radiation induction:* tumors which show statistically significant differences in incidence between an irradiated and a comparable control population, and (3) *proof of radiation induction:* tumors which show a positive correlation between dose and incidence.

Human tumors with satisfactory evidence of radiation induction include bone sarcomas, soft-tissue sarcomas, cavitary mesothelioma, paranasal sinus tumors, skin carcinoma (basal and squamous), pulmonary carcinoma, esophageal carcinoma, gastric carcinoma, colonic carcinoma (except rectum), thyroid carcinoma, leukemia, breast carcinoma, liver tumors, and multiple myeloma. The majority of these tumors noted in humans are secondary to irradiation from atomic bomb exposure. Colonic cancer followed irradiation for benign gynecologic disorders in women. Thyroid cancer followed irradiation for benign conditions of the head and neck. Leukemia has been noted following ankylosing spondylitis irradiation and occupational exposure to and systemic use of ^{32}P for polycythemia. Recent literature seems to indicate that a small percentage of patients developed leukemia after irradiation for cancer of the cervix. Breast cancer is reported to occur following multiple fluoroscopies or irradiation for acute postpartum mastitis. Liver tumors developed following thorotrast deposition for diagnostic procedures.

Human tumors with possible radiation induction include lymphomas, leukemias (usually granulocytic), bone sarcomas, osteochondromas, second neoplasms in childhood, bone and soft-tissue sarcomas, thyroid and malignant tumors in childhood, salivary gland tumors, pharyngeal cancers, pancreatic cancer, kidney tumors, urinary bladder tumors, uterine sarcomas, and brain tumors. Numerous reports in the literature have appeared for many years reporting on malignancies following radiotherapy. One of the more recent reports is that by Penn [27] in which he listed childhood malignancies, bone sarcomas, soft-tissue sarcomas, skin cancers, leukemia, brain tumors, thyroid tumors, breast cancers, liver tumors, osteosarcomas, thyroid cancer, squamous cell cancer, etc.

Time and space do not permit us to discuss, in detail, more than a few specific areas of radiation carcinogenesis. Before we look at radiation carcinogenesis per se, it is worth noting that the carcinogenesis due to other neoplastic agents is a complex and confused area. In view of the known carcinogenic chemotherapeutic agents, careful analysis of all claims of carcinogenesis due to irradiation must be carried out to rule out the effect of other carcinogens [30].

One of the areas in which we have been interested is radiation breast carcinogenesis. The evidence for this is based on atomic bomb data, fluoroscopy data, patients treated for postpartum mastitis with orthovoltage irradiation, patients treated with irradiation for cystic disease, and patients treated with irradiation for cancer of the contralateral breast [3, 5, 15, 16, 2–24, 31]. Boice et al. [3] noted in 1979 that radiation-induced breast cancers do not appear in any of these groups until the ages of breast cancer risk, thus suggesting that the development is influenced by hormonal or other age-related factors occurring later in life. This latency, however, is apparently unrelated to dose; for example, radiogenic breast cancers induced by large doses do not appear to occur earlier than those induced by lower doses.

We have evaluated many of the trials related to radiation breast carcinogenesis and come to the conclusion that there are a number of problems in each of these studies. We have reported on our findings at a previous San Francisco Cancer Symposium and in other papers [23, 24]. We have concluded that breast cancer in women is a complex disease with predisposing and epidemiologic factors involved. We have noted that there is no doubt that radiation is a carcinogenic agent and no question that the incidence of breast cancer is increased in individuals who are treated during the perimenarche at the age of 10–19 years. However, based on the evidence from the studies, we noted that current clinical studies do not appear to show a markedly increased risk of second primary contralateral breast cancer. Since many of the studies are only recently completed, and there is a delay from 5 to 10 years following irradiation for the relevent breast cancer, some of the data might not be available at this time. We have frequently stressed the point that we feel that there is no apparent significant increased risk based on the clinical studies at this time. We have noted that the major studies implicating a significant risk of breast cancer secondary to irradiation suffer from one or more methodological flaws: the absence of appropriate comparison groups, the greater diagnostic surveilances in the irradiated group, the overinterpretation of relative risks, and the inability to separate the risk of breast cancer associated with the original disease from the additional risks of irradiation. We also noted that in none of the studies it had been possible to accurately evaluate the effect of other known risk factors in breast cancer including geographic areas of residence, social class, age at first birth, history of benign breast disease, family history of cancer, menstrual history, etc. [23, 24].

Confirming our hypothesis are a number of recent reports. A study on a large number of patients [1] reported 14,000 women with breast cancer treated between 1946 and 1982. Of these patients, 194 developed a second primary tumor in the contralateral breast more than 1 year after diagnosis of the first primary tumor. When groups with and without irradiation were compared, there was no evidence for radiation-induced carcinogenesis in the contralateral breast [1].

To further substantiate our viewpoint, recent reports from the United States [8] and from Denmark [32] evaluated the radiation risk of chest fluoroscopy exposures for the indication of breast cancer and found no increased risk evident with exposure to any type of fluoroscopy.

Other reports [29, 31] attempted to evaluate the potential biases on the risk of breast cancer among those who received radiotherapy for acute postpartum mastitis. These studies did not assess all potential biases, but did note that the patients who had mastitis and *did not* receive irradiation developed a similar incidence of nonneoplastic breast tumors to patients who did receive irradiation. They also noted that the relative risk for neoplastic breast tumor secondary to irradiation declined to 2.0

(95% CI 1.1–4.0) from a higher previous estimate of the same patient material.

We [23] noted that if we assume the highest excess risk and approximate six-fold increase from 1 to 300 rad to the opposite breast, 36 cases of breast cancer per 1 million women would result from exposure to radiation following a 10-year latent period. Therefore, among the 20,000 patients usually undergoing radiation therapy in our country per year, fewer than 1 additional case of breast cancer would occur after 10 years. Furthermore, this risk is probably overestimated, since exposure to irradiation at an older age is associated with lower risks than exposure at an early age.

It is also worth noting at this juncture that despite claims to the contrary [9, 11, 20, 36], mammography provides an infinitely small risk for women to develop breast cancer due to the amount of radiation involved in the procedure. Boice [2] has estimated that there would be approximately an additional 52 cancer cases per 100,000 women receiving mammography. Thus, this author predicted that medical exposure would increase a woman's lifetime risk of breast cancer from 9.09 to only 9.14.

We have also looked at the details of second neoplasms in children who were irradiated for malignant neoplasms at the University of Minnesota. We noted that although there was an increased risk of second neoplasm, a number of these were out of the radiation field, and the majority of these were benign. The incidence of development of second neoplasms was lower in our group than in the Boston orthovoltage group [25]. Using an actuarial approach, we found an incidence of secondary neoplasms to be 2% with a malignant neoplasm rate of 1.0% with megavoltage irradiation which contrasts with the 17% incidence of secondary neoplasms reported by Li et al. [25] from Boston using orthovoltage. We noted a number of biases inherent in other studies including the types of tumor and chemotherapy. We concluded that up to 10% of the long-term survivors may develop a second neoplasm within 30 years of the initial therapy. These may be benign or malignant and within or out of the areas treated. Interestingly, there was no difference in the rates of malignant tumors in the irradiated and unirradiated areas. Because of the time span of the study, it was impossible to evaluate the oncogenic role of chemotherapy. We noted that the incidence of malignant neoplasms in the irradiated areas in our study developed relatively slowly, but we also noted the need to maintain vigilance [28]. A recent report [34] of bone sarcomas related to radiotherapy and chemotherapy in children noted a relative risk of 2.7% for radiotherapy-treated patients and one of 4.7% for chemotherapy-treated patients. Tucker et al. [34] also noted an increased risk with increased dose of radio- or chemotherapy, and they also reported that it seemed likely that heritable factors contributed to the constellations of multiple childhood cancers including bone sarcoma.

Insofar as leukemia is concerned, Boice [2] has noted that the lifetime risk of leukemia from diagnostic X-ray exposure is similar to that of dying from cardiopulmonary disease after smoking about 200 cigarettes or the risk of dying from any cause during a single day in the life of a 60-year-old man. We have also reported on the incidence of ANLL after treatment of Hodgkin's disease. In another report [21] we noted that in review of the literature the incidence of Hodgkin's disease patients who develop leukemia was, for the most part, negligible for patients treated with radiation only, but was statistically significant in patients who received chemotherapy or combinations of chemotherapy and irradiation. This relation existed whether it was given alone or combined with radiation therapy either as salvage or as initial treatment. We have also noted that all combinations of chemotherapy will produce an increased risk of leukemia in patients given radiotherapy plus chemotherapy. This includes the ABVD combination which has been reported not to produce a significant increase in incidence of ANLL.

Until recently, almost every report in the literature had substantiated the fact that the incidence of ANLL in patients with Hodgkin's disease treated with radiation therapy is not significant. A recent report from Stanford [33] on 1,500 patients followed for 15 years or more did note an increased relative risk for patients with Hodgkin's disease treated with radiation therapy to develop both leukemia and other second malignancies. This risk, however, was reported to be far less than that of chemotherapy or chemotherapy/radiotherapy combination. As we have noted, this incidence of ANLL secondary to irradiation alone for Hodgkin's patients has not been substantiated by other studies and the findings of the Stanford Group need to be carefully evaluated [7, 19, 21].

Malignancies other than leukemia occur after treatment of Hodgkin's disease [6, 7, 19, 26]. These include lung cancer, melanomas, non-Hodgkin's, lymphoma, thyroid cancer, etc. [7, 19, 33]. One report noted that patients who had intensive radiotherapy, but not intensive chemotherapy, did not have an increased incidence of second cancers, whereas patients who had intensive chemotherapy or intensive chemotherapy plus radiotherapy had a significantly increased incidence of second cancers.

Until recently, it has been thought that irradiation for cancer of the cervix did not induce leukemia. A recent paper by Boice et al. [4], however, reports a risk of leukemia following irradiation for cervical cancer. More than 150,000 women were evaluated. Radiation was found to have a relative risk of 2.0 (Cl 1.0–4.2) for all forms of leukemia other than chronic lymphocytic leukemia. The risk increased with increasing irradiation dose, until the average doses of 500 rad were reached, at which point the risk decreased with increasing dose to the bone.

Conclusion

This essay is a brief overview of the problems of radiation carcinogenesis. That radiation is and can be a carcinogen cannot be disputed. This risk in regard to the healing arts is, as we have noted, overestimated.

Nevertheless, this risk should lead, all involved in the medical use of irradiation, to limit exposure, insofar as possible, to minimize exposures, to use irradiation-involved procedures only when suitably less carcinogenic methods are not available, and to use irradiation as carefully and accurately as possible and only when indicated. We must be aware of the risks involved with combined use of chemotherapy and radiation therapy. When we consider the use of ionizing radiations in the diagnosis and/or treatment of malignant neoplasm, we must be as sure as possible that these risks are outweighed by the benefits. However, we must not let undocumented and/or exaggerated concerns that prevent us from using one of the most effective anti-cancer agents when and where indicated.

References

1 Basco, V.; Coldman, A.; Elwood, J.; Young, M.: Radiation dose and second breast cancer. Br. J. Cancer *52:* 319–325 (1985).

2 Boice, J. D., Jr.: The danger of X-rays – real or apparent? New Engl. J. Med. *315:* 828–830 (1986).

3 Boice, J. D., Jr.; Land, C. E.; Shore, R. E.; Norman, J. E.; Tokunaga, M.: Risk of breast cancer following low-dose radiation exposure. Radiology *131:* 589–597 (1979).

4 Boice, J.; Blettner, M.; Kleinerman, R.; Stovall, M.; Moloney, W.; Engholm, G.; Austin, D.; Bosch, A.; Cookfair, D.; Krementz, E.; Latourett, H.; Peters, L. J.; Schulz, M.; Lundell, M.; Pettersson, F.; Storm, H.; Bell, C.; Coleman, M.; Fraser, P.; Palmer, M.; Prior, P.; Choi, N.; Hislop, T.; Koch, M.; Robb, D.; Robson, D.; Spengler, R.; Fournier, D. von; Frischkorn, R.; Lochmuller, H.; Pompe-Kirm, V.; Rimpela, A.; Kjorstad, K.; Pejovic, M.; Sigurdsson, K.; Pisani, P.; Kucer, H.; Hutchinson, G.: Radiation dose and leukemia risk in patients treated for cancer of the cervix. J. natn. Cancer Inst. *79:* 1295–1311 (1987).

5 Boice, J.; Fraumeni, J.: Progress in cancer research and therapy; in radiation carcinogenesis: epidemiology and biological significance, No. 26 (Raven Press, New York 1984).

6 Coleman, C.: Secondary malignancy after treatment of Hodgkin's disease: an evolving picture. J. clin. Oncol. *4:* 821–924 (1986).

7 Coleman, M.; Easton, D.; Horwich, A.; Peckham, M.: Second malignancies and Hodgkin's disease. The Royal Marsden Hospital experience. Radiother. Oncol. *11:* 229–238 (1988).
8 Davis, F. G.; Boice, J. D.; Jr.; Kelsey, J. L.; Monson, R. R.: Cancer mortality after multiple fluoroscopic examinations of the chest. J. natn. Cancer Inst. *78:* 645–652 (1987).
9 Evans, J. S.; Wennber, J. E.; McNeil, B. J.: The influence of diagnostic radiography on the incidence of breast cancer and leukemia. New Engl. J. Med. *315:* 810–815 (1986).
10 Fajardo, L. F.: Ionizing radiation and neoplasia; in Fenoglio-Preiser, Weinstein, Kaufman, New concepts in neoplasia as applied to diagnostic pathology, pp. 97–125 (Williams & Wilkins, Baltimore 1986).
11 Gohagan, J. K.; Darby, W. P.; Spitznagel, E. L.; Monsees, B. S.; Tome, A. E.: Radiogenic breast cancer effects of mammographic screening. J. natn. Cancer Inst. *77:* 71–76 (1986).
12 Hall, E. J.: Radiobiology for the radiologist, pp. 357–383 (Harper & Row, London 1978).
13 Hankey, B. F.; Curtis, R. E.; Naughton, M. D.; Boice, J. D.; Flannery, J. T.: A retrospective cohort analysis of second breast cancer risk for primary breast cancer patients with an assessment of the effect of radiation therapy. J. natn. Cancer Inst. *70:* 197–204 (1983).
14 Hatlinghus, S.; Rode, L.; Shristensen, I.; Vaage, S.: Sarcoma following irradiation for breast cancer. Acta radiol. oncol. *25:* 239–242 (1986).
15 Hislop, T. G.; Elwood, J. M.; Coldman, A. J.; Sinelli, J. J.; Worth, A. J.; Ellison, L.G.: Second primary cancers of the breast: incidence and risk factors. Br. J. Cancer *49:* 79–85 (1984).
16 Ivins, J. C.; Taylor, W. F.; Wold, L. E.: Elective whole-lung irradiation in osteosarcoma treatment: appearance of bilateral breast cancer in two long-term survivors. Skeletal Radiol. *16:* 133–135 (1987).
17 Jablon, S.; Bailar, J. C.: The contribution of ionizing radiation to cancer mortality in the United States. Prev. Med. *9:* 219–226 (1980).
18 Jablon, S.: Epidemiologic perspectives in radiation carcinogenesis; in Boice, Fraumeni, Radiation carcinogenesis: epidemiology and biological significance, vol. 26, pp. 1–8 (Raven Press, New York 1984).
19 Koletsky, A. J.; Bertino, J. R.; Farber, L. R.; Prosnitz, L. R.; Kapp, D. S.; Fischer, D.; Portlock, C. S.: Second neoplasms in patients with Hodgkin's disease following combined modality therapy: the Yale experience. J. clin. Oncol. *4:* 311–317 (1986).
20 Law, J.: Cancers induced and cancers detected in a mammography screening programme. Br. J. Radiol. *60:* 231–234 (1987).
21 Levitt, S. H.; Lee, C. K. K.; Aeppli, D. M.; Bloomfield, C. D.: Radical tratment of Hodgkin disease with radiation therapy: results of a 15-year clinical trial. The 1985 Erskine Lecture. Radiology *162:* 623–630 (1987).
22 Levitt, S. H.; Mandel, J.: Benefits versus risk sin conservation surgery with irradiation for breast cancer. Am. J. Med. *77:* 93–100 (1984).
23 Levitt, S. H.; Mandel, J. S.: Breast carcinogenesis: risk of radiation. Int. J. Radiat. Oncol. Biol. Phys. *11:* 1421–1423 (1985).
24 Levitt, S. H.; Mandel, J.: Breast irradiation and future risk of carcinogenesis; in Vaeth, Front. Radiat. Ther. Onc., vol. 17, pp. 131–142 (Karger, Basel 1982–1983).
25 Li, F. P.; Cassidy, J. R.; Jaffe, N.: Risk of second tumors in survivors of childhood cancer. Cancer *35:* 1230–1235 (1975).

26 McHenry, C.; Jarosz, H.; Calandra, D.; McCall, A.; Lawrence, A. M.; Paloyan, E.: Thyroid enoplasia following radiation therapy for Hodgkin's Lymphoma. Archs Surg. *122:* 684–686 (1987).

27 Penn, I.: Second neoplasms following radiotherapy or chemotherapy for cancer. Am. J. clin. Oncol. *5:* 83–96 (1982).

28 Potish, R. A.; Dehner, L. P.; Haselow, R. E.; Kim, T. H.; Levitt, S. H.; Nesbit, M.: The incidence of second neoplasms following megavoltage radiation for pediatric tumors. Cancer *56:* 1534–1537 (1985).

29 Prince, M. M.; Hildreth, N. G.: The influence of potential biases on the risk of breast tumors among women who received radiotherapy for acute postpartum mastitis. J. chron. Dis. *39:* 553–560 (1986).

30 Rieche, K.: Carcinogenicity of antineoplastic agents in man. Cancer Treat. Rev. *11:*–67 (1984).

31 Shore, R. E.; Hildreth, N.; Woodard, W.; Dvoretsky, P.; Hempelmann, L.; Pasternack, B.: Breast cancer among women given X-ray therapy for acute postpartum mastitis. J. natn. Cancer Inst. *77:* 689–696 (1986).

32 Strom, H. H.; Iversen, E.; Boice, J. D.; Jr.: Breast cancer following multiple chest fluoroscopies among tuberculosis patients. Acta radiol. oncol. *25:* 233–238 (1986).

33 Tucker, M. A.; Coleman, C. N.; Cox, R. S.; Varghese, A.; Rosenberg, S. A.: Risk of second cancers after treatment for Hodgkin's disease. New Engl. J. Med. *318:* 76–81 (1988).

34 Tucker, M. A.; D'Angio, G. J.; Boice, J. D.; Jr., Strong, L. C.; Frederick, P. L.; Stovall, M.; Stone, B. J.; Green, D. M.; Lombardi, F.; Newton, W.; Hoover, R. N.; Fraumeni, J. F., Jr.: Bone sarcomas linked to radiotherapy and chemotherapy in children. New Engl. J. Med. *317:* 588–593 (1987).

35 Upton, A.; Albert, R.; Burns, F.; Shore, R.: Radiation carcinogenesis (Elsevier, New York 1986).

36 Vinocur, B.: The breast cancer battle: screening with mammography. Diagnostic Imaging 1986:84–91

Seymour H. Levitt, MD, Department of Therapeutic Radiology-Radiation Oncology, School of Medicine, University of Minnesota Hospital and Clinics, Box 436, Harvard Street at East River Road, Minneapolis, MN 55455 (USA)

Vaeth JM, Meyer JL (eds): Radiation Tolerance of Normal Tissues.
Front Radiat Ther Oncol. Basel, Karger, 1989, vol 23, pp 417–418

Discussion

Dr. Chauser: Dr. Levitt, on carcinogenisis related to breast cancer, is there any influence of age in any of the statistics that you were reviewing?

Dr. Levitt: There is theoretically an age-related incidence: younger women have a higher incidence per dose. We are dealing with older women, for the most part so the estimated risk is probably far less than what people have calculated. The relative risk per rad is greater in younger than in older women – we are talking about women at about the time of puberty.

Dr. Yatvin: Dr. Levitt, on the ANLL data that you had, was there any contribution of the number of survivors with just radiation alone compared to the combined modality that might have influenced the data, or that you might see more tumors developing because of the chemotherapy?

Dr. Levitt: No, that wasn't a factor. These are patients that we followed for 10 years.

Dr. Yatvin: But the total number that were treated in each case. In other words, the numbers varied; the radiation dose was generally slightly less, but there were others to whom chemotherapy alone was given. If you took the total number of treatments and the number of survivors . . . I don't know if you could get that information from the data that you had available to you.

Dr. Levitt: I honestly don't know, but I think that the experience has been pretty much been what we have reported, if you look at the number of patients irradiated that have survived over a period of years. Although I must say that one of my colleagues (Clara Bloomfield) maintains that there is a very small incidence of radiation-induced ANLL, we really haven't seen it. I think that almost every institution comes out with the same data.

Dr. Chauser: Dr. Parker and perhaps Dr. Fajardo would like to comment as well. Is there any difference, morphologically, in the changes that you have seen in these tissues with particle irradiation?

Dr. Parker: Not being a pathologist, I don't think there is anything qualitatively differently, maybe differently quantitavely, I don't think that you can look at something under a microscope and say that it was treated by neutrons.

Dr. Fajardo: I have examined only a few tissues that have suffered from irradiation, and I have not seen any qualitative difference. The ones that impressed me the most were the pituitaries that were irradiated with neutrons or particles. And there the destruction of the organ was remarkable. But I could not have made a differential diagnosis. I agree with Dr. Parker.

Dr. Parker: There might be one implied exception. When we irradiated whole brain, there was massive change throughout the brain that our pathologist had never seen with any other form of treatment. Once they knew that it was neutron, I suppose that they will always know that. But there was nothing qualitatively different.

Dr. Fajardo: I mentioned that I have only examined a few tissues irradiated with heavy particles or with neutrons specifically, and I don't see any qualitative difference, so I agree with Dr. Parker. I was struck by the effectiveness of neutrons in destroying the pituitary.

Dr. Parker: The energy absorption in bone per unit dose delivered is considerably less than it is for photons, which would make you predict that for equal physical doses you should get into less trouble. The problem is that the soft tissues around the teeth apparently didn't get that message, so we are having some problems which are quite unique. The bone looks normal.

Dr. Fajardo: Does that translate into any morphologic difference?

Dr. Parker: No, except that the soft tissues supporting structures around the teeth disappear.

Vaeth JM, Meyer JL (eds): Radiation Tolerance of Normal Tissues.
Front Radiat Ther Oncol. Basel, Karger, 1989, vol 23, pp 419–427

Conference Summary

S. Dische

Marie Curie Research Wing, Regional Center for Radiotherapy and Oncology, Mount Vernon Hospital, Northwood, Middx., UK

In the treatment of any disease, the benefit must be measured against any harm caused, and nowhere is this more important than in oncology; we must recognize that when radiation therapy is employed, the task of observing that morbidity is a demanding one, for here the pattern differs from that associated with other modalities in that the most serious events occur long after the course of treatment is completed. It was important, therefore, that 'The Radiation Effects on Normal Tissues: Clinical Tolerance Levels' was the subject of the 23rd Annual San Francisco Cancer Symposium.

In a broad and comprehensive overview, Philip Rubin spoke on many themes and developed many ideas, but dominant was the need to abandon simple concepts held 20 years ago of tolerance doses for each site in the body and replace with a much more complex system, for we now recognize that there are many factors associated with the radiotherapy, and the patient, which affect normal-tissue responses, and there is the further complication of combined modalities. William Moss described the development of our knowledge, of the major advances and, too, of the errors which have occurred. An awareness of past experience is essential to those planning to advance the field. Radiation therapy is privileged to be based upon the well-developed basic science of radiobiology, and Elizabeth Travis and Emmanuel van der Schueren detailed the development of laboratory models for early- and late-reacting tissues and told us of their latest findings. This work has particular relevance to the exploration of dose fractionation effects in humans.

Luis Fajardo shared with us his deep understanding of the pathology of radiation change, and he and John Hopewell showed, in a detailed review, the function of the endothelial cell and the complexity of the processes involved in normal function and in response to radiation. Howard Thames took us through the clinical data regarding fractionation, pointing out the patterns which are now discernible in the results of clinical trials. This is probably the most exciting area of development in radiation therapy at the moment and was the subject of last year's Cancer Symposium. Have we learned the lessons of our history and are we basing our current studies securely upon laboratory and clinical science?

Eric Hall described *in vitro* work in the laboratory and put the oncogenic potential of radiation in the context of that induced by cytotoxic chemotherapy; there was the fascinating possibility of a reversal by drug and hormonal manipulation.

The scientific basis of our clinical science was again demonstrated by Tim Kinsella when he reported the large-animal studies which were followed by human application of intra-operative radiation therapy. Richard Hoppe showed the complex changes in immune status which may be caused by radiation therapy and showed, too, how this could be taken advantage of in the management of some non-malignant conditions. James Fontanesi reviewed the evidence indicating a marked increase in radiosensitivity of normal tissues of patients with AIDS. This obviously has a very practical application, but is also important to human radiobiology. We know that rare cases of congenital and collagen disease may also be associated with this higher sensitivity, but perhaps other conditions are associated with lesser changes which may, nevertheless, be important in increasing the risk of radiation injury. Sarah Donaldson's task was the important area of paediatric radiation therapy. Nothing is more distressing to the radiation therapist than to see gross impairment of development and induction of neoplasms in children as a result of the treatment given, and their recognition is obviously of extreme importance in deciding the best management of new cases of paediatric malignancy.

John Mayer and Ted Phillips quantified the increase in normal-tissue change which was to be associated with hyperthermia, radiosensitizers, radioprotectors, and cytotoxic chemotherapy, whilst Seymour Levitt examined radiation carcinogenesis. It was reassuring to see the figures suggesting a low incidence following conventional treatment for carcinoma of breast and Hodgkin's disease. Neutrons differ from photon therapy in the distribution of the changes seen; Robert Parker showed that with the worldwide experience of over 9,000 patients much has been learned. However, much more needs to be established. Bernard Pierquin discussed brachytherapy and low dose rate effects based essentially on his own careful, and extensive, clinical observations.

We then went through the regions of the body with many distinguished contributors. Each paper reflected the problems associated with the site, the pattern of morbidities seen, and the personal approach of the speaker; certain common themes emerged:

(1) In each area there had been a slow build up of knowledge based upon careful clinical observation and in most situations laboratory experiment.

(2) In nearly all sites there were steep dose-effect curves. The dose per fraction was of great importance, and differences of 10% or less could lead to considerable differences in the incidence of late radiation effects.

(3) The volume of tissue irradiated was always important, especially when associated with high dose.

(4) The addition of a cytotoxic agent was associated with an increased morbidity making the pattern much more complex.

(5) There was always the unexpected finding, and there must be continued clinical vigilance. An individual might show an unusual sensitivity, generally or only with one system. There was always the possibility of technical error which may be discovered because of a surprising early reaction.

(6) Some speakers discussed the possibility of use of predictive markers in order to reverse or avoid morbidity.

The importance of all the knowledge discussed in this 2-day Symposium can be considered in two ways: its impact upon the clinical science of radiation oncology and then upon practical everyday clinical radiation therapy.

It is for clinical science to advance knowledge, and this greatly depends upon the careful observation of patients which must be prolonged over many years of follow-up. A recent example is found in the long-term follow-up of patients included in an overview of randomized trials of radiotherapy in breast cancer reported by Cuzick et al. [1, 2]. An increased number of deaths has been observed among those receiving radiation therapy 15 or more years after treatment, and this has reached significant levels. The original data did not include detailed information regarding the radiotherapy given to enable a full analysis to be made, and so this must now be added many years after the original treatment. There is some suggestion that the increased deaths are due to cardiac disease and neoplasms at all sites, and so the scattered radiation associated with older techniques of orthovoltage radiation may be incriminated. A full and careful analysis is required of these data.

The clinical scientist must gather precise data. A further common theme in all presentations has been the difficulty in comparing one study with another because there is no common language with regard to radiation morbidity.

We looked at reports of trials in radiation therapy to see how morbidity is described and examined 58 consecutive papers in 7 issues of the *International Journal of Radiation Oncology, Biology, Physics.* The papers described the results of radiation therapy covering all sites where such treatment is employed. Forty-five described the results of treatment in sequentially presenting patients, while in 6 the results were compared with those of a previously treated group, and, finally, in 7 the study was a prospective, randomized controlled one. It was of interest that radiation morbidity was not mentioned in 11, and, although it was considered in a further 8, no real data were given. In 19 of the remaining 39, individual case descriptions of patients who suffered morbidity were given, but there was no overall calculation as to the incidence. In 12 further papers incidence figures were given, but there was no scale of severity employed. There were just 8 papers where morbidity was graded and incidence figures carefully given. In 2 of these, the EORTC/RTOG scale was employed, in another a previously published scale was employed, while in the remaining 5 papers the authors described the morbidity using their own grading systems. A review of similar publications in European journals revealed much the same pattern. [Dische et al., unpubl. data].

The situation can be contrasted with that in medical oncology where the WHO booklet on the recording of results of chemotherapy of cancer treatment is fairly widely accepted and commonly used. The system, unfortunately, is not suitable for radiation therapy, for its scales cannot easily be applied to the conditions under which radiation therapy is given. Further, the WHO booklet is essentially concerned with acute morbidity, devoting only one short paragraph to late effects [3].

The EORTC/RTOG classification has been used for many years and covers nearly all systems dealing with both acute and late reactions. It has been used by the EORTC/RTOG groups and some others. However, some studies performed under the auspices of these same organizations have not employed it. Why has such a system, advocated by such important research organizations on both sides of the Atlantic, not been accepted generally? If we look at the advised systems for early and late radiation morbidity in the lower gastro-intestinal tract, including the pelvis (table I), we note that the grades suggested for the recording of such reactions include a consideration of symptoms, complications, investigations, and treatment employed for the complication. With all these different elements to consider, judgement must be made in order to decide grading.

The grading system has obviously failed to achieve wide acceptance, and yet all must be agreed that a system for grading of morbidity, which would be accepted by all working in the field, would lead to great advance. Not only would all new studies be based on similar criteria, but it might then be possible to make some comparison between studies, and a considerable advance in human radiobiology would result.

Table I. RTOG/EORTC early and late radiation morbidity scoring system

Early morbidity – lower gastro-intestinal tract, including pelvis	
Grade 0	no change
Grade 1	increased frequency or change in quality of bowel habits not requiring medication/rectal discomfort not requiring analgesics
Grade 2	diarrhoea requiring parasympatholytic drugs (e.g. Lomotil)/mucous discharge not necessitating sanitary pads/rectal or abdominal pain requiring analgesics
Grade 3	diarrhoea requiring parenteral support/severe mucous or blood discharge necessitating sanitary pads/abdominal distention (flat-plate radiograph demonstrates distended bowel loops)
Grade 4	acute or subacute obstructions/fistula or perforation gastro-intestinal bleeding requiring transfusion/abdominal pain or tenesmus requiring tube decompression or bowel diversion
Late morbidity – small and large intestine	
Grade 0	none
Grade 1	mild diarrhoea/mild cramping/bowel movement five times daily/slight rectal discharge or bleeding
Grade 2	moderate diarrhoea and colic/bowel movement >5 times daily/excessive rectal mucus or intermittent bleeding
Grade 3	obstruction or bleeding requiring surgery
Grade 4	necrosis/perforation/fistula

Another system simply modifying the EORTC/RTOG scheme would obviously run into the same problems already encountered. As with the TNM system, modifications would lead to incomparability with the results observed in previous studies.

If we look again at the EORTC/RTOG system on the grading of early and late radiation damage to bowel and list all the features which are included, we find that there are many common to both (table II). We are here looking at the elements that make up the morbidity. Each one of these elements can be separately assessed and recorded, and so one can devise a proforma which will ask for just this information (table III). It does have a formidable number of boxes, but most of the data which would be required at any one time would be limited. During radiotherapy it is merely the frequency of stool, its consistency, the treatment required for the diarrhoea, the type of pain, and its management which would feature. The rest of the boxes would only exceptionally be required. Much of the required information is simple and straightforward and such data could be gathered by a nurse or technician for most of the judgement is taken away.

This way towards an internationally agreed system has been the subject of a Workshop which was convened by the Medical Research Council in London, February 25–26, 1988. For 2 days an international group

Table II. Items featuring in RTOG/EORTC morbidity scoring schemes

	Acute	Chronic
Symptoms		
Blood	0	+
Mucous	0	+
Stool		
frequency	+	+
consistency	+	+
Discomfort (cramp)	+	+
Pain	+	+
Complications		
Bowel obstruction	+	+
Fistula	+	+
Perforation	+	+
Investigation		
X-ray abdomen	+	0
Treatment		
Medication		
diarrhoea	+	0
pain	+	0

made up of 14 radiation oncologists, 3 radiobiologists, and 3 medical statisticians considered the situation and as a result have proposed a dictionary of elements making up morbidity in all sites of the body and are proposing for each site a list of (1) desirable and (2) optional elements. The final version of this will be considered at a further meeting of the Members of the Workshop in The Hague in September 1988 and will then be passed to all interested for study for test. It is hoped a system will result which will be widely applicable in the assessment of morbidity in clinical trials and which will allow an international language and the gathering of valuable human radiobiological data. What of the importance of this meeting for the everyday practice of clinical radiation oncology?

(1) With regard to the acceptable risk of morbidity, it is obvious that a simple tolerance table can do no more than give a broad guidance to the radiation oncologist. Not only must we consider all the contributing factors, but the acceptable level of risk of morbidity must differ according to the situation. For example, a young woman receiving therapy after lumpectomy for an early carcinoma of the breast must be exposed to the minimum of risk, while with a man with an advanced laryngeal carcinoma, anxious to preserve his larynx, a much higher risk of morbidity will be reasonable. Many have stressed that the risk of morbidity must be acceptable to patients, but this is not simple to apply. Can a patient in the

Table III. Proforma for the elements to be considered when assessing bowel morbidity (lower gastro-intestinal tract).

Frequency of bowel action/24 h			1 ... 8, 9 = 9 or more
Consistency of faeces			1 formed, 2 formed/liquid, 3 liquid
Dehydration			0 nil, 1 mild, 2 moderate, 3 severe
Medication			0 nil, 1 intermittent, 2 regular, 3 narcotics used
Parenteral fluids/feeding			0 no, 1 yes
Blood loss			0 no, 1 intermittent, 2 daily
Bleeding	Volume		0 nil, 1 slight, 2 moderate, 3 gross haemorrhage
Stricture	Diagnosis		0 no, 1 clinical, 2 radiological
	Management		0 none, 1 conservative, 2 surgical
Perforation	Diagnosis		0 no, 1 clinical, 2 radiological confirmation
	Management		0 none, 1 conservative, 2 surgical
Fistula	Diagnosis		0 no, 1 clinical, 2 radiological confirmation
	Management		0 none, 1 conservative, 2 surgical
			2 surgical
Rectal discharge	Type		0 nil, 1 intermittent, 2 persistent
	Management		0 none, 1 local introduction, 2 colostomy, 3 diarrhoea, 4 resection, 5 other
Wound healing	Delayed		0 no, 1 yes
Anastomotic breakdown			0 no, 1 yes
Radiological findings:			
Loss of bowel distensibility			0 no, 1 yes
Stricture			0 no, 1 single, 2 multiple
Shortening of rectum/sigmoid			0 no, 1 yes
Loss of normal rectal curves			0 no, 1 yes
Increase of presacral space			0 no, 1 yes
Mucosal pattern change			0 no, 1 patchy, 2 confluent
Ulceration			0 no, 1 isolated, 2 multiple
Fistula			0 no, 1 yes
Perforation			0 no, 1 yes

highly emotional situation of having recently been told that he or she has cancer really put into perspective the risks involved, particularly those which may extend over 20, 30, or more years? The weight of responsibility must still lie with the responsible radiation oncologist.

(2) The steep dose-response curves with differences of 10% or less in dose, making significant differences in the incidence of morbidity, demands that we keep a very high standard of clinical practice. However, we know that a 10% variation in dose across the target volume is often

found acceptable. We obviously must strive to reduce such variations to the minimum possible. While remaining open to improvements, the consistent practice of well-tried schemes of treatment must be encouraged. We must be alert to the errors which may occur when new practices are introduced or different schemes for notation of dose are used. For any one patient the maximum, the modal, and the dose at the intersection of beams will all be different and may extend over a range which can make differences in the incidence of morbidity.

(3) The fractionation of radiation therapy and radiation morbidity are very closely related, and in many of the contributions the danger of large dose fractions was stressed. In the pursuit of cure this must obviously lead to the adoption of multifraction techniques to avoid late morbidity, but hypofractionation has still an important place in management. Palliative radiotherapy for a patient who has a limited expectation of life should be given with a limited number of treatments over a short period of time, and so a judicious use of hypofractionation is most appropriate. Even in curative or long-term palliative work, the giving of large dose fractions has a place. We see it being employed in intraoperative radiation therapy and in half-body radiotherapy. We need to employ the whole range of fractionation schemes which are available to give the best and the most suitable treatment to all our patients.

(4) How can we minimize morbidity? (i) We must make careful case selection. A patient not treated is a patient not exposed to hazard, and this particularly applies to our young patients. However, not to treat or to use too low a radiation dose so as to minimize morbidity may prejudice the patient's chance of cure. (ii) We must use strictly defined protocols based on trial and experience. Changes should not be made casually and, in particular, the addition of chemotherapy made with caution and only in a trial situation until the limits of tolerance are well defined. (iii) We must use all the techniques now available for localization of tumour and of areas of spread and make meticulous planning. (iv) We must keep our volumes for irradiation to exactly the right size to control disease, and the high-dose regions must be particularly well defined and kept as small as possible. (v) We must make sure that the plan of treatment is realized in all its aspects and the highest technical standard maintained and errors avoided. There must be careful clinical observation during radiation therapy, looking for unexpected problems for we know, unfortunately, that sometimes this may be the first indicator of a technical breakdown.

Encouraged by the increasing success of cancer treatment, the society we serve not only expects cure of cancer, but a life expectation for those patients which is normal in length and quality. It is necessary for radiation oncologists to rise to this challenge and do their best to achieve it.

References

1 Cuzick, J.; Stewart, H.; Fisher, B., et al.: Overview of radomized trials comparing radical mastectomy without radiotherapy against simple mastectomy with radiotherapy in breast cancer. Cancer Treat. Rep. 1987; *71:* 7–14.

2 Cuzick, J.; Stewart, H.; Peto, R.; et al.: Overview of randomized trials of postoperative adjuvant radiotherapy in breast cancer. Cancer Treat. Rep. 1987; *71:* 15–29.

3 WHO Handbook for Reporting Results of Cancer Treatment. Geneva, World Health Organisation, 1979.

S. Dische, MD, Marie Curie Research Wing, Regional Center for Radiotherapy and Oncology, Mount Vernon Hospital, Northwood, Middx. HA6 2RN (UK)

Subject Index